T0344659

**Essential
Angioplasty**

Companion website

This book is accompanied by a website:
www.wiley.com/go/essentialangioplasty.com

The website contains additional resources including:
- PowerPoint presentations
- Details of key meetings
- Further useful publications list
- Additional images and captions

Further resources and updates to follow publication.

Essential Angioplasty

E. von Schmilowski, MD, PhD
Specialist Registrar Cardiologist
The Heart Hospital
London, UK

R. H. Swanton, MD, FRCP, FACC
Consultant Cardiologist
The Heart Hospital
London, UK

WILEY-BLACKWELL
A John Wiley & Sons, Ltd., Publication

Library of Congress Cataloging-in-Publication Data
von Schmilowski, Eva.
  Essential angioplasty / Eva von Schmilowski, Howard Swanton.
      p. ; cm.
  Includes bibliographical references and index.
  ISBN-13: 978-0-470-65726-3 (hard cover : alk. paper)
  ISBN-10: 0-470-65726-X (hard cover : alk. paper)
    1. Angioplasty. I. Swanton, Howard. II. Title.
  [DNLM: 1. Angioplasty–instrumentation. 2. Angioplasty–methods. 3. Intraoperative Complications–prevention & control. 4. Postoperative Complications–prevention & control. WG 166.5.A3]
  RD598.35.A53S65 2012
  617.4'13–dc23
                            2011015324
A catalogue record for this book is available from the British Library.

Wiley also publishes its books in a variety of electronic formats. Some content that appears in print may not be available in electronic books.

Set in 9.5/12 pt Palatino by Toppan Best-set Premedia Limited
Printed and bound in Malaysia by Vivar Printing Sdn Bhd

1   2012

Contents

Companion website

This book is accompanied by a website containing additional resources:

www.wiley.com/go/essentialangioplasty.com

Foreword

Coronary angioplasty has become one of the great interventions in modern medicine. Over the last three decades since Gruentzig first introduced this procedure in 1977 the technique has developed to an astonishing degree and its application has spread worldwide. It has avoided the need for coronary bypass surgery in hundreds of thousands of patients with angina, and is increasingly managed as a day case procedure.

The plain old balloon designed by Gruentzig is still used in a design very similar to his original one. To it has been added firstly the bare metal stent, then the drug-eluting stent and now the fully absorbable stent which is entering trials. Remarkable improvements in intracoronary imaging have paralleled these advances.

The result is that almost all cases of coronary disease can be managed wholly or in part by coronary angioplasty. The question becomes not "Can I do this procedure?", but "Should I do it?"

This guide book for the trainee starting coronary angioplasty goes through the procedure in a step by step fashion, and deals with all the modern technology available. It also answers the question fundamental to good practice: "Should I take this case on, or should I refer the patient for surgery?" The answer so often lies in trial data which are included in every section dealing with techniques. We have all struggled with a procedure and got into difficulties because we tried to do too much. The book's motto "keep it simple" will stand the trainee in good stead. Although the technology is increasingly sophisticated this phrase must be in the operator's mind with every case. This very helpful guide book will keep it there!

John Ormiston
MBChB, MD, FRACP, FRACR, FCSANZ, ONZM
Medical Director
Mercy Angiography
Auckland, New Zealand

Preface

It is hoped this book will be of help to the cardiologist starting out in coronary intervention. Standing at the catheter table for the first time as an assistant operator at a coronary angioplasty case can be a daunting experience however many coronary angiograms you have performed previously. A vast choice of techniques and technology confronts the beginner. This book is designed to guide you through the procedure, avoiding potential pitfalls and complications. It has been written to provide a solid basic background and allow you to develop your own personal approach in interventional cardiology. Our principle was to follow the motto "keep it simple," to provide selected, practical knowledge with a full range of useful tools and tips and to avoid increasing amounts of useless information. The book also deals in detail with more complex intervention, which we hope will help the more experienced interventionist.

It is 35 years since Andreas Grüntzig performed the first balloon coronary angioplasty in man in 1977. Since that time there have been huge advances in pharmacology, technology, and imaging – both X-ray and intracoronary imaging.

This book will help you apply all these advances with each stage of the coronary intervention. A section on angiographic projections will help in the selection of the best view of a lesion in any coronary segment. Radiation doses to patient, operator, and laboratory staff are higher in coronary angioplasty than in diagnostic coronary angiography and the radiation section will help remind the operator how to minimize the radiation dose. There are sections on choice of vascular access and closure devices. Pharmacology is covered in detail. The bewildering choice of guiding catheters, wires, balloons, and stents are dealt with in individual sections. All chapters are illustrated by diagrams, charts, and tables as well as angiographic pictures.

Even with the correct selection of equipment, the story has just started. Every common coronary lesion is dealt with in a step-by-step fashion with caveats listed. Included are sections on primary coronary angioplasty in acute myocardial infarction, the thrombotic lesion, bifurcation lesions, ostial lesions, graft lesions, and left main stem stenosis. There is a section on intracoronary imaging. Complications are covered and include contrast-induced nephropathy.

Cardiology is right at the forefront of medical specialties in its evidence base. We have literally hundreds of trials to guide our practice. The best relevant trials in coronary intervention are included at the end of each chapter with a full list at the back of the book. We would welcome and be very grateful for any suggestions and feedback on gaps in the subject or topics which you feel have been dealt with inadequately.

An integral and very important part of the book is a website, www.wiley.com/go/essentialangioplasty.com. This will provide you with regular updates on topics or content covered in the book, updates on relevant clinical trials, news of new equipment, techniques, and technologies, and reports from key interventional meetings. Additionally, you will benefit from many downloadable color images and illustrations which will cover the most important areas of interventional cardiology. Also included are PowerPoint presentations and clinical cases with video clips which will, we hope, be both entertaining and instructive.

Finally, we encourage you to use this book in the catheter lab on a regular basis. We believe it will help you develop excellent standards in your daily interventional practice.

Good luck!

E. von Schmilowski
R. H. Swanton

Acknowledgments

We would like to thank all our mentors, teachers, friends and colleagues in the numerous catheter laboratories in which we have worked. We are very grateful for all their help, wise advice and shared knowledge. Thank you to the radiographic staff at the Heart Hospital for their great goodwill in helping access angioplasty cases.

A special thanks to John Ormiston for his continuing support and supervision over the years. His angioplasty experience and ideas have been invaluable.

We owe a massive debt to Osamu Yamamoto for his amazing illustrations in the book. A big thank you for all the long hours working together on initial drafts and sketches and bringing these/them to reality. His patience with endless corrections has been extraordinary.

A huge thank you to Diana Simich for her support, patience and understanding. Our enriching conversations were always inspiring and gave much needed motivation. Without her the book would never be the same. To Kerry Spackman for sharing his great thoughts and ideas and for his strong belief in this project. To Lucie and Dominic Sleeman for their encouragement and support on the final stages of the writing. Thank you for your wonderful friendship.

Thank you to a great team of editors who have been so patient and understanding. A special thank you to Tom Hartman who showed immediate interest in the project and shared our enthusiasm for the book and the companion website. We are most grateful for his loyalty and priceless editorial suggestions. We are equally grateful to Kate Newell, Ruth Swan, Cathryn Gates and Kevin Fung for their encouragement and uncomplaining assistance with the final preparations of the manuscript.

Finally and most especially we would like to thank our families for their unconditional love, patience and endless faith in us.

E. von Schmilowski
R. H. Swanton

List of Abbreviations

AA, arachidonic acid
ACS, acute coronary syndrome
ACT, activated clotting time
AP, anteroposterior
APTT, activated partial thromboplastin time
ARC, Academic Research Consortium
ARU, aspirin reaction unit
BMS, bare metal stents
CAD, coronary artery disease
CART, controlled antegrade and retrograde subintimal tracking
CIN, contrast-induced nephropathy
CMR, cardiac magnetic resonance
CPR, cardiopulmonary resuscitation
CSA, cross-sectional area
CTFC, corrected TIMI frame count
CTO, chronic total occlusion
DAPT, dual antiplatelet therapy
DEB, drug-eluting balloons
DES, drug-eluting stent
DS, digital subtraction (angiography)
EEM, external elastic membrane
FFR, fractional flow reserve
GPI, glycoprotein inhibitor
GTN, glyceryl trinitrate
HPPR, high post-clopidogrel platelet reactivity
IABP, intra-aortic balloon pump
IC, intracoronary
IM, intramuscular(ly)
IMA, internal mammary artery
IMC, internal mammary artery catheter
IRA, infarct-related artery
IV, intravenous(ly)
IVUS, intravascular ultrasound
JVP, jugular venous pulse/pressure
LA, left atrium
LBBB, left bundle branch block

LCB, left coronary bypass
LIMA, left internal mammary artery
LM, left main
LV, left ventricle, left ventricular
LVEDP, left ventricular end-diastolic pressure
MACE, major adverse cardiac events
MBS, myocardial blush score
MLA, minimum luminal cross-sectional area
MLD, minimum luminal diameter
MVD, multivessel disease
NAC, N-Acetylcysteine
NSTEMI, non-ST-elevation myocardial infarction
NURD, nonuniform rotational distortion
OMB, obtuse marginal branches
OTW, over the wire
PA, posteroanterior; pulmonary artery
PCI, percutaneous coronary intervention
PEA, pulseless electrical activity
PGA, polyglycolic acid
PLLA, poly-L-lactic acid
PO, per orem
POBA, plain old balloon angioplasty
PTT, partial thromboplastin time
QCA, quantitative coronary angiography
RCB, right coronary bypass
RPFA, rapid platelet function assay
RSV, right sinus of Valsalva
RWMA, regional wall motion abnormalities
SBP, systolic blood pressure
STAR, subintimal tracking and re-entry (technique)
STEMI, ST-elevation myocardial infarction
SVR, systemic vascular resistance
TAVI, transcatheter aortic valve implantation
TIMI, thrombolysis in myocardial infarction
TLD, thermoluminescent dosimeter
TLF, target lesion failure
TLR, target lesion revascularization
TOE, transesophageal echocardiography
TT, thrombin time
TVF, target vessel failure
TVR, target vessel revascularization
UFH, unfractionated heparin
VASP, vasodilator-stimulated phosphoprotein
VASP-P, VASP phosphorylation
VSD, ventricular septal defect

1 Fundamentals

Standards of Excellence in Interventional Cardiology

As you are reading this, interventional cardiology has become an important part of your life. After a demanding training and long hours in hospital cardiology practice you have become a member of the interventional community. You undoubtedly have great potential, strong motivation, and a determination to learn and master your profession.

Interventional cardiology is not only about how educated, intelligent, or skilled you are. Good qualifications are indeed important, but being an excellent operator does not necessarily make you an excellent interventional cardiologist. There is much more to it than educational achievements and manual skills.

A skilled angioplasty operator should select patients appropriately and use the best and most up-to-date techniques, equipment, and pharmacotherapy. An interventional cardiologist, on the other hand, should in addition to these skills have a wide knowledge base, common sense, and the ability to cooperate and communicate effectively with both colleagues and patients.

Much of what follows is about being a first-class doctor rather than being a skilled technician. It may be taken for granted by the patient and medical colleagues that the conduct described below is to be expected as part of a first-class service. However, we have all seen how pressure of time and work and the stress of a difficult procedure can erode these standards. It is important that good standards of practice should develop from the very

Essential Angioplasty, First Edition. E. von Schmilowski, R. H. Swanton.
© 2012 John Wiley & Sons, Ltd. Published 2012 by John Wiley & Sons, Ltd.

beginning of training. You will make a positive impact on both patients and the people you work with, and in a few years time your younger colleagues will learn from you.

We hope these few practical thoughts will help you see interventional cardiology from a more human perspective and will make your profession more worthwhile, rewarding, and enjoyable.

Take Care of the Patient
- You are a physician and cardiologist, not just an interventionist. Treat the whole patient, not just the lesion in the coronary artery. Try to imagine what it must be like facing up to a coronary angioplasty.
- Meet the patient and the patient's family before and after the procedure. Explain what will be done and what has been done.
- Be available, kind, and keen to talk. Be honest, quietly confident, and do not hide anything. In getting consent, be realistic about the risks involved. These should be the risks in your hands in your hospital, not national risks.
- During the procedure, mind your language and be careful with comments you make. Don't forget that most patients are awake during a percutaneous coronary intervention (PCI), and sedation does not necessarily stop them hearing or remembering remarks.

Treat the patient, not the lesion.

Quality and Respect Are Essential
- Be humble and respect the people you work with. You are not the master of the universe. Don't act in a superior way.
- Be professional. Build your reputation as a professional physician and a decent human being, not a pop star.
- Dress properly. Have clean hands and fingernails.
- Be available and well organized. Keep your desk clean, keep your files in order, manage your time effectively by planning ahead.
- Be reliable, honest, and truthful. We all want to work with people whom we can trust and rely on.
- Be effective, but not arrogant.
- Be decisive. Don't dwell on problems, solve them. A good decision made quickly is ideal, but when you are stuck, any decision is better than no decision.
- Be strong and determined. Do not give up because things are getting difficult.
- Be adaptable as well as decisive. Be prepared to change strategy if your initial plan is not working out.
- Be a good speaker. Express your opinions in sentences rather than in paragraphs.
- Don't argue with anyone. Accept constructive criticism.
- Be calm and peaceful. Control your emotions when things go wrong. Do not raise your voice.

• Be well balanced. Keep your mind and body in healthy shape. Your mind is like a parachute. It only works when open.

Any decision is better than no decision.

Communicate Effectively
• Cooperate with your medical colleagues and catheter lab staff.
• Present results of the procedure to your referring doctor.
• Be careful when you present your opinions about PCI performed by others and avoid disparaging or disdainful remarks.
• Consider and respect others' views. If you disagree, disagree gracefully.
• A healthy and friendly atmosphere in the catheter lab is very important.
• Maintain a good relationship with catheter lab staff. Help them and teach them, but do not patronize them. Many of them will be highly experienced. Discuss cases with them, particularly when things go wrong.
• Remember each nurse and technician by name and thank them at the end of the procedure.
• Do not make people feel intimidated by your knowledge, experience, skills, achievements, etc. The greatest people will never make you feel intimidated.

Build bridges, not walls.

Don't Overestimate Your Skills
• Courage is important. However, there is a thin line between courage and stupidity. The only hero in a heroic procedure is the patient. Be very cautious, particularly in the first few months of your training.
• If in doubt, ask your more experienced colleagues for their opinion. Discuss the problem with others.
• In complex cases, ask one of your colleagues to scrub in with you, even if you think you don't need help.
• There is no failure. Only feedback. When complications occur, stay calm, manage the patient appropriately, and do not leave the bedside until the situation is under control. Once the patient is stable, immediately contact your more experienced colleague to explain the case and review the patient in detail. Always tell the truth.
• Being told you are competitive may be a compliment or an insult. PCI is not a rugby game and it is not about winning, beating others, or proving you are the best.
• Avoid "Let me show you…" situations. Compete when it is yourself you are competing against.

Skill is successfully walking a tightrope over Niagara Falls.
Intelligence is not trying.

Learn, Learn, Learn
• Learn every day. Enjoy it and share your knowledge. Learn before you start practicing. Manual skills are extremely important, but without a solid theoretical background you can only be good, never great.

• Attend and participate in interventional meetings at least once a year. Euro PCR in Europe, ACI in the UK, and TCT in the USA are invaluable meetings and will broaden your horizons and inspire you. You will learn from the greatest and most experienced interventionists in the world.
• Keep up to date with interventional technology, new equipment, and new trials.

Good judgment comes from experience and experience comes from bad judgment.

Above all keep it simple. Simplicity is the ultimate sophistication.

Introduction to Interventional Procedures

• **Coronary Angioplasty, 4**
• **Coronary Angiography, 5**

Coronary Angioplasty

When Andreas Grüntzig introduced coronary angioplasty in man in 1977, he introduced a technique which proved to be one of the great advances in modern medicine. Major advances in technology coupled with great improvements in both X-ray and intracoronary imaging have enabled cardiologists to tackle more and more complex coronary lesions. This has saved hundreds of thousands of patients a year worldwide from the need for coronary artery bypass surgery (CABG). Coronary angioplasty has been of value in the management of patients who develop angina years after CABG and has extended treatment options in elderly or frail patients who are considered unsuitable for coronary surgery.

Coronary angioplasty has revolutionized the treatment of acute myocardial infarction (MI), replacing thrombolysis in many areas reducing hospital mortality and mortality in cardiogenic shock. It has proved its superiority over thrombolysis in acute MI, preventing postinfarct angina and recurrent infarction.

With these extraordinary advances has come an understanding of the indications for PCI. It is primarily a technique for the relief of anginal symptoms which have not responded to medical treatment. Not all patients with refractory angina should be advised to have a PCI as CABG may still be an alternative treatment option in certain groups of patients: particularly those with complex, diffuse three-vessel disease and diabetes. PCI can be of value as part of a hybrid procedure: e.g., stenting of a coronary lesion before a transcatheter aortic valve implantation (TAVI). The points below indicate some common clinical situations where PCI should be considered:

• Stable angina resistant to medical treatment
• Symptomatic one-, two-, or three-vessel disease (based on the result of the stress test and suitable coronary anatomy)

- Angina with a poor exercise test result: e.g., ST depression at low workload with symptoms, or inadequate BP response
- ST elevation MI (STEMI)
- Unstable angina / non Q wave MI / NSTEMI
- Angina in patients with severe LV dysfunction and heart failure if ischemia has been demonstrated
- Recurrent angina after coronary bypass surgery

Coronary Angiography

Coronary angiography is a diagnostic procedure for assessing the severity of coronary lesions. The result determines the choice of treatment. The majority of patients undergoing angiography are symptomatic with confirmed angina, and they often require prompt further interventional treatment. Angiography is also performed in patients with congenital heart disease, aortic dissection, a large area of ischemia, and new onset of left ventricular dysfunction or heart failure, as well as in those who require valve surgery. Finally, in some patients the diagnosis of coronary disease is uncertain and cannot be excluded by noninvasive testing. In this situation angiography is needed to decide treatment strategy. Patients with acute coronary syndrome (ACS) require urgent angiography (see pp. 133–162). Coronary angiography is contraindicated in the following situations:

- *No consent:* The patient refuses consent
- *Active:* Bleeding, infection
- *Acute:* Stroke, renal failure, endocarditis
- *Severe:* Anemia, coagulopathy, electrolyte disturbances
- *Heart failure:* If decompensated
- *Hypertension:* If uncontrolled

Interventional Tools
The standard diagnostic table contains the following equipment:
- Sterile cups
- Sterile syringes
- Sterile introducing needle
- 1% lidocaine (lignocaine)
- Intracoronary glyceryl trinitrate (GTN), adenosine, nitroprusside, verapamil, atropine
- Coronary manifold
- Sheath for vascular access
- Diagnostic coronary catheter
- Guide wire 0.035″
  In addition if proceeding to angioplasty:
- Inflation device
- Contrast media (50% contrast/50% saline)
- Hemostatic valve (e.g., Ketch or Touhy–Borst)

- Coronary guiding catheter
- Coronary guide wire 0.014″

Basic Principles
In a procedure probably proceeding to PCI, limit the use of contrast as much as possible. Use only selected projections, focusing on stenotic segments and potential involvement of side branches. This will help you choose the best working projection. In the patient who has had coronary bypass surgery, angiography is usually only a diagnostic procedure and there is less restriction on contrast use. As well as the native vessels, focus on the state and number of bypass grafts and their proximal and distal anastomoses. Distal runoff into the native vessel is important. The angiogram must be reviewed with a cardiothoracic surgeon to decide on the best treatment strategy.

There is no such thing as routine angiography. Every individual procedure requires care and attention:

- Proceed gently; never force wires, sheaths, or catheters.
- Start angiography with an initial injection of 100–200 µg intracoronary GTN.
- Assess coronary anatomy: significant narrowing, vessel dominance, coronary anomalies, coronary collaterals, coronary blood flow.
- Are there any missing areas, or absent vessels? If so, consider the possibility of a severe lesion, complete total occlusion (CTO) lesion, or thrombus.
- Standard projections usually provide complete information about major vessels. Sometimes, however, these do not fully display coronary arteries, and multiple projections with steeper angles are needed to avoid overlaps.
- Do not finish before you are sure all vessels including side branches have been identified and shown properly.
- Think about a treatment strategy: medical therapy, angioplasty, or bypass surgery. Review the patient with a more experienced colleague or with a cardiothoracic surgeon for a final decision.

Pitfalls in the Interpretation
Misinterpretation or underestimation of severe stenoses, e.g., due to diffuse disease, tortuosities, etc., may have serious clinical implications. A few points may help in the assessment of the angiogram:

- *Adequate contrast injection* is important for good opacification of the coronary arteries. This can be improved by use of a larger-size catheter or a power injector.
- *Poor opacification* is a common problem. This results in streaming and may be misinterpreted as an ostial lesion, a missing side branch, or thrombus. An adequate-sized diagnostic catheter may help overcome it.
- *Subselective injection.* If the left main is short or double-barreled, a standard contrast injection may selectively opacify only one vessel – either the left anterior descending artery or the left circumflex artery. If the left circumflex artery is opacified clearly, the left anterior descending artery may be misinterpreted as totally occluded, and vice versa. Sometimes a rapid contrast

injection may reveal the missing vessel. In other cases, separate injection in the left anterior descending and in the left circumflex may be necessary to opacify both vessels satisfactorily.

• *Coronary spasm.* Catheter-tip-induced spasm is usually caused by too deep catheter engagement, which results in mechanical trauma and arterial constriction. Administration of intracoronary 100–200 µg GTN will relieve the spasm and help identify whether the vessel is occluded or in spasm. If there is concern about blood pressure, a smaller dose of 100 µg can be given. Sublingual nitroglycerin may be ineffective in relieving spasm. Catheter-induced coronary spasm is most common during engagement of the left main coronary artery or the right coronary artery (RCA) and may be misinterpreted as an ostial lesion (see below).

• *Ostial stenosis.* The first sign of an ostial stenosis is damping or partial ventricularization of the arterial pressure as soon as the diagnostic catheter engages the coronary ostium. There is absence of contrast reflux into the aorta with a coronary injection (see Figure 5.20). In the left main stem this may be difficult to recognize due to the variability of the left main anatomy and the risk of catheter-induced spasm. Use left anterior oblique (LAO) cranial or LAO caudal view to check the left main ostium, and steep LAO view for the RCA ostium. Injection during gradual catheter withdrawal from the ostium may help confirm an ostial lesion.

• *Occlusion at the origin* of the vessel may be difficult to recognize, particularly if no stump is visible. Late filling from distal collaterals helps confirm the vessel track.

• *Unusual anatomic variants*, such as coronary collaterals, myocardial bridge, or congenital coronary anomalies, are rare. Before a congenital variant is accepted as a diagnosis, an occlusion or collateral channels should be excluded.

Although the overall complication rate of coronary angiography is low, the elderly, patients with diabetes, renal failure, left ventricular dysfunction, obesity, congestive heart failure, anemia, coagulopathy, peripheral vascular disease, severe comorbidities, and higher risk of bleeding are all at higher risk from the procedure.

Key Learning Points

• Coronary angiography is a diagnostic procedure for assessing the extent and severity of coronary lesions.
• There is no such thing as routine angiography. Every individual procedure requires care and attention.
• Every coronary angiogram should start with an initial intracoronary injection of 100–200 µg nitroglycerin.
• Standard projections usually provide complete information about major vessels; however, additional projections may be needed.
• Always review the angiogram before finishing the procedure.

Vascular Access

Femoral Access
Introduction
In many centers worldwide femoral access is well established and is the most popular puncture technique, but the world is changing and the radial approach is now becoming dominant. The femoral approach permits good guide catheter control, easy access with larger devices, and a low rate of thrombotic complications. The overall complication rate, however, is still significant and the most common problem is major bleeding at the puncture site. The correct puncture technique and optimal antithrombotic and antiplatelet therapy may reduce the risk, but bleeding complications may still occur despite a textbook procedure. Advantages and disadvantages of the femoral access are listed in Table 1.1.

Outcomes from the randomized ACUITY trial (see below under "Trials") suggest that in patients with acute coronary syndromes undergoing proce-

Table 1.1 Advantages and disadvantages of femoral access.

Advantages	Disadvantages
Well-established technique	Higher risk of local complications
Easy technically	Higher risk of bleeding
Allows the use of larger caliber equipment	Longer recovery time (4–6 hours)
Good catheter control	Longer time to ambulation
Low risk of thrombosis	Risk with peripheral arterial disease
Shorter radiation time	Risk with abdominal aortic aneurysm
All vessels, grafts, and both internal mammary arteries accessible from one puncture site	Less favored by patients than radial approach
Access artery spasm uncommon	

dures via the femoral route, the use of bivalirudin during the procedure or the use of closure devices or both resulted in a lower rate of major bleeding from the access site.

Femoral Artery Anatomy

Femoral artery access is a blind puncture as the path of the artery is invisible. The optimal puncture site should be located by certain landmarks: the iliac crest, the inguinal skin crease, and the symphysis pubis. First locate the level of the inguinal ligament, which has a variable relationship to the inguinal skin crease, but lies along a line from the pubic tubercle to the anterior superior iliac spine. The femoral artery crosses beneath the inguinal ligament and lies in the floor of the femoral triangle (Figure 1.1). You will feel the pulse if you put two fingers perpendicular to the long axis of the femoral artery. Note that too low a puncture increases the risk of local complications (overt bleeding, hematoma, false aneurysm) whereas a puncture that is too high (above the inguinal ligament) can result in an unrecognized and large retroperitoneal hematoma. Femoral artery anatomy can vary, and in case of difficulties in advancing a wire, a quick fluoroscopic assessment with contrast injection may be helpful. The best view to display the femoral artery is the right anterior oblique (RAO) 20°. The ideal puncture should be approximately 1 cm below the inguinal ligament and above the origin of the profunda femoris.

Before the procedure, review the patient's medical history and focus on previous procedures, access problems, what shaped catheters engaged the

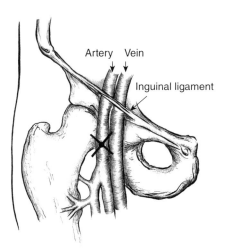

Figure 1.1 Femoral artery anatomy. The level of the inguinal ligament has a variable relationship to the inguinal skin crease, but lies along a line from the pubic tubercle to the anterior superior iliac spine. The femoral artery crosses beneath the inguinal ligament and lies in the floor of the femoral triangle. The ideal puncture site (*marked by a cross*) is below the inguinal ligament but above the origin of the deep femoral artery (profunda femoris). The femoral artery lies lateral to the femoral vein.

coronary artery, use of closure devices, and signs of peripheral vascular disease. Does the patient have a history of intermittent claudication?

Physical examination is mandatory:

- Check the femoral pulses in both groins.
- If the femorals are weak, listen for a bruit over the femoral artery and then press the stethoscope firmly in both iliac fossae for an iliac bruit.
- Check the color and temperature on both legs.
- Check the pulses in both feet.
- Examine the groin for hematoma, swelling, fibrosis, or infection.

Femoral Puncture Using the Seldinger Technique

Equipment Selection

An 18-gauge 7-cm needle, a 6–7F sheath, guide wire, and catheter (and, optionally, scalpel) are required. Some operators use a scalpel routinely, others do not unless using a very large sheath. A 9F sheath or smaller can pass through the skin without a scalpel cut. A scalpel cut in the skin tempts one to keep using it even if the needle is in the wrong place. The patient also requires lidocaine for local anesthesia.

The vascular introducer sheath allows access to the femoral artery, facilitates the passage of catheters, and helps maintain hemostasis at the puncture site (an example of a femoral sheath is shown in Figure 1.2). In general the sheath size should be the same size as the catheter and the most commonly used length is 11 cm. After successful puncture, advance the sheath over the wire by gently pushing with a rotating motion. If resistance is felt, look for the reason rather than continue pushing. Resistance may occur due to spasm, occlusion, tortuosity or abnormal take-off. If the patient has previously had coronary angiography via the femoral route the resistance is usually due to extensive fibrosis around the artery. A quick fluoroscopic view may be helpful. If the femoral artery is tortuous, select a longer sheath (25–35 cm) to improve catheter support and manipulation. For radial access hydrophilic sheaths 5–6F are optimal. A longer sheath (23 cm) is preferred to reduce the risk of spasm of the radial artery. When the sheath is placed in the artery, withdraw

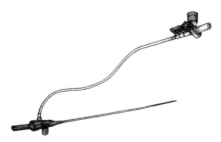

Figure 1.2 Femoral sheath.

the dilator, aspirate and inject saline to remove fibrin form the tip of the sheath leaving a clean connection tube.

Femoral Puncture Technique (Figure 1.3)
In most cases the right femoral artery is chosen for access.
• Make sure that the puncture site is below the inguinal ligament.
• Find the point of maximal pulsation.
• Apply adequate local anesthesia using a 25-gauge needle and 10–20 ml 2% lidocaine. Inject small volumes slowly and aspirate each time before the next injection. The final aliquot of lidocaine should be just on the top surface of the femoral artery, but not inside it.
• Feel the pulse on the femoral artery with your fingers.
• If you want to use a scalpel, make a small 2.0-mm skin incision with the scalpel at the intended entry site. As mentioned above, scalpel use is not essential
• Advance the needle slowly until its tip reaches the top of the artery; feel the pulse with needle tip.
• Insert the needle deeper, puncture the artery, and observe the pulsating arterial blood flow .
• If the puncture fails, withdraw the needle, flush it, and compress the puncture site briefly before resuming.
• After a successful puncture, reduce the angle of the needle (more horizontal and more in line with the vessel lumen) and start advancing the J-shaped wire into the needle. There should be pulsatile blood flow out of the needle as you do this. If you feel resistance, do not push the wire, but check progress and the site of the wire on fluoroscopy.
• Once the wire has been successfully advanced up the artery, remove the needle, pressing gently on the puncture site.
• Advance the sheath over the wire by pushing and rotating.
• If you feel resistance, this may be due to fibrosis around the artery from previous punctures. Keep the introducing sheath flat/horizontal. If it will not advance, check the wire position and entry track with quick fluoroscopy. If the wire looks straight and not kinked, switch to a smaller dilator. Then retry with the original dilator and sheath, but check before reusing it that the tip of the dilator and the sheath tip are not buckled, but taper nicely.
• Remove dilator and wire simultaneously.
• Aspirate to remove potential clot from the sheath and inject saline, leaving a clean side arm connection tube.

Difficulties with Advancing the Wire
If attempts to pass the wire meet with resistance, consider possible reasons:
• If the needle is too close to the posterior wall (poor pulsatile blood flow out of the needle), pull or rotate the needle very slightly and try to insert the

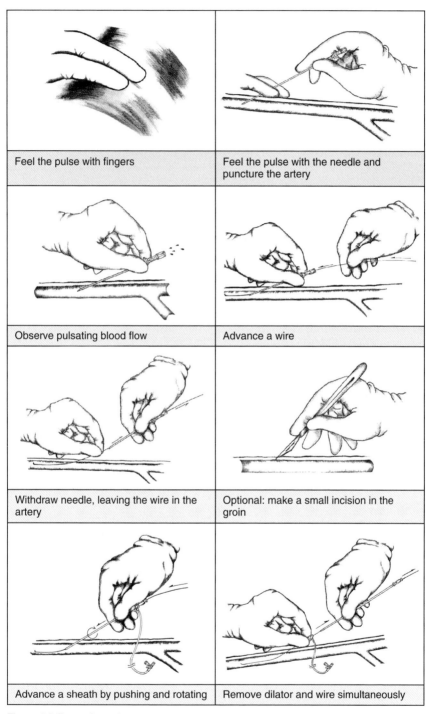

Figure 1.3 Femoral puncture.

wire again. If this does not work, withdraw the needle, flush it, and puncture the artery again.

• If the iliac artery is tortuous, the wire may initially pass easily through the needle for a few centimeters and then stop. Inject a small amount of contrast and check the arterial anatomy under fluoroscopy. This may reveal why there is obstruction to wire advancement.

• If the patient has a femoral bypass graft, the risk of bleeding, hematoma, catheter damage, or kinking is higher. Try to avoid catheterizing through a graft. Use the other leg or the radial route. If a patient has had a femoro-femoral crossover graft, elect to use the radial route also. To avoid complications, if there is no alternative, puncture the artery as close to the inguinal ligament as possible. Use a dilator size 1F larger than the selected sheath size.

• At no time should the patient experience any pain. If pain is felt, the wire and/or sheath may not be truly intraluminal or initial local anesthesia was inadequate.

Puncture of an Apparent Pulseless Artery

Apparent pulselessness of an artery may be caused by previous local surgery, severe calcification, or gross obesity. It may also be caused by a very low stroke volume in cardiogenic or hypovolemic shock. Detection of the pulseless artery is based on anatomical landmarks. The femoral artery is located 1.5–2.0 cm lateral to the point of posterior depression. This should be found lateral to the pubic tubercle and inferior to the inguinal ligament. In patients with previous catheterization, finding the previous puncture site may be helpful. Use the pressure line on the end of the needle to detect phasic arterial pressure as soon as the artery is punctured.

Fluoroscopy just below the inferior border of the femoral head is often necessary to detect vessel calcification and the wire track.

Previous Local Surgery

Fibrosis and scarring from previous local surgery increase the risk of local bleeding and may cause difficulties with the puncture. The best option is to assess previous angiograms if possible. If in doubt, use the radial artery approach.

Arterial and Venous Access

There are no clear rules as to which vessel should be punctured first. From a practical point of view it is often easier to puncture the vein first. A wire can be placed in the vein first to secure access. This is followed by the arterial puncture, inserting the sheath into the artery, and finally inserting the vein sheath. Placing a wire and sheath inside the vein does not change the anatomy of the common femoral artery, but helps stabilize it for a puncture. Although the femoral vein usually lies medial to the artery, occasionally it may lie more beneath it, increasing the risk of an arteriovenous fistula.

When Can the Sheath Be Removed?

After diagnostic angiography, remove the sheath just after the procedure and use manual compression or a closure device. If you proceed with PCI, the timing of sheath removal depends on which anticoagulant has been used:

• After heparin, check activated clotting time (ACT) and wait until activated clot time is less than 150 seconds.
• After bivalirudin, the sheath can usually be removed immediately at the end of the procedure, as the half-life of bivalirudin is short. Some interventionists remove the sheath after 90 minutes from the end of the procedure.
• After enoxaparin, wait 6–8 hours from the last dose.
• After fondaparinux, wait at least 8 hours from the last dose.
• If the patient is on glycoprotein inhibitors (GPIs), check the platelet count before sheath removal.

It is very important to remember that delayed sheath removal outside the laboratory will be painful as the local anesthetic will have worn off. Sedation and atropine 0.6 mg IV are recommended to avoid vagal reactions. Always check the blood pressure at the time of sheath removal, and assess pulses when finished. Be prepared for a vasovagal reaction.

Many operators prefer to remove the sheath in the laboratory using a closure device with additional manual pressure or a Femostop device if necessary.

Trials
ACUITY

In subgroup analysis of the ACUITY (Acute Catheterization and Urgent Intervention Triage Strategy) trial, 11,621 patients with acute coronary syndromes were randomized to undergo angiography with or without PCI by femoral access. In all, 37.1% of the patients received a vascular closure device. Major bleeding was defined as bleeding requiring interventional or surgical correction, hematoma greater than 5 cm at the access site, retroperitoneal bleeding, or hemoglobin drop of more than 3 g/dL with ecchymosis or hematoma less than 5 cm, oozing blood, or prolonged bleeding (>30 minutes) at the access site. At 30 days, major vascular complications were significantly reduced among the patients who received a closure device. The lowest rate of access site bleeding (<1%) was reported in patients who were treated with bivalirudin monotherapy and a vascular closure device. A vascular closure device and bivalirudin monotherapy were both independent determinants of freedom from major bleeding.

- Always examine the patient and assess the groin before the procedure.
- Optimal antithrombotic and antiplatelet therapy minimize the risk of bleeding.
- Good puncture technique is essential to avoid entry site complications.
- Feel the pulse with your fingers and with the needle tip.
- Do not puncture the posterior wall of the femoral artery.
- Do not puncture the femoral artery above the inguinal ligament.
- If in doubt, a fluoroscopy check will help avoid complications.
- If still in real doubt, remove everything and start again.

Radial Access
Introduction
The radial approach has become increasingly popular in the last few years, though it is still not the access route of choice in many countries. Many operators remain unconvinced, mostly due to technical difficulties with the procedure and the longer learning curve.

Radial artery cannulation is more demanding technically than femoral puncture. Radiation exposure and procedure time tend to be longer than with femoral access, with the initial learning curve and anatomical variations causing delays. In spite of this, however, successful radial access is achieved in over 95% of patients, and the risk of postprocedural occlusion is less than 5%. The radial approach also reduces the rate of minor access site complications such as large hematoma or pseudoaneurysm. Hospital stay and ambulation times are shorter and outcomes better compared with the femoral approach. Advantages and disadvantages of the radial access are listed in Table 1.2.

Table 1.2 Advantages and disadvantages of radial access.

Advantages	Disadvantages
Lower bleeding complication rate	Steeper learning curve
The radial artery is superficial and easy to identify	Risk of unsuccessful puncture, radial artery spasm, or occlusion
Suitable for obese patients	The radial artery is smaller than the femoral
Suitable for patients with peripheral vascular disease	Somewhat higher radiation dose and longer procedural time
Rapid ambulation time and early discharge	Variations in radial or brachial anatomy
Shorter recovery time: 1–2 hours	Possible entry site failure
Allows immediate sheath removal despite use of heparin and GPIs	Not possible in patients with anomalous palmar arch
Preferred by patients	Inability to use catheters larger than 7F, although these are rarely used for PCI nowadays

GPIs, glycoprotein inhibitors; PCI, percutaneous coronary intervention.

Most transradial procedures are performed with 5F or 6F diagnostic catheters or 6F guide catheters. There are no limitations regarding device options and even complex procedures such as bifurcation lesions, CTO or thrombectomy can be performed safely using 6F or, in larger patients a 7F guide. Alternatively, a sheathless 5F guide catheter with a larger internal lumen (7F) can be used.

Radial Artery Anatomy

The aorta gives rise to the innominate (brachiocephalic) artery, the left common carotid artery and the left subclavian artery. The innominate artery becomes the subclavian artery after giving off the right common carotid artery. It then becomes the axillary artery in the shoulder and the brachial artery in the upper arm. At or just below the elbow, the brachial artery divides into the radial and ulnar arteries. The radial artery is more superficial than the femoral artery, separated from the major veins and nerves, and is not an end artery. As it is not an end artery and there are anastomoses through the palmar arch with the ulnar artery, in most patients radial occlusion will not result in ischemic complications. At the wrist the radial artery lies just on the scaphoid bone.

Palmar Arch Patency

Before attempting transradial puncture, it is important to confirm adequate dual arterial supply to the hand.

Allen's Test

This is a simple and quick test for ulnar artery collateral flow and assessment of palmar arch patency. Allen's test is performed routinely in all patients undergoing radial artery puncture. An abnormal (positive) Allen's test occurs with inadequate or absent collaterals from the ulnar artery, which can lead to acute ischemia in the case of radial artery occlusion or, in extreme cases, even amputation of the hand. These complications are exceptionally rare.

Proceed as shown in Figure 1.4:
- Feel the radial and ulnar artery pulses simultaneously.
- Compress both the radial and ulnar artery at the wrist by pressing them.
- Observe hand ischemia.
- Ask the patient to clench and unclench the fist several times, keeping pressure on both arteries.
- Ask the patient to extend the fingers, and release the pressure on the ulnar artery.
- Observe the result. Blushing should appear within 10 seconds as the circulation returns to the hand,
- If the color of the hand does not return within 5–10 seconds, Allen's test is considered positive and arterial puncture CANNOT be attempted on that side.

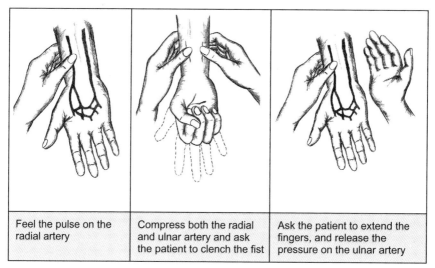

| Feel the pulse on the radial artery | Compress both the radial and ulnar artery and ask the patient to clench the fist | Ask the patient to extend the fingers, and release the pressure on the ulnar artery |

Figure 1.4 Allen's test.

Modified Allen's Test with Oximetry and Barbeau Score

If in doubt interpreting Allen's test, check ulnar arch patency with oximetry using the Barbeau score. Proceed as follows (Figure 1.5):

• Feel the radial artery and ulnar artery pulses.

• Place a pulse oximeter probe on the thumb and compress the radial and ulnar arteries at the wrist. Observe the oximetry pulse tracing.

• After 2 minutes release the ulnar artery, keeping the radial compressed, observe the oximetry pulse tracing, and assess the results of radial artery compression using the Barbeau score.

• The presence of an arterial wave on pulse oximetry, even with reduced amplitude, confirms the presence of adequate blood flow in the palmar arch. If the pulse tracing is negative both initially and after 2 minutes' compression – which means that the Barbeau score is D – the patient is NOT SUITABLE for radial access (Figure 1.5; Table 1.3).

Reverse Allen's Test

This should be performed in patients undergoing a second procedure through the same radial artery as previously. The test helps assess radial artery patency in case of an asymptomatic occlusion. Proceed as in the normal Allen's test with one exception: release compression over the radial artery only and observe the result.

When Radial Puncture Cannot Be Performed

There are a few situations in which the radial artery cannot be punctured:

• Absence of radial pulsation

• Abnormal (positive) Allen's test

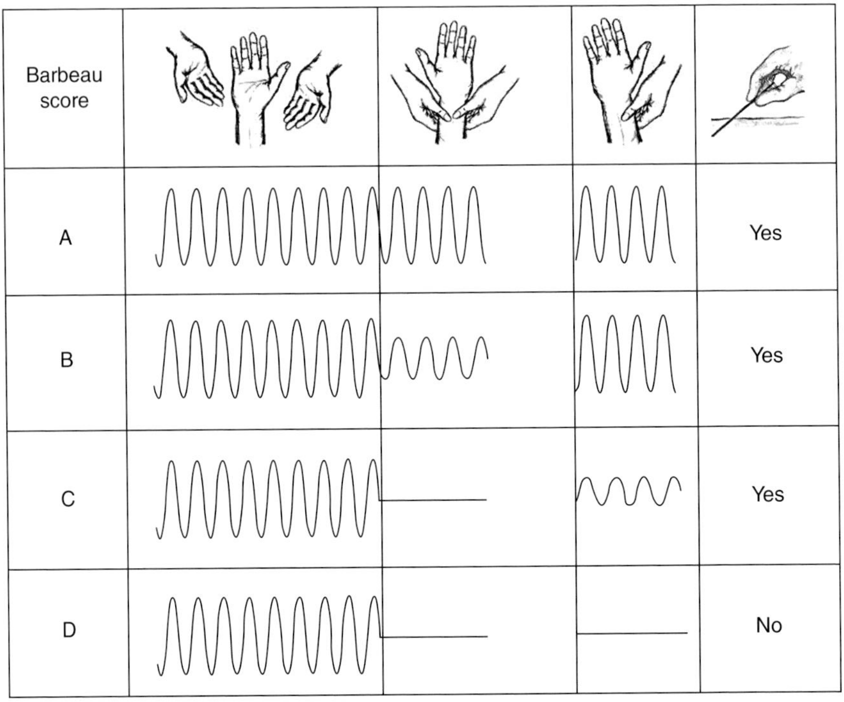

Figure 1.5 Modified Allen's test with oximetry and Barbeau score. A–C confirm palmar arch patency and radial puncture can be performed safely. With D, radial puncture is contraindicated. (Adapted from Baim DS, *Grossman's Cardiac Catheterization Angiography and Intervention*, 7th edition. Lippincott Williams & Wilkins, Philadelphia, 2006.)

Table 1.3 Modified Allen's test and Barbeau score interpretation based on oximetry.

Barbeau Score	Pulse Tracing	Pulse in Oximetry at Start	Pulse in Oximetry After 2 Minutes	Radial Puncture
A	Normal	Positive	Positive	Suitable
B	Damping	Positive	Positive	Suitable
C	Loss of pulse with recovery within 2 min	Negative	Positive	Suitable
D	Loss of pulse without recovery	Negative	Negative	Not suitable

- Potential need for an intra-aortic balloon pump (IABP) during the procedure, e.g., during emergency cases
- Use of catheters or devices larger than 7F
- Presence of a severely calcified or tortuous radial artery
- Presence of upper peripheral vascular disease, e.g., Raynaud's disease
  There are a few pitfalls in the transradial approach that one should be aware of:
- Radial access
- Radial spasm

- Anatomical variability
- Aberrant right subclavian artery
- Inadequate catheter control and back-up

Radial Puncture

For a standard transradial procedure, right hand access is preferable. Access through the left hand is more difficult and, secondly, should be avoided in patients likely to need bypass surgery (the surgeon may need to use the radial artery from the nondominant hand as a graft).In patients with a LIMA graft the left radial or femoral routes are preferable.

Equipment Selection
Dedicated equipment is preferable: a 21-gauge 4-cm needle, a 5–7F short (<10 cm) hydrophilic sheath, and a guide wire. The patient also requires lidocaine, GTN, verapamil, and heparin.

Radial Puncture Technique
Proceed as follows:
- Supernate the hand with wrist hyperextended.
- Feel the radial pulse.
- The optimal puncture site is 1–2 cm proximal to the radial styloid process (Figure 1.6).

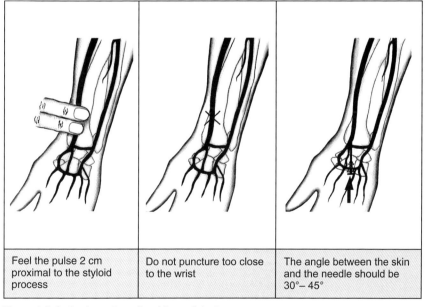

Feel the pulse 2 cm proximal to the styloid process	Do not puncture too close to the wrist	The angle between the skin and the needle should be 30°– 45°

Figure 1.6 Optimal puncture site of the radial artery.

- Do not puncture too close to the wrist. as below this point the artery is tortuous; puncturing too close to the wrist is the most common mistake.
- Start with local anesthesia using 2% lidocaine and a short needle. Do not infiltrate the radial artery, as this may cause radial spasm. Remember that the angle between the skin and the needle should be approximately 30°–45°.
- Puncture the artery accurately on the first attempt.
- If you fail, wait for a while to allow the spasm to relax, then attempt the puncture again.
- After successful puncture, and if the flow is good, slowly insert a wire through the needle with gentle rotation of the needle.
- If the flow is poor, withdraw the needle slowly until it is in the artery lumen.
- If wire passage is smooth, insert a hydrophilic sheath over the guide wire.
- Inject vasodilators through the sheath to reduce the risk of artery spasm.
- Administer IV heparin 50 U/kg (which is usually 3000–5000 U) to avoid thrombosis.

This is the classic bare needle puncture, which is the standard technique in many centers. Some operators, however, prefer to use a venous cannula (butterfly) with the puncture set. This can be more difficult technically, but gives access to the artery before sheath insertion. The cannulation puncture technique requires the following steps:

- The needle is inserted until blood flow appears.
- Then the needle is advanced through the posterior wall of the artery.
- The needle is removed and the cannula is withdrawn slowly until arterial blood flow confirms an intraluminal position of the cannula.
- The guide wire can then be gently advanced.

Catheter Selection

Commonly used catheters for the femoral approach, such as Judkins left (JL), Judkins right (JR), or EBU (Extra Back-Up), are also suitable for the left radial intervention. The general rule is, however, that for the right radial approach the catheter should be 0.5 size smaller than would be selected for a femoral procedure, e.g., JL3.5 (instead of the JL4) for left coronary engagement and JR4 for the right coronary artery. In some cases Amplatz left may be useful. For left ventriculography use a standard pigtail catheter.

If the subclavian artery is tortuous, ask the patient to take a deep breath in to lower the heart. If this does not help, switch to an Amplatz catheter. It is also safer to keep the J wire in the catheter during manipulation and ensures better control. Asking the patient to take a deep breath in followed by anti-clockwise catheter rotation can also be helpful if the wire goes into the descending aorta.

Radial Access Problems and Complications

Sometimes either the wire or the catheter cannot be advanced smoothly. This is often caused by radial spasm, but may also be due to anatomical variations such as tortuosities in the subclavian system, radioulnar loops, short ascending aorta, or anomalous origins of the great vessels. It is important to become familiar with these problems as most of them can be negotiated using simple maneuvers.

A few issues should be considered:

- Radial artery spasm, subintimal tracking, and local pain remain the major problems of radial access.
- Puncture itself as well as sheath insertion and wire manipulation are often uncomfortable and may cause hypotension and a vasovagal reaction.
- Adequate sedation and analgesia are an important part of the procedure and should be used routinely (e.g., fentanyl 25 µg in divided doses up to 100 µg IV). Pulse oximetry on a finger of the other hand is mandatory.
- Bleeding as a complication is very rare.

If resistance is felt passing the wire or catheter up the arm, check the position under fluoroscopy and consider:

- Radial artery spasm
- Radioulnar loop
- Radial artery occlusion
- Radial artery stenosis
- Subintimal tracking
- Tortuosity, e.g.. due to too distal puncture site
- Small side branches
- Aberrant right subclavian artery with late takeoff

Subintimal Tracking and Tortuosities

Subintimal tracking and tortuosities always carry a risk of dissection or perforation. It may be necessary to remove the wire and to confirm arterial flow. Consider repuncture more proximally or switch to the other radial or femoral approach.

Radial Artery Spasm and Management

The radial artery is very sensitive and prone to spasm. Spasm may be caused by too large a catheter size, wire manipulation, or during J-wire exchanges. Although spasm is often short-lived and may resolve spontaneously, it causes pain and difficulties with catheter manipulation. Rarely with severe persistent spasm the wire or sheath may be trapped and immovable. Very rarely general anesthesia may be required to remove the equipment.

To limit the risk of spasm, inject standard intra-arterial vasodilators of three routinely used agents: verapamil, lidocaine and GTN (the doses are listed in Table 1.4). Always use a hydrophilic sheath and wire. A long sheath helps protect the artery wall during catheter manipulation. Inject GTN through the arterial sheath, wait a while, and continue with the hydrophilic wire. Give a GTN tablet sublingually and inject vasodilators again. If spasm still persists, reinject analgesics and wait. Sometimes application of a warm compress to

Table 1.4 Vasodilators in spasm management.

Vasodilators	Dose
Verapamil	2 mg
Lidocaine 2%	20 mg aliquots
Glyceryl trinitrate	100–200 μg

the arm may help relieve the spasm. If spasm still persists, the sheath must be removed.

In summary: Spasm can be avoided by adequate local anesthesia and sedation, successful first puncture and cannulation, selection of correct catheter size, injection of vasodilators, and use of a long sheath.

Tortuosities in the Subclavian System
Subclavian tortuosities are more common in females, in patients with hypertension, and in the elderly. Deep inhalation may be help elongate and straighten out the bends a little, allowing the catheter to advance smoothly. A hydrophilic wire may also be useful.

Radioulnar Loop
Although this occurs in approximately 2% of patients, the complete loop is the commonest case of access failure and if not recognized carries a potential risk of vessel perforation during insertion of the wire. Dealing with radial loop requires skill and patience. Sometimes the loop may be negotiated successfully using a J wire with guiding catheter support and a soft hydrophilic wire to straighten the loop. In some cases it is just impossible to cross the loop.

Radial Occlusion
Radial artery occlusion is more likely if the diameter of the artery is small, the sheath is too large, anticoagulation during the procedure is inadequate, or cannulation is prolonged. This should not be a problem clinically, as ulnar collaterals supply blood to the whole hand and ischemic necrosis is very rare. Radial artery occlusion can be avoided with adequate procedural anticoagulation: give intra-arterial heparin bolus 50 U/kg during diagnostic angiography and 100 U/kg during angioplasty. The activated clotting time should be maintained above 250 seconds. Bivalirudin is an alternative, but the added expense seems unjustified as control of bleeding from the radial access site is usually straightforward. Always perform Allen's test to check patency of the palmar arch. An occluded artery can usually be crossed with a wire and reopened.

Arterial Perforation
Although perforation is very rare, vigorous wire manipulation, particularly in tortuous or calcified segments or radial loops, is always risky. Any

resistance during wire insertion should result in wire withdrawal and a fluoroscopy check. If advancing the wire and catheter is difficult, it is better to switch to a smaller catheter or use a femoral approach than to keep manipulating.

If the perforation is within the sheath area, the sheath can seal it and prevent further extravasation. In this case the procedure can be continued from this site. After the procedure either a compression bandage or an inflated blood pressure cuff should be placed over the perforated area and maintained for a couple of hours. This will prevent compartment syndrome.

If the perforation is proximal and cannot be sealed by the sheath, the arm above the elbow should be compressed by either a compression bandage or an inflated blood pressure cuff during the rest of the procedure and for a couple of hours afterwards to ensure adequate hemostasis.

Compartment Syndrome

A compartment syndrome is most commonly caused by perforation and excessive bleeding into the deep compartments of the forearm. Increased pressure within the compartment following arterial perforation limits arterial blood supply and leads to ischemia. The early signs of compartment syndrome are pain, increased tension and tightness in the forearm, sometimes extending proximally to the elbow, swelling in the compartment, and altered hand sensation. Nerve palsies are possible as well as ischemic necrosis. The patient may have difficulties with fist closure. Ulnar pulses are usually present and Allen's test is normal and negative. Because compartment pressure may cause nerve damage, a decompression fasciotomy is an emergency.

Aberrant Right Subclavian Artery

This is the most common congenital aortic arch anomaly, and is usually asymptomatic, although it may present with dysphagia. The aberrant subclavian artery arises from the distal and posterior part of the aortic arch at its junction with the descending aorta and forms a vascular ring round the esophagus. When difficulties occur with catheter manipulation, contrast injection may confirm the presence of an aberrant artery. In LAO projection the wire enters the origin of the aberrant subclavian artery pointing towards the left and a sharp angle has to be negotiated into the ascending aorta.

Vasovagal Reaction

Bradycardia and hypotension may occur during insertion of the sheath, but less commonly than with femoral access. This is usually a transient reaction and treatment is with atropine 0.6–1.2 mg and intravenous fluid.

Persistent Pain

Vascular or neurological complications are very rare but may occur as a result of prolonged hemostatic compression.

Hemostasis

ACT monitoring is not necessary before sheath removal as the radial artery is easily compressible and the sheath can be removed immediately after the procedure. Hemostasis can be obtained using a Hemoband or similar device to compress the artery. This is a transparent band that allows direct visualization of the puncture site and ensures effective hemostasis. The band should compress the artery without obstructing venous return. The risk of bleeding is low and the band can be removed after 2–4 hours if hemostasis is secure. If bleeding occurs the balloon should be reinflated.

The patient can be mobilized immediately after the procedure but should be told to rest the arm for 24 hours and keep it dry and clean. Complications with closure devices such as arterial occlusion are extremely rare.

Trials
OCTOPUS

In this prospective multicenter study, 377 patients were randomized to coronary angiography and PCI using either the femoral or the radial approach. In this analysis, the incidence of vascular complications was significantly reduced in the radial group (1.6% vs. 6.5%; $P = 0.03$), with all vascular complications except for one occurring in the femoral group.

RAPTOR

The RAPTOR study was designed to see if operators experienced in femoral access could switch immediately to radial access. A total of 410 patients were included to study patient safety, radiation exposure, patient comfort, duration of procedures, and staff involvement. The trial demonstrated that experienced interventional cardiologists can easily quickly change their practice towards radial access. It took significantly more time to puncture the radial artery and to perform coronary angiography, but the PCI procedure time was similar in both femoral and radial groups. Radiation times and radiation doses were also higher in patients undergoing angiography treated with the radial approach, but overall there were no differences between the two groups of patients undergoing PCI.

MORTAL

In this study 38,872 patients were randomized for PCI using either femoral access (79.5%) or radial access (20.5%). The need for a periprocedural transfusion was almost 50% lower using the radial approach in comparison with the femoral approach. In the femoral group, 2.8% of the patients required a periprocedural transfusion, but only 1.4% in the radial group needed a transfusion. This reduction in the need for transfusions was related to a significant mortality benefit at 30 days and 1 year.

- Get familiar with variations of radial anatomy to deal with loops and tortuosities.
- Always perform Allen's test before radial artery puncture.
- Proceed carefully and use a hydrophilic sheath and wire.
- Prevent spasm, occlusion, and pain.
- Always give a vasodilator cocktail and sedation.
- Smaller is better: use the smallest size catheter you can.

Coronary Anatomy and Projections

Introduction

A comprehensive knowledge of coronary anatomy and of the common anatomical variations is absolutely fundamental to successful coronary angiography and angioplasty. In addition, each vessel and each segment of each vessel is best visualized in certain radiographic projections to avoid vessel overlap and foreshortening. These standard projections may need to be modified slightly in individual cases. Exact visualization of a lesion in the correct projection is crucial to successful angioplasty.

Coronary Artery Anatomy

The origins of the normal coronary arteries are located in the center of the left and right sinuses of Valsalva above the aortic valve. The posterior sinus of the aortic valve is the noncoronary sinus.

Left Coronary Artery

The left coronary artery (LCA) originates from the left coronary sinus of Valsalva initially as the left main coronary artery. This is of variable length and may even be absent, with the LCA bifurcating immediately at its origin. There may even be a double-ostial LCA. The left main coronary artery divides into the left anterior descending (LAD) and left circumflex (LCx) coronary artery branches. The LAD runs towards the cardiac apex in the anterior interventricular groove. It gives rise to several diagonal branches running superficially and several septal perforator branches which run in parallel and at right angles to the main vessel. The LAD supplies blood to the anterior wall through its diagonal branches, the anterior two-thirds of the interventricular septum through its septal perforator branches, and the cardiac apex by its terminal branches. In some cases the left main trifurcates, giving rise to another vessel, the intermediate coronary artery, which supplies the free anterior wall and runs between the LAD and LCx. The LCx coronary artery courses in the left atrioventricular groove and has two or more obtuse marginal branches (sometimes known as posterolateral circumflex arteries) and through them supplies blood to the posterior and lateral walls.

Right Coronary Artery

The right coronary artery (RCA) originates from the right coronary sinus of Valsalva and runs in the right atrioventricular groove to the junction of the atrioventricular groove and the posterior interventricular sulcus, called the crux. The dominant RCA supplies blood to the inferior wall, to the inferior one-third of the interventricular septum, including blood supply to the posterior papillary muscle, and through its marginal branches to the free right ventricular wall. The posterior descending branch (PDA) supplies the inferior one-third of the interventricular septum, and the posterolateral branch supplies the posterolateral wall of the left ventricle.

Smaller branches from the RCA (down which a wire sometimes tracks, but not usually amenable to angioplasty) include the sinus node branch and the conus branch arising proximally and the atrioventricular nodal artery arising from the RCA at the crux.

Dominant, Nondominant, or Codominant?

By definition, the term *dominance* applies to the artery that supplies the posterior diaphragmatic part of the interventricular septum, i.e., the PDA. The dominant artery can be either the RCA or the LCx. Sometimes both the RCA and the LCx reach the crux and give rise to the posterior descending coronary artery. In these situations the arterial system is codominant. Coronary artery dominance is determined by the origin of the atrioventricular nodal artery at the crux. In almost 85% of cases the atrioventricular nodal artery originates from the RCA so the RCA is dominant, and only in 15% does it originate from the LCx. The dominant coronary artery gives off the PDA, which provides septal branches to the inferior one-third of the interventricular septum.

Quality of Angiographic Images

Catheter position and adequate contrast injection are two factors which help determine the quality of angiographic images. There are a few basic principles:

• The catheter should be positioned deeply enough and engage the artery without causing reverse contrast flow. Good selection of catheter size is crucial. Poor catheter engagement with nonselective contrast injection will result in a poor-quality angiographic image.

• The catheter tip must be as coaxial as possible with the origin of the coronary artery. Avoid contrast injection if the catheter tip is at right angles to the vessel wall (a possibility if too small a Judkins catheter is selected for the LCA) as this may cause a main stem dissection.

• Contrast injection should be adequate, sufficient, and rapid to fill the arteries properly during at least one cardiac cycle. Inadequate contrast volume or injection rate will result in poor visualization and may cause misinterpretation and incorrect assessment of the coronary anatomy and lesions.

• The first injection to the LCA and RCA should be preceded by a small contrast test in case there is an ostial lesion in either or these vessels.

• Too vigorous a contrast injection will cause pressure damping or vessel dissection and must be avoided.

• Contrast can be injected either using an automated injector or manually with a standard syringe. Automated injections are very practical, are easy to use, and help reduce the volume of contrast and radiation time.

Radiation Dose (see Radiation Safety p. 58)

This will be monitored by the radiographer; screening times of more than 45 minutes should be avoided except in emergency situations. Most angioplasty procedures need less than half this screening time. Remember that radiation dose to the operator is greatest when the X-ray tube is nearest to the operator (i.e., LAO cranial or LAO projections) and least when it is furthest away (i.e., RAO and RAO caudal projections). Minimizing radiation takes practice and experience. Good operators can perform routine coronary angiography in under 2 minutes screening, with a patient radiation dose of 5 mSv or less.

Coronary Images

Optimal visualization using the correct radiographic projection is the clue to good angiography. The anatomy of the coronary arteries as well as segments with lesions should always be assessed in several standard views. Generally, every coronary artery segment should be assessed in at least two orthogonal projections. This includes standard RAO, LAO, and anteroposterior (AP) cranial and caudal images.

A few routine projections should be used initially. This will save time, radiation dose, and contrast dose. Nevertheless, the majority of patients, particularly those with complex lesions, will require additional views – slight modifications of standard projections. These will be needed to visualize lesions which overlap or are foreshortened in standard views.

The aim is to "open" the view avoiding overlapping and foreshortening. With overlapping arteries a lesion may be masked, may look less significant, or may even not be recognized at all. Beware the foreshortened projection which makes a lesion shorter and appear more severe.

Visualization of small branches and collaterals is also very important. This helps identify the correct course for the guide wire and helps avoid complications such as perforation or dissection. It also identifies retrograde filling of a distal vessel via collaterals in cases of complete total occlusion.

Summary of general principles that can be helpful during the procedure:
• The catheter tip should be co-axial with the vessel.
• Ask the patient to take a deep inhalation, and to hold it, with every injection.
• Avoid too powerful a contrast injection with the risk of vessel dissection or catheter recoil.
• Ensure that contrast injection is adequate to complete coronary artery filling in one cardiac cycle.
• Identify missing vessels, coronary anomalies, and grafts. Missing arteries may be filled by septal collaterals.
• Generally all caudal views with the image intensifier or flat plate tilted towards the patient's feet offer best image of the LCx, while cranial views with projection tilted toward the patient's head are best for the LAD.
• Avoid vessel overlapping and foreshortening.
• Take at least two orthogonal views of the same segment.
• Often slight additional angulation – caudal, cranial, RAO, or LAO – is needed to "open" the view to avoid overlapping and to visualize the segment of interest.

The most important landmarks related to the LAO/RAO view are summarized in Table 1.5.

Table 1.5 Orientation points of important landmarks in the left/right anterior oblique (LAO/RAO) view.

Landmark	LAO View	RAO View
Image intensifier	To the left	To the right
Spine	On the right	On the left
Apex	To the left	To the right
LAD	On the left	On the right
LCx	On the right	On the left

Right Anterior Oblique Views

In RAO projections the spine is located to the left of the view with the LAD coursing smoothly from the left to the right and the LCx running down to the bottom of the screen (Table 1.6; Figure 1.7).

• *RAO cranial* view offers a good view of the middle and distal segments of LAD and distal LCx. All proximal segments, however, are overlapped and

Table 1.6 RAO angiographic projections of coronary arteries.

	RAO Cranial	Straight RAO	RAO Caudal
LCA	LAD mid and distal LCx distal	–	LM and LAD proximal LCx with marginal branches
RCA	–	RCA mid with PDA Distal collaterals	–

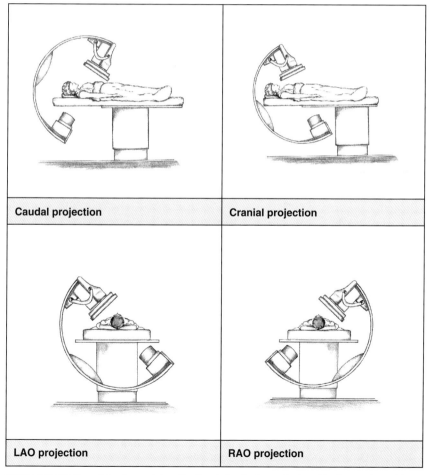

Caudal projection — Cranial projection

LAO projection — RAO projection

Figure 1.7 Position of the image intensifier in relation to the patient and to the angiographic projections.

foreshortened. Shallow RAO cranial (RAO 15°, cranial 30°) is a good view to display the left main and the entire length of the LAD.
• *RAO caudal* projection offers a good view of the left main and proximal LAD but a very good view of the LCx with marginal branches pointing downwards. The distal LAD in this view is overlapped by diagonal branches.
• *Straight RAO* projection is not very useful for LCA visualization because of overlap and foreshortening, but it offers good views of the RCA. RAO 30° is commonly used to display the RCA with the PDA and potential distal collaterals.

Left Anterior Oblique Views
LAO projections display the spine on the right side of the view and the LAD pointing down and to the left (Table 1.7; Figure 1.7).
• *LAO cranial* projection shows the middle and distal segments of the LAD with diagonals and the distal LCx. All proximal segments including the left main, however, are overlapped and foreshortened. LAO cranial projection offers a good view of the distal RCA with the PDA.
• *LAO caudal or spider* view offers great trifurcation delineation. It is best for the left main, proximal LAD, but particularly for the proximal LCx with marginal branches pointing downwards. The image is usually overlapped by the diaphragm and the spine and the quality may be poor. Deep inhalation can be helpful for better visualization.
• *Straight LAO* view. Be aware that the straight LAO view commonly used as LAO 30° or 60° is not suitable for LAD visualization because of overlap and foreshortening. It shows the middle segment of the LCx better and is of great value for RCA visualization, displaying the ostium and its middle segment.

Posteroanterior Views
The main disadvantage of this projection is that the spine is positioned in the middle of the image and interferes with the coronary arteries. However, in some cases, particularly if standard views are difficult to obtain, posteroanterior (PA) projections help to display the ostial left main coronary artery (Table 1.8; Figure 1.7).

Table 1.7 LAO angiographic projections of coronary arteries.

	LAO Cranial	Straight LAO	LAO Caudal
LCA	LM ostium LAD mid and distal LCx distal	LCx mid/distal	LM and proximal LAD LCx with marginal branches
RCA	RCA distal/crux and PDA	RCA ostium/mid/distal	LIMA anastomosis

LIMA, left internal mammary artery.

Table 1.8 Posteroanterior (PA) angiographic projections of coronary arteries.

	PA Cranial	Straight PA	PA Caudal
LCA	LM ostium LAD mid/distal LCx distal	LM ostium	LM bifurcation LAD proximal LCx proximal and marginal branches bifurcation
RCA	RCA distal and PDA	–	–

LCA, left coronary artery; RCA, right coronary artery; LM, left main coronary artery; LAD, left anterior descending coronary artery; LCx, left circumflex coronary artery.

Table 1.9 Optimal angiographic projections of the left main coronary artery. Views in bold type are the initial standard views.

Segment of Artery	Projection
Ostial	**PA, cranial 40°** LAO 30°–45°, cranial 30° LAO 45°, caudal 35° (spider)
Body	**RAO 30°, caudal 30°** PA, caudal 30°
Distal	**LAO 45°, caudal 35° (spider)** PA, caudal 30° RAO 30°, caudal 30°

- *PA cranial* exposes the entire length of the LAD all the way down to the diagonals.
- *PA caudal* shows the distal left main coronary artery and proximal parts of the LAD and LCx.
- *Straight PA* shows the left main coronary artery ostium.

Optimal Angiographic Projections
LM: Left Main Coronary Artery
The course of the left main coronary artery is downward, forward, and slightly to the right. Anatomically, the left main may be short or long, straight or curved. Different views are needed to visualize its proximal, body, and distal segment. RAO or LAO caudal views offer the best images (Table 1.9).

LAD: Left Anterior Descending Coronary Artery
The LAD should be assessed in at least two projections. The middle segment is best visible in the LAO cranial projection. This is also a good projection for the origin of diagonal branches and therefore a very good projection for bifurcation procedures. However, the image may be overlapped by the distal segment of the LCx or left posterolateral vessels. Foreshortening of the proximal segment is also possible, which gives an impression of a shorter and more

Table 1.10 Optimal angiographic projections of the left anterior descending artery. Views in bold type are the initial standard views.

Segment of Artery	Projection
Ostial	**RAO 30°, caudal 30°**
	LAO 45°, caudal 35° (spider)
	LAO 50°, cranial 30°
	PA, caudal 30°
	PA, cranial 40°
Body	**PA, cranial 35°–45°**
	RAO 30°, cranial 30°
	LAO 50°, cranial 30°
	Lateral with caudocranial 20°
Distal	**RAO 30°, caudal 30°**
	Lateral with caudocranial 20°
	RAO 30°–45°
LAD/diagonal	**LAO 50°, cranial 30°**
	PA, cranial 35°–45°
	LAO 45°, caudal 35° (spider)
Diagonals	RAO 30°, cranial 30°

Table 1.11 Optimal angiographic projections of the left circumflex coronary artery. Views in bold type are initial standard views.

Segment of Artery	Projection
Ostial	**LAO 45°, caudal 35°**
	PA, caudal 30°
	RAO 30°, caudal 30°–40°
Body	**LAO 30°**
	RAO 30°, caudal 30°PA caudal 30°
Distal	**LAO 45°–60°**
	LAO 50°, cranial 30°
	RAO 30°, caudal 30°
OM/bifurcation	**PA, caudal 30°**
	LAO 45°, caudal 35° (spider)
	RAO 30°, caudal 30°

OM, obtuse marginal branch.

severe lesion than it really is. Deep inhalation can be helpful in improving visualization (Table 1.10).

LCx: Left Circumflex Coronary Artery

Generally for LCx visualization, caudal views are the most useful. The RAO caudal and PA caudal views display the LCx without foreshortening in the proximal segments and without overlapping of the LAD. Deep inhalation can help expose the whole length of the LCx (Table 1.11).

Table 1.12 Optimal angiographic projections of the RCA.
Views in bold type are the initial standard views.

Segment of Artery	Projection
Ostial	**LAO 50°, cranial 30°,**
	PA caudal
	LAO 45°–60°
Body	**LAO 45°–60°**
	Lateral with caudo-cranial 20°
	RAO 30°–45°
Distal/PDA	**PA, cranial 35°–45°**
	LAO 50°, cranial 30°
	RAO 30°–45°

Table 1.13 Optimal angiographic projections of left internal mammary artery graft.

Segment of Graft	Projection
Ostial segment	Shallow RAO, LAO 60°
Mid vessel	Shallow RAO, lateral
Insertion to LAD junction	RAO cranial, lateral view
Insertion to RCA junction	LAO, RAO, lateral view
Origin from the left subclavian	PA, RAO cranial

RCA: Right Coronary Artery

The LAO cranial offers the best view of the RCA as its major branches are the posterior descending and the posterolateral branch, which have a downward course. The RAO projection, however, displays the mid segment of the artery, foreshortening the proximal and distal parts (Table 1.12).

LIMA: Left Internal Mammary Artery

The left internal mammary artery (LIMA) originates from the first part of the left subclavian artery, just distal to the origin of the left vertebral artery. As a graft it is anastomosed to the mid LAD and the RAO 40° projection offers optimal visualization. However, the lateral view can also be helpful. LAO 60° gives the best view of the LIMA ostium (Table 1.13).

SVG: Saphenous Vein Grafts

A preoperative angiogram should be assessed before the procedure if possible. Generally projections used for visualization of the bypass graft are similar to those for the same segments of the native vessels. The best view for an ostial lesion is a shallow RAO or PA caudal to see the origin of the vein graft, and this is also optimal for an RCA vein graft. Sternal wires are also helpful in localizing the graft origin and its track (Table 1.14).

Table 1.14 Optimal angiographic projections of saphenous vein graft.

Segment of Graft	Projection
SVG – LAD	LAO caudal
SVG – LCx	RAO caudal
SVG – native LAD	LAO cranial
SVG – native OM	PA caudal
SVG – PDA	LAO cranial

If the requisite number of vein grafts cannot be identified, perform aortography in the LAO 30° projection.

Standard Projections

The best projection for engagement of both the left and the right coronary artery is LAO 50°. This view displays the origin of the LCA and the RCA and should be used routinely.

Left Coronary Artery Views (Figure 1.8)

LAO 50° Cranial 30° View

Although the sinus of Valsalva on the proximal LAD in this view is superimposed, this projection offers the best view of the left main, mid LAD, and further all along down to the diagonals and septals. Diagonals are well displayed and clearly separated. Deep inhalation is very helpful in avoiding overlap with the diaphragm and liver. Foreshortening and overlapping may occur in the distal segments of the LCx.

RAO 45° Cranial View

This offers the best view of the middle and distal segments of the LAD and distal LCx. This is also a great projection for diagonal branches and septal collateral visualization. This may be particularly useful in PCI of chronic total occlusion, where septal collaterals are used in the retrograde approach.

RAO 30° Caudal 30° View

This projection displays the mid and distal left main, proximal LAD, and most of the LCx with obtuse marginal branches pointing downwards and showing the profile of the whole length of the proximal LAD. It has to be noted that the middle and distal segments of the LAD are usually overlapped by diagonal branches.

PA Caudal 30° View

This gives the best view for visualization of the distal left main and ostial LAD and LCx. This is also the best working projection for intervention. Note that sometimes shallow RAO or LAO angulation may be needed to uncover the coronary arteries from the dense image of the vertebrae and catheter

View of the coronary arteries	Image intensifier position	
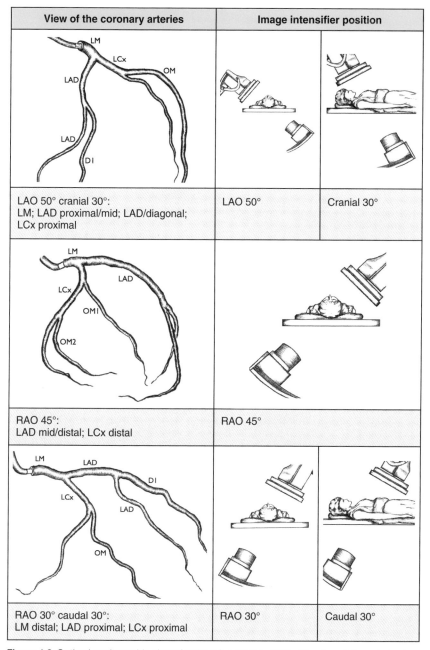		
LAO 50° cranial 30°: LM; LAD proximal/mid; LAD/diagonal; LCx proximal	LAO 50°	Cranial 30°
RAO 45°: LAD mid/distal; LCx distal	RAO 45°	
RAO 30° caudal 30°: LM distal; LAD proximal; LCx proximal	RAO 30°	Caudal 30°

Figure 1.8 Optimal angiographic views for the left coronary artery. The view of the arteries is shown on the left with the corresponding table position on the right. LAD, left anterior descending coronary artery; LAO, left anterior oblique; LCA, left coronary artery; LCx, left circumflex coronary artery; LM, left main coronary artery; PA, posteroanterior; RAO, right anterior oblique.

View of the coronary arteries	Image intensifier position
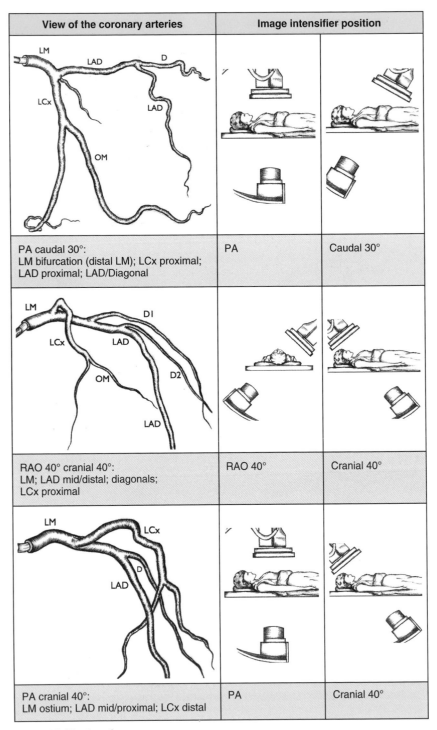	
PA caudal 30°: LM bifurcation (distal LM); LCx proximal; LAD proximal; LAD/Diagonal	PA Caudal 30°
RAO 40° cranial 40°: LM; LAD mid/distal; diagonals; LCx proximal	RAO 40° Cranial 40°
PA cranial 40°: LM ostium; LAD mid/proximal; LCx distal	PA Cranial 40°

Figure 1.8 (*Continued*).

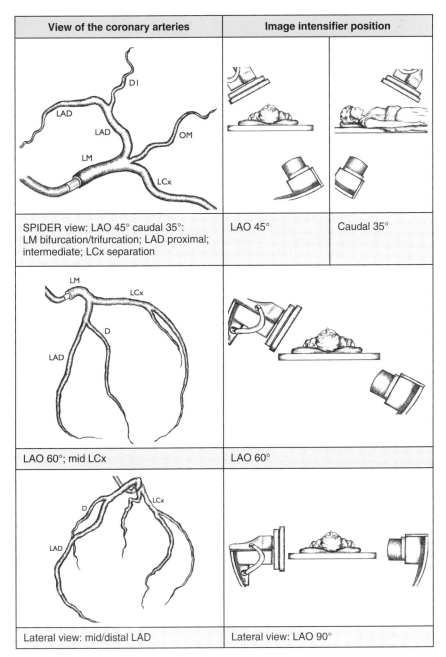

View of the coronary arteries	Image intensifier position
SPIDER view: LAO 45° caudal 35°: LM bifurcation/trifurcation; LAD proximal; intermediate; LCx separation	LAO 45° — Caudal 35°
LAO 60°; mid LCx	LAO 60°
Lateral view: mid/distal LAD	Lateral view: LAO 90°

Figure 1.8 (*Continued*).

placed in the aorta. The great advantage of this projection is the reduced dose of operator radiation.

RAO 40° Cranial 40° View
This is an excellent view for mid and distal LAD lesions. The circumflex tends to overlap the main LAD. It is not usually of much help for proximal circumflex lesions.

PA Cranial 40° View
This view shows best the proximal and mid segments of the LAD and is the best projection for an LAD bifurcation procedure.

LAO 45° Caudal 35° View (Spider)
This projection offers the best view of trifurcation of the LAD, the intermediate, and the LCx arteries. The left main is usually well visualized. However, aortic cusp overlap may obscure its proximal segment. This is the projection of choice if there are difficulties crossing the proximal segment of the LAD and LCx.

LAO 60°
The steep LAO view is best for the main circumflex. Distal circumflex vessels may overlap and the LAD is foreshortened. The high radiation dose to the operator with this view can be reduced by adding caudal tilt.

Lateral View
This view offers great separation of LAD and LCx and best visualization of the mid and distal LAD. There is a foreshortening of the left main and proximal LAD. This projection is of great value in showing the LIMA anastomosis to LAD.

Right Coronary Artery Views (Figure 1.9)
- *LAO 50° view.* This is the best projection of the ostial and mid segments of the RCA. PDA and posterolateral branches are foreshortened.
- *LAO 30° cranial 20° view.* This image provides a view of the entire length of the RCA particularly, displaying the proximal and mid RCA and PDA with crux and the right posterolateral branch. Deep inhalation is needed to separate the artery from the diaphragm.
- *PA cranial 40° view.* Usually this image shows the mid and distal segment of the RCA and its bifurcation into the PDA and left ventricular branch. However, it also offers a good view of the ostium of the RCA. This is an excellent projection for visualization of distal collaterals from the RCA to the mid and distal LCx artery. This helps localize the origin of an occluded LCx artery. Simultaneous contrast injection through the right and the left coronary arteries may be needed.

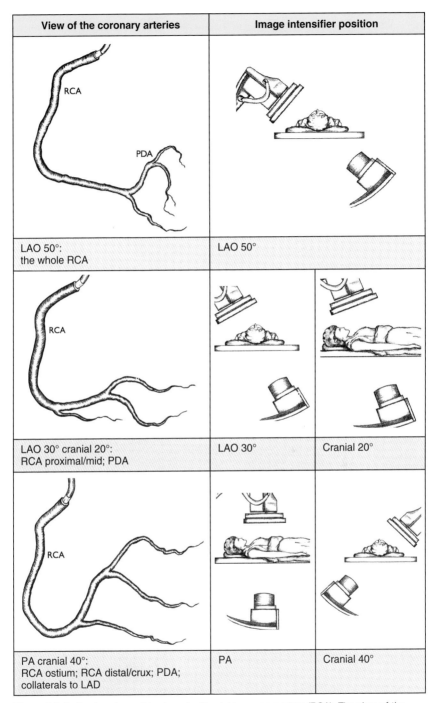

View of the coronary arteries	Image intensifier position
LAO 50°: the whole RCA	LAO 50°
LAO 30° cranial 20°: RCA proximal/mid; PDA	LAO 30° Cranial 20°
PA cranial 40°: RCA ostium; RCA distal/crux; PDA; collaterals to LAD	PA Cranial 40°

Figure 1.9 Optimal angiographic views for the right coronary artery (RCA). The view of the arteries is shown on the left with the corresponding table position on the right.

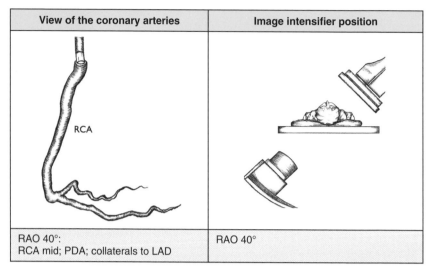

View of the coronary arteries	Image intensifier position
RAO 40°: RCA mid; PDA; collaterals to LAD	RAO 40°

Figure 1.9 (*Continued*).

Table 1.15 Best views for bifurcation lesions.

Bifurcation	Best View
Left main bifurcation	RAO caudal, spider
LAD/diagonal bifurcation	LAO cranial
LAD/diagonal bifurcation proximal	Spider
LCx bifurcation	RAO caudal, spider
LCx bifurcation distal	LAO cranial
RCA/PDA bifurcation	PA cranial

• *RAO 40° view.* This view allows visualization of the mid segment of the RCA as well as all the length of the long PDA with its septal branches directed upwards. This view also offers good view of distal collaterals to the LAD.

Projections for Bifurcation Lesions

Optimal visualization of the bifurcation is an important part of a successful procedure. The left main bifurcation is best displayed in the RAO caudal and spider view. Sometimes a steeper spider view is very useful. The best projection for an LAD/diagonal bifurcation lesion is the LAO cranial view. However, a proximal bifurcation should be assessed in the spider view. RAO caudal and spider projections also offer a great view of the proximal circumflex artery. Distal lesions of the circumflex artery, however, are displayed adequately in the LAO cranial view. A RCA distal bifurcation is well visualized in the PA cranial projection. The best views for bifurcation lesions are shown in Table 1.15.

- The dominant artery supplies the PDA and is either the RCA or the LCx.
- Avoid overlapping and foreshortening.
- The first injection in the LCA and RCA should be preceded by a small contrast test.
- Establish a few routinely used projections. Use additional views if needed.
- Be alert to missing vessels, coronary anomalies. and grafts.
- Minimize screening time and radiation dose.

Anomalies

Introduction

Although congenital abnormalities of the coronary arteries found in adults are uncommon, knowledge of the most common anomalies is important for successful angiography and for planning further treatment.

Congenital abnormalities of the coronary arteries may involve the origin, course, number, structure, and/or termination of the vessel. Normally, the left main coronary artery arises from the left coronary sinus of Valsalva and divides into the left anterior descending artery and the circumflex artery. The right coronary artery originates from the right coronary sinus of Valsalva. Sometimes, however, there is a single coronary artery arising from the right or the left coronary sinus. In other cases there are two or three separate origins of the anomalously arising coronary arteries. Accurate delineation of the origin and the course of the vessel is important, as an anomalous origin of an artery can be mistaken for an occlusion or an absent artery when problems are encountered trying to identify its origin.

Table 1.16 The commonest coronary artery anomalies at coronary angiography.

Absent left main artery – separate ostia of the left anterior descending and left circumflex arteries
Anomalous origin of the left circumflex artery arising from the proximal right coronary artery
Anomalous origin of the left circumflex artery arising from the right sinus of Valsalva
Leftward origin of the right coronary artery nearer the left main than usual
Anomalous origin of the left main artery arising from the right sinus of Valsalva – four possible courses of the artery to reach the left ventricle (see Fig 1.12)

Less Common Coronary Anomalies at Angiography
Single coronary artery. Complete absence of either the right or the left coronary artery. Extreme dominance.
Origin of left coronary artery from pulmonary trunk
Coronary fistulae, e.g., left anterior descending to pulmonary artery; left or right coronary artery to coronary sinus, right atrium, or right ventricle

A coronary artery arising from the wrong coronary sinus occurs in 0.64% of all births. Those anomalies that are present at birth may cause no cardiac symptoms at all provided myocardial blood supply is satisfactory. Some anomalies, however, are hemodynamically significant and are associated with abnormalities of myocardial perfusion, with a higher risk of myocardial ischemia or sudden death (usually on exercise). Symptoms include syncope, arrhythmias, myocardial infarction, heart failure, or endocarditis. In general, life-threatening anomalies are usually associated with the origin of the left main coronary artery from the opposite sinus of Valsalva.

The most commonly diagnosed anomalies are separate origins of the LAD and the LCx from the left sinus of Valsalva, and the LCx arising from the right sinus of Valsalva adjacent to or directly from the RCA itself. Also relatively common is the RCA arising more leftward than usual and sometimes near the origin of the LCA. This is a common reason for the inability of inexperienced angiographers to find the RCA. Common coronary anomalies are listed in Table 1.16.

Anomalies at Angiography
Absent LM: Separate Origin of the LAD and the LCx from the Left Sinus of Valsalva
Separate origination of the LAD and the LCx from the left sinus of Valsalva (absent LM) is one of the most commonly seen coronary anomalies (1% population). Absent LM is benign, although failure to recognize this may cause problems with coronary artery cannulation and perfusion during cardiac surgery.

Cannulation of Separate Origin of the LAD and the LCx
When there is an absent left main coronary artery, there are two possible catheter engagements. Sometimes the tip of the catheter (JL4) engages the LAD and contrast injection opacifies the LAD, and the LCx is also opacified enough by nonselective contrast injection to obtain adequate visualization.

Sometimes, however, spillover is inadequate and the LCx has to be cannulated separately to provide optimal opacification and delineation of disease. In this situation a standard JL4 should be swapped for a larger curve (e.g., JL5) or alternatively an Amplatz left catheter (AL1 or AL2).

Sometimes the LCx is selectively engaged by, for example, a JL4 catheter. To engage the LAD selectively, the JL4 can be swapped for a smaller curve, e.g., JL3.5.

Anomalous Origin of the LCx from the RCA or the Right Sinus of Valsalva

The LCx originating from the RCA or from the Right Sinus of Valsalva is another frequent anomaly and is benign. The initial course of the LCx is usually posterior to the aorta (Figures 1.10 and 1.11).

Cannulation of the Anomalous Origin of the LCx Arising from the RCA
The RCA can be engaged using a JR4 catheter with a standard contrast injection that will also opacify the anomalous LCx. If the visualization is poor, separate cannulation of the LCx is required either with the JR4 with further torque or using an Amplatz left catheter. Sometimes a straighter catheter, e.g., a right coronary bypass graft shape (RCB), is useful.

Cannulation of the Anomalous Origin of the LCx Arising from the Right Sinus of Valsalva
The best working projection is usually LAO 50°, but RAO 40° can be useful. Although engagement with JR4 may be successful, the best choice of catheter is often a right coronary bypass shaped catheter (RCB).

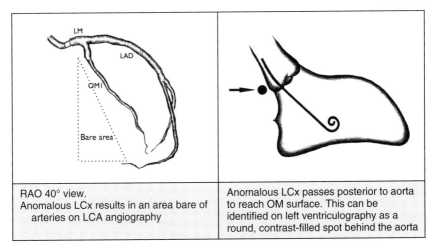

RAO 40° view. Anomalous LCx results in an area bare of arteries on LCA angiography	Anomalous LCx passes posterior to aorta to reach OM surface. This can be identified on left ventriculography as a round, contrast-filled spot behind the aorta

Figure 1.10 Anomalous LCx arising from the right coronary sinus.

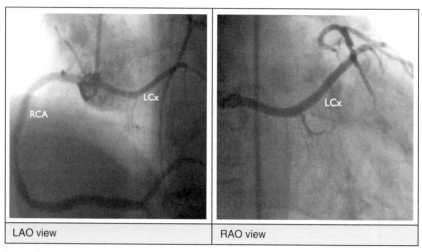

| LAO view | RAO view |

Figure 1.11 Anomalous origin of the LCx arising from the RCA.

Anomalous Origin of the LM Arising from the Right Sinus of Valsalva (RSV): Both Coronaries from the RSV

This anomaly is more important clinically, depending on the course the artery takes to reach the left anterior and left circumflex distribution. An interarterial course (between the aorta and pulmonary artery) may cause chest pain, a positive exercise test, and a higher risk of sudden cardiac death. Ischemia is usually triggered by exercise due to compression of the LM between the aorta and pulmonary trunk, but may also be caused by acute angulation, kinking, or spasm of the LM.

The classification is dictated by the course of the left main coronary artery (Figure 1.12). This course, as the artery passes from the right sinus of Valsalva to the left ventricle, can be deduced using the information in Figure 1.12. CT angiography is useful for defining the course separation of the normally positioned aorta and pulmonary artery; or, alternatively, ventriculography may be used.

• *Interarterial course:* The LM passes between the aorta and the pulmonary trunk. This course can be associated with severe ischemic symptoms and sudden death, but fortunately is very rare.

• *Anterior course:* The LM passes anterior to the pulmonary trunk or to the right ventricular outflow tract. Benign condition.

• *Retroaortic course:* The LM passes behind the aortic root. At angiography the LM (posterior to the aorta) is seen as a dot. Patients are asymptomatic. Benign condition.

• *Septal course:* The LM goes within or through the interventricular septum beneath the right ventricular outflow tract, then dividing into the LAD and LCx. Benign condition.

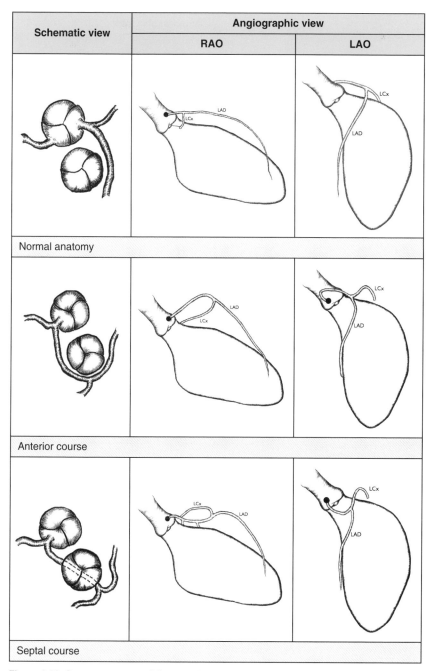

Figure 1.12 Common courses of the normal and anomalous left main coronary artery.

Schematic view	Angiographic view	
	RAO	**LAO**

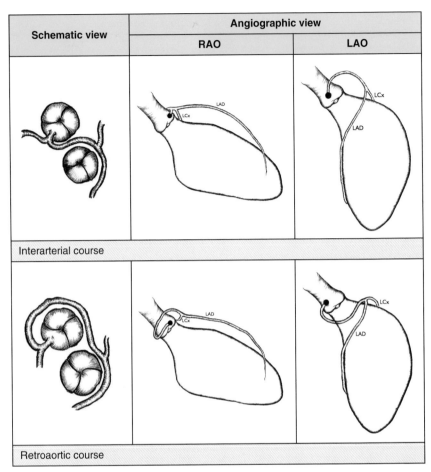

| Interarterial course | | |
| Retroaortic course | | |

Figure 1.12 (*Continued*).

The least commonly seen LM course is the interarterial course, with the LM located between the aorta and the pulmonary artery or between the aortic valve and the right ventricle adjacent to the pulmonary valve. These patients require careful assessment with exercise testing, myocardial perfusion imaging, and magnetic resonance imaging.

Anomalous Origin of the RCA Arising from the Left Sinus of Valsalva (LSV): Both Arteries from the LSV

This is generally a benign condition; its main importance is that inexperienced angiographers may not be able to find it. This origin is the commonest reason for angiographers having difficulty finding the RCA. The anomaly is a spectrum, from an origin that is mildly leftward but still in the right sinus, to the extreme case of the RCA arising from the LCA.

An RCA that arises more leftward than usual appears on CT angiography to pass between the aorta and pulmonary artery, but is generally a benign condition. Rarely, symptoms, particularly chest pain, may be triggered by exercise. Physical effort or stress increases blood flow through the aorta and pulmonary artery, causing transient occlusion or compression of the aberrant RCA between the aorta and pulmonary trunk. Ischemia may also occur from acute angulation of the RCA or its narrow ostium.

Anomalous origin of the RCA may coexist with ectopic origin of the LM from the noncoronary sinus of Valsalva. The Judkins left catheter is the best for successful cannulation.

Schematic and angiographic views of common coronary anomalies are illustrated in Figure 1.13. An echocardiographic short axis view is useful in screening the origins of the coronary arteries.

Fistulae: Anomalous Termination

Fistulae are rare conditions resulting in abnormal termination of a coronary artery either into the coronary sinus or the pulmonary trunk or directly into a cardiac chamber. Consequently, there is an arteriovenous communication between the coronary artery and the right side of the heart or, sometimes, the central veins (a small left-to-right shunt). The majority of fistulae originate either from the LCA or from the RCA systems, but in rare cases the originate from both. Most coronary fistulae involve the RCA and terminate in the right heart (the right ventricle, right atrium, or coronary sinus). The small left-to-right shunt created can cause an early diastolic murmur resembling mild aortic regurgitation.

Fistulae may coexist with congenital heart diseases (tetralogy of Fallot, patent ductus arteriosus, or atrial septal defect). Although most fistulae are associated with small shunt flow, and these patients are asymptomatic, large, high-flow fistulae may cause symptoms. This is due to decreased perfusion in the area of the myocardium supplied by the arterial flow of the fistula. As a result, a hemodynamic steal phenomenon occurs, causing symptoms such as angina, arrhythmia, dyspnea, or mitral regurgitation (both ischemic and functional due to ventricular dilatation). Whereas small fistulae may be ignored, medium or large symptomatic fistulae causing chronic volume overload should be closed. Either an interventional procedure using embolization coils or covered stents can be used, or, with large fistulae, surgery may be required.

If fistulae are treated by embolization or surgery, there is a chance that new fistulae will form.

Coronary cameral fistula is a rare condition in which coronary flow drains directly into the ventricular chamber without passing through a coronary venous system.

Fistulae are usually asymptomatic. Rarely they can be involved with endocarditis.

Anomaly	Schematic View	Angiographic View
RCA arising from the LSV	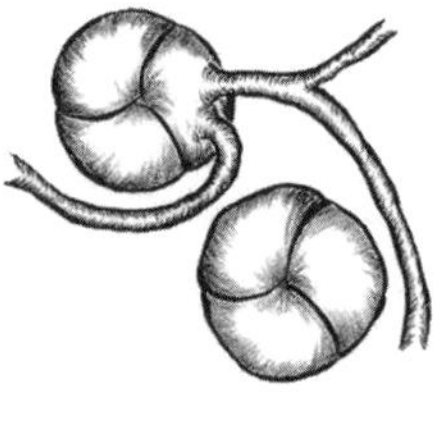	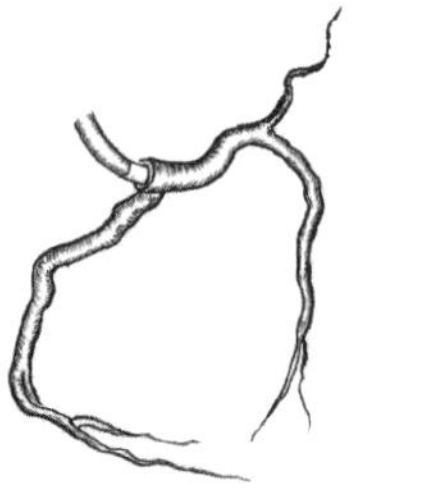
Absent LM. Separate origin of the LAD and LCx from the left coronary sinus of the aorta	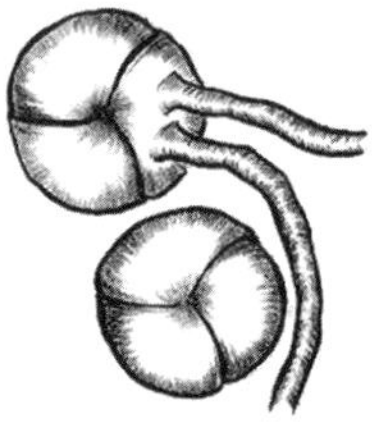	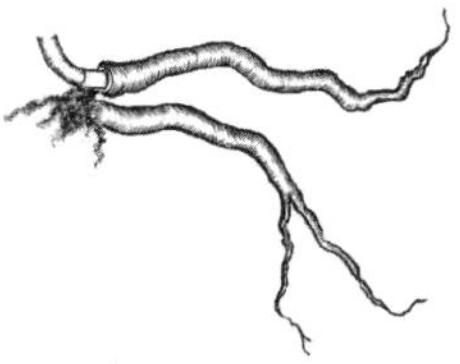
Origin of the LCx arising from the RCA	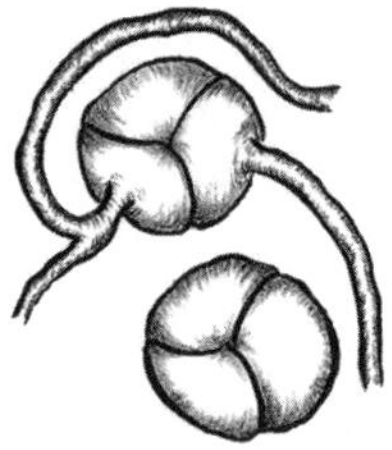	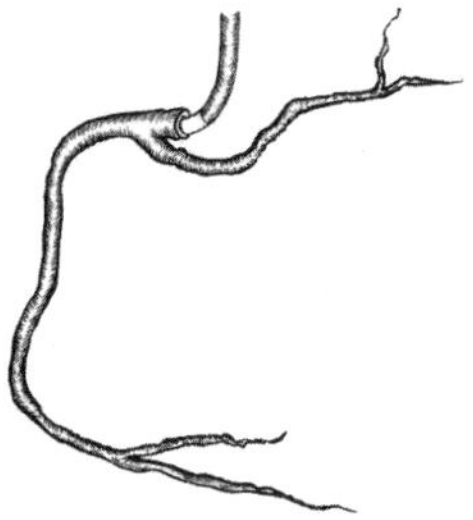
Origin of the LCx arising from the RSV	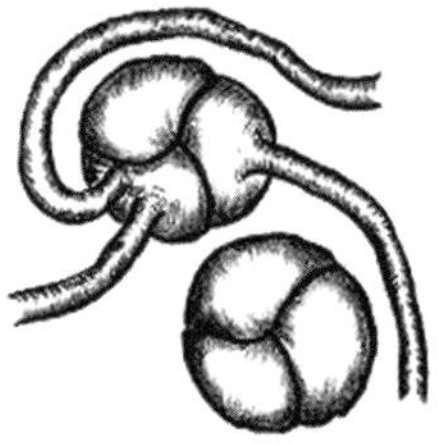	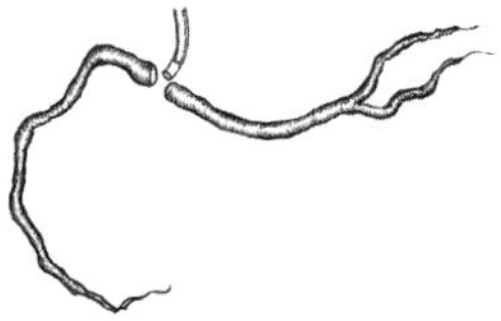

Figure 1.13 Common coronary anomalies.

A few points may be helpful in recognizing fistulae at angiography:
1. Fistulae tend to involve the RCA and drain into the right heart: the right ventricle, pulmonary artery, right atrium, or coronary sinus (see Figure 1.14).
2. Shunts are usually small and do not compromise coronary flow.
3. Multiple fistulae may be associated with polymyositis.

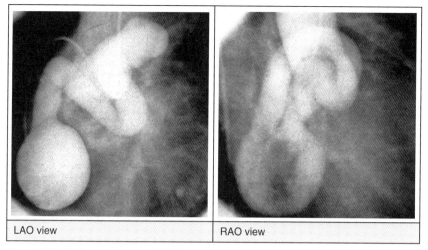

| LAO view | RAO view |

Figure 1.14 Right coronary artery fistula to the right atrium.

Anomalies at Ventriculography

Pseudoaneurysm

Pseudoaneurysm of the left ventricle is most commonly caused by myocardial infarction, but rarely occurs from infection, trauma, or cardiac surgery. Common symptoms include angina, left ventricular failure, ventricular arrhythmias, or systemic emboli from mural thrombus. Surgery is required for enlarging aneurysms or if the patient is symptomatic on medical treatment.

Diverticulum

This is a very rare congenital defect associated with abnormality of muscles of the abdomen wall, diaphragm, or sternum. The presence of a left ventricle diverticulum and abdominal wall defect has been described as Cantrell syndrome.

Tako-Tsubo (Octopus Bottle Heart)

This is a cardiomyopathy, more commonly seen in women with acute coronary syndrome with ST elevation and sudden onset of chest pain, heart failure, or cardiogenic shock. There are dynamic ST/T ischemic changes in the ECG and transient left ventricular dysfunction. Coronary angiography is usually normal with transient apical left ventricular dysfunction (apical ballooning), and basal hypercontractility. Tako-tsubo is often caused by emotional or physical stress, probably due to excess sympathetic adrenergic activity or acute coronary vasospasm (transient stunning).

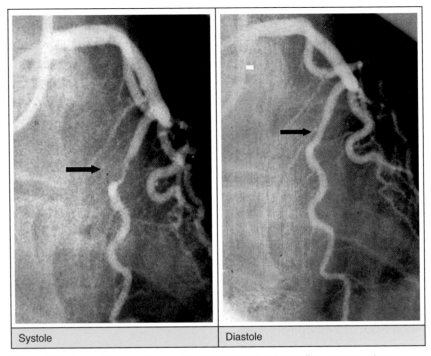

| Systole | Diastole |

Figure 1.15 Myocardial bridge (arrowed) in the left anterior descending coronary artery.

Anatomical Variants at Angiography
Myocardial Bridge
A myocardial bridge refers to a short segment of the coronary artery (usually LAD) running an intramyocardial course. In consequence, during systole the segment of the artery within the myocardium is compressed. At angiography this appears as a transient narrowing which returns to normal during diastole (Figure 1.15). Bridges are often associated with hypertrophic cardiomyopathy and are related to the severity of left ventricular hypertrophy. There used to be a vogue for stenting or surgical resection of a myocardial bridge, but coronary flow is mostly diastolic. Hence they should be regarded as a physiological variant and left alone.

Coronary Collaterals
Collaterals are anastomoses between major coronary arteries which develop over time if a coronary narrowing is greater than 90% or the vessel is totally occluded. Collateral flow can be either antegrade (forward flow) or retrograde (backward flow); it plays an important role in myocardial oxygen supply and helps visualization of the recipient artery.

Severely stenosed or totally occluded arteries fill with contrast during angiography later than normal arteries. Large functional collaterals are usually

Table 1.17 Rentrop classification for coronary collaterals.

Rentrop Grade	Distal Collateral Filling
0	No distal filling from collaterals
1	Filling from side branches, very weak opacification
2	Partial filling of the distal epicardial segment, dense opacification
3	Complete filling of the distal epicardial segment, very dense opacification

well visualized at angiography and are capable of maintaining myocardial viability in the collateral-fed segment. All occluded arteries have collateral filling except when they become acutely occluded in the acute phase of myocardial infarction. If a vessel appears to be absent and is not filled by collaterals even with a long cine acquisition, and the study is not in the acute phase of myocardial infarction, the most likely explanation is an anomalous origin for the artery.

Collateral opacification and density can be assessed using the Rentrop grading system, which describes different degrees of collateral filling of the recipient artery as shown in Table 1.17.

Key Learning Points

- The majority of coronary anomalies cause no symptoms.
- Separate origins of the left anterior descending artery and the left circumflex artery from the left sinus of Valsalva are the most commonly seen coronary anomalies.
- An anomalous left circumflex artery may arise from the right sinus of Valsalva or from the right coronary artery.
- A large coronary fistula can cause myocardial ischemia.
- Myocardial bridges are most common in the left anterior descending artery.

Left Ventriculography and Aortography

- **Left Ventriculography, 51**
  Procedure
  When Not to Proceed
  Complications of Ventriculography
  Mitral Regurgitation
- **Aortography, 56**
  Procedure
  When Not to Proceed
  Aortic Regurgitation

Left Ventriculography

Contrast ventriculography is not an obligatory part of angiography in ischemic heart disease as most information about the left ventricle (LV) can be obtained

from noninvasive tests. In some patients, however, ventriculography is necessary, and it provides valuable information. It is used:
• To assess global and regional wall motion abnormalities. Abnormal wall motion suggests ischemia, infarction, hypertrophy, or aneurysm.
• To assess LV volume, shape, size, and ejection fraction.
• To assess calcification in the aortic and mitral valves and in the LV wall (pericardial or infarct scar).
• To assess the severity of mitral regurgitation based on the density of contrast opacification of the left atrium compared to opacification of the ventricle, the size of the atrium, and the number of cardiac cycles required for opacification of the left atrium by the regurgitant jet.
• To identify and assess the severity of a ventricular septal defect (VSD), left ventricular hypertrophy, subaortic obstruction, pseudoaneurysm, or LV thrombus.
• To assess myocardial mass.

Left ventricular angiography is performed using a pigtail catheter and power injector. If crossing the valve with a pigtail catheter is difficult, an Amplatz left 1 or Judkins RCA catheter may be helpful using a long exchange wire. The standard procedure is performed in RAO 30° projection which provides a good view of the lateral, anterior, apical, and inferior walls. These segments are most frequently affected by ischemia, but assessment of the LV function based only on this view alone can be misleading. LAO 60° with cranial angulation gives the best view for the lateral and septal LV walls allowing evaluation of VSD and septal wall motion.

Procedure

Before the procedure check the arterial pressure on the monitor. If the pressure is elevated (>180 mmHg) administer GTN, or give a nifedipine 10 mg capsule orally – to be crushed in the mouth.

Advance the pigtail catheter carefully round the arch to the aortic root. Remember the pigtail loop should be pointing to the patient's left toward the front of the mitral valve. The ventricle can be entered either using the J wire or the catheter itself (Figure 1.16).
• *When using the J wire to cross the valve:* On reaching the aortic root, withdraw the catheter a few centimeters, advance the J wire, and rotate the catheter slightly, trying to enter the ventricle by probing the aortic valve with the wire. While probing, rotate the catheter gently, each time changing the catheter position. Then advance the pigtail over the wire and obtain a stable position in the LV.
• *When using the pigtail itself to cross the valve:* Slightly rotate or withdraw the catheter slightly to achieve a suitable position. Push the catheter down to the valve, cross the valve, and enter the ventricle. Withdraw the catheter a fraction and rotate it anticlockwise up to 90°. Once the pigtail is in the left ventricle, try to ensure a stable catheter position just short of the apex and free of the mitral chordae. The catheter tip should not be pushed against the ventricular

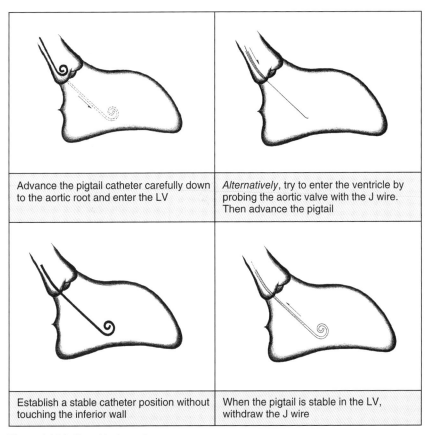

Advance the pigtail catheter carefully down to the aortic root and enter the LV	*Alternatively*, try to enter the ventricle by probing the aortic valve with the J wire. Then advance the pigtail
Establish a stable catheter position without touching the inferior wall	When the pigtail is stable in the LV, withdraw the J wire

Figure 1.16 Left ventriculography.

wall as this causes ventricular arrhythmias. If arrhythmias are caused by the catheter touching the inferior wall, rotate it clockwise. If it is touching the anterior wall, rotate it anticlockwise. The best pictures will be obtained if the rhythm is stable when the patient takes a deep inspiration (gets the diaphragm off the LV image). When the catheter is stable in the left ventricle, withdraw the wire, aspirate blood, and connect the catheter to the power injector. It is important to make sure that all bubbles in the pressure injection syringe have been removed before injection.

• *Set up the pressure injector.* A higher injection pressure is needed if you use a smaller-size catheter. Normal settings for power contrast injections for a 6F pigtail are as follows:

Flow rate 12–15 ml/s,
Total contrast volume 30–50 ml
Rate of rise 1.0 s
Pressure limit 600 psi

• *Monitor the arterial pressure.* LV systolic pressure should be <180 mmHg before a contrast injection. Patients with impaired LV function and elevated left ventricular end-diastolic pressure (LVEDP) require a bolus of 200 µg GTN intraventricularly. Low-osmolar contrast is recommended, especially if the serum creatinine is raised.

• *Contrast volume.* In selecting the contrast volume, the estimated LV volume and presence of mitral regurgitation are important. Minimize the volume if the creatinine is above 200 µmol/l. For a normal LV , use 0.5 ml/kg, i.e., approx. 35 ml for the average patient. Larger volumes, up to 50 ml, are required for a dilated LV or for additional mitral regurgitation.

• *Contrast injection.* Inform the patient that the injection may cause a warm sensation spreading down through the body, and a sensation that they are urinating. Ask the patient to take in a deep breath and hold it just before the injection. During contrast injection, observe the monitor to detect ventricular ectopy and potential problems such as ventricular tachycardia or contrast staining. If complications occur, withdraw the catheter immediately.

• *After the injection* reconnect the catheter to the pressure monitor. Record the LV pressure, concentrating on the LVEDP. Wait for a short while to stabilize any ectopics, then pull back the catheter firmly into the aortic root, just above the aortic valve, and observe any pressure gradient across the aortic valve.

When Not to Proceed
Left ventriculography should be avoided in the following situations:
• Known left ventricular thrombus on echocardiography
• Severe calcific aortic stenosis (risk of cerebral microemboli on crossing the valve with a catheter)
• Severe chronic renal failure: creatinine above 300 µmol/l
• Recent left ventricular failure or pulmonary edema
• Dye load already used (e.g., at PCI) more than 5 ml/kg body weight
• Mechanical aortic valve prosthesis
• Endocarditis of aortic or mitral valves

Complications of Ventriculography
Complications are rare and often of no clinical importance. Cardiac arrhythmias, particularly ventricular tachycardia and ventricular fibrillation, may occur, and if sustained require cardioversion. Ventricular ectopy during contrast injection is very common and does not require treatment. Air embolization should be avoided by proper catheter flushing before the procedure. Staining injection of contrast in the myocardium is usually transient and is rare with a pigtail catheter; it is more of a risk with an end hole catheter (e.g., coronary diagnostic catheters which should not be used for ventriculography). In some rare cases, contrast allergy with transient hypotension may also occur.

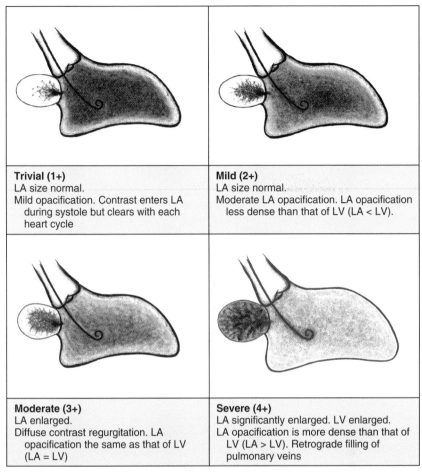

Trivial (1+) LA size normal. Mild opacification. Contrast enters LA during systole but clears with each heart cycle	**Mild (2+)** LA size normal. Moderate LA opacification. LA opacification less dense than that of LV (LA < LV).
Moderate (3+) LA enlarged. Diffuse contrast regurgitation. LA opacification the same as that of LV (LA = LV)	**Severe (4+)** LA significantly enlarged. LV enlarged. LA opacification is more dense than that of LV (LA > LV). Retrograde filling of pulmonary veins

Figure 1.17 Severity of mitral regurgitation.

Mitral Regurgitation

The severity of mitral regurgitation can be assessed using a four-degree scale as follows (Figure 1.17):

• *Trivial* (1+): A small regurgitant jet. Although contrast enters the left atrium during systole, it clears with each heart cycle and does not fill the entire left atrium (LA).

• *Mild* (2+): Contrast opacification of the left atrium is less dense than that of the left ventricle.

• *Moderate* (3+): Contrast opacification of the left atrium is the same as that of the left ventricle. The left atrium does not clear with each cardiac cycle.

• *Severe* (4+): Contrast opacification of the left atrium is more dense than that of the left ventricle. The left atrium fills in one cardiac cycle and there is retrograde filling of the pulmonary veins.

Aortography

Usually aortography is performed to assess the aortic valve, degree of aortic regurgitation, and anatomy of the aortic root. CT and magnetic resonance imaging (MRI) give valuable additional information about the aortic root anatomy and pathology. Indications for ascending aortography are:
- Evaluation of the aortic valve in aortic stenosis or regurgitation
- Aortic root or arch aneurysm
- Evaluation of the great vessels
- Bypass graft identification if in coronary angiography graft engagement proves impossible or inadequate
- Aortic coarctation
- Subvalve or supravalve aortic stenosis
- Assessment of central shunts (Waterston, Blalock, etc.)
- Thromboembolic and inflammatory disease

Procedure

The standard procedure is performed in the LAO 30° projection. This gives the best visualization of the ascending aorta and the aortic arch, with clear views of the innominate artery, carotid arteries, and left subclavian arteries.

The power injector settings are different from left ventriculography as a faster flown rate is needed:
- Flow rate 18–25 ml/s
- Total contrast volume 30–60 ml
- Rate of rise 0.5s
- Pressure limit 1000 psi

Use a pigtail catheter. Advance the catheter carefully. Go down to the aortic valve and then withdraw the catheter about 3–5 cm. The catheter will jump down towards the valve with the onset of the injection, and it is important that it does not touch the valve during contrast injection as this may cause spurious aortic regurgitation. The loop of the pigtail catheter must not be in a sinus of Valsalva at the start of the injection. Once again, ensure all air bubbles are removed before connecting the catheter to the injector, and ask the patient to take in a deep breath and hold it just before contrast injection. Inject contrast and assess the aortic valve and root, great vessels, and the aortic arch. This may mean moving the table during injection.

When Not to Proceed

It is important to note that aortic dissection is not an indication for aortography. This diagnosis should be made by either transesophageal echocardiography (TOE) or MRI. Aortography may be hazardous in dissection, as the rapid rise in intra-aortic pressure with a contrast injection may extend the dissection, antegradely into the great vessels or retrogradely around the coronary ostia, and cause acute infarction or sudden death.

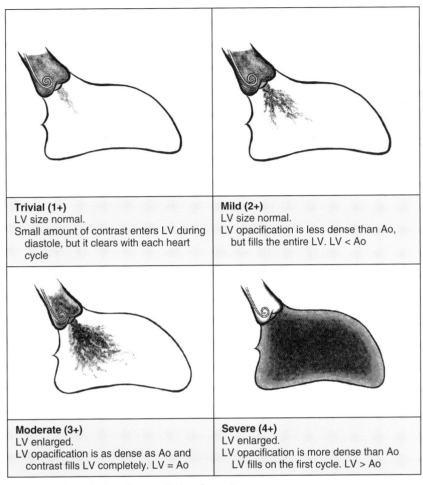

Trivial (1+) LV size normal. Small amount of contrast enters LV during diastole, but it clears with each heart cycle	**Mild (2+)** LV size normal. LV opacification is less dense than Ao, but fills the entire LV. LV < Ao
Moderate (3+) LV enlarged. LV opacification is as dense as Ao and contrast fills LV completely. LV = Ao	**Severe (4+)** LV enlarged. LV opacification is more dense than Ao LV fills on the first cycle. LV > Ao

Figure 1.18 Severity of aortic regurgitation. Ao, aorta.

Aortic Regurgitation

The severity of aortic regurgitation is also graded 1–4, or described as trivial, mild, moderate, or severe, depending on the opacification of the ventricle after the third cycle following contrast injection (Figure 1.18).

• *Trivial* (1+): Although a small amount of contrast enters the LV during diastole, it clears with each heart cycle and contrast never fills the LV.

• *Mild* (2+): Contrast opacification of the LV is less dense than that of the ascending aorta. The LV just fills completely but is cleared with each cycle. LV size is normal.

• *Moderate* (3+): LV opacification is persistent and as dense as that of the aorta. Contrast fills the LV completely and is not cleared with each cycle. LV is usually dilated.

• *Severe* (4+): LV opacification is persistent and denser than that of the aorta. Contrast fills the LV completely on the first cycle. LV is usually dilated.

Key Learning Points

• Ventriculography is not an obligatory part of diagnostic coronary angiography.
• Use a pigtail catheter, RAO 30° view. Depending on LV cavity size and mitral regurgitation, 30–50 ml of contrast should be used.
• LV pressure should be monitored carefully before and after contrast injection.
• All bubbles from the catheter and the syringe must be expelled.
• Mitral and aortic regurgitation assessment is based on the degree and extent of contrast opacification.
• In aortic dissection, avoid aortography.

Radiation Safety

Introduction

Every interventional cardiologist must have a sound knowledge of the basic principles of radiation safety in order to obtain the best possible images and to protect the patient, operator, and staff from unnecessary radiation exposure. All radiation carries some risk, and X-ray dosage must be minimized.

Although there is no official limit to the radiation dose for a PCI procedure, the use of radiation should be reasonable and clinically justified on the basis of a risk/benefit balance. According to the ALARA concept ("as low as reasonably achievable"), the dose must be reduced where possible to avoid unnecessary radiation and prevent potential long-term complications. During the procedure, the operator should try to reduce the radiation dose by minimizing exposure time, maximizing the distance from the X-ray tube, and using protective shields routinely.

Basic Principles

A few basic principles will help reduce radiation dose to patient and staff:
- Radiation is present in the catheter lab only when the foot pedal is pressed.
- Press the pedal only when looking at the monitor.
- Do not use fluoroscopy when someone is standing on the left side of the table.
- Stand as far from the radiation source as possible.
- Use the ceiling-mounted glass shield; it will protect the upper body and eyes.
- Ensure the lead skirt attached to the lower edge of the table is positioned correctly to protect operators from the X-ray tube.
- Keep the table as high as you comfortably can.
- Keep the detector or image intensifier as close to the patient's chest as possible – this is particularly important with cranial angulation.
- Use cine reasonably and sparingly – low-dose fluoroscopy gives 27 nGy/pulse, standard-dose fluoroscopy 38 nGy/pulse, but cine fluoroscopy 200 nGy/pulse! Pulsed fluoroscopy is now standard, but the frame rate per second can be chosen by the operator and should be as low as possible (e.g., 12 frames per second rather than 25 per second for PCI cases).
- Do not use cine acquisition when fluoroscopic image quality is good enough.
- Minimize the number of cine acquisition shots: e.g., are three different projections of a nonculprit vessel in primary PCI really necessary?
- Avoid the use of magnified images unless essential (e.g., for critical stent positioning).
- Radiation scatter causes image degradation, with loss of contrast and unwanted radiation dosing in staff. Good collimation is important and reduces radiation dose from scatter.
- Use biplane fluoroscopy only if necessary.
- Use freeze frame images for reference rather than repeated fluoroscopy.
- Monitor radiation dose to both patient and operators. Monitor screening time.
- Document your actual radiation dose by wearing two radiation detector (thermoluminescent dosimeter, TLD) badges: one under the lead apron, and one outside the lead apron on the left shoulder.
- Keep a maximum distance from the X-ray beam, especially if just observing: radiation intensity is inversely proportional to the square of the distance from the source.
- Wear the heaviest lead apron you can manage: 0.5 mm if possible. A two-piece apron may be more comfortable, with a tight belt resting on the hips holding the skirt up.

- Check that the operator's left chest is well covered by lead (especially in female operators).
- Wear a thyroid collar.
- Learn about radiation dose to the operator with different tube positions by wearing a portable electronic dosimeter: the intensity of the noise produced in higher-dose tube positions rapidly sharpens "radiation hygiene."
- Very heavy patients (>150 kg) and steep angles increase radiation dose.
- Radial procedures tend to need larger radiation doses than femoral, but result in fewer vascular complications.

Minimize Time

Prolonged angioplasty inevitably leads to increased exposure to radiation; the risk occurs when exposure time is longer than 120 minutes. The more complex the procedure, the longer the exposure time and the higher the risk of skin damage. A simple single-vessel PCI usually lasts approximately 15 minutes, but complex procedures need prolonged fluoroscopy time (multivessel PCI at least 25 minutes; CTO more than 40 minutes). Radiation-induced complications are normally apparent a few weeks after PCI, and the patient should be informed of the potential risk associated with prolonged radiation dose before the procedure.

Maximize Distance

There is a relation between radiation dose and distance from the detector, and the catheter lab staff should stay as far from the detector as possible. Exposure decreases rapidly with distance; the dose rate follows the inverse square law (see Figure 1.19).

Use a Shield

Shielding absorbs radiation between you and the detector, reducing the radiation dose, and it should be used on regular basis. Ceiling-mounted transparent shields protect the operator's head and thorax. The operator's lower trunk and legs are protected by the table-mounted lead skirt, which must be positioned correctly.

Position Table and Detector Properly

The distance between table and detector affects the radiation dose both to the patient and to the operator. The lowest radiation dose and the optimal position are achieved if the table is kept at a practical and convenient height and the detector as close to the patient as possible (Figure 1.20). The dose is much higher if the space between the patient and the detector is too large, the detector is too high, or the table is too low.

Parameters and Units
Radiation Parameters

Peak kilovoltage (kV_p) identifies X-ray photon penetrating power. Increasing kV_p increases the penetration of the beam passing through the patient. The

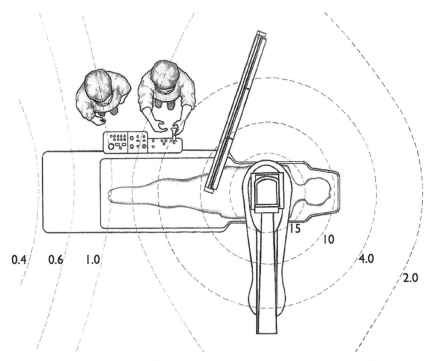

Figure 1.19 Relation between radiation exposure and distance from the detector. Figure shows scattered radiation isodose curves (mR/hour).

beam is not attenuated and the patient dose is lower, but the image is lower in contrast.

Milliamperage (mA) determines the number of X-ray photons produced per unit time.

Pulse width (ms) determines the duration of the X-ray pulse associated with an image frame (usually 5–8 ms).

Radiation Units

The Gray (Gy) is a unit of absorbed energy per unit volume; this estimates the risk of a damaging effect to the exposed tissue.

The Sievert (Sv) is a dose quantity that factors in the relative biological damage caused by the particular type of radiation. It is the unit which defines the absorbed dose (effective dose), which includes a measure of radiation risk and enables comparisons between investigations.

Dosimetric Quantities

There are four basic measurements shown in Table 1.18. The first three are a measure of the energy of the X-rays. The fourth, the effective dose, is

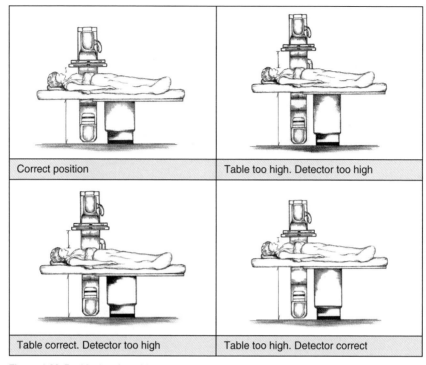

| Correct position | Table too high. Detector too high |
| Table correct. Detector too high | Table too high. Detector correct |

Figure 1.20 Positioning the table and the detector for lowest radiation dose and optimal imaging.

Table 1.18 Dosimetric quantities.

Dosimetric Quantity	Unit
Entrance surface dose (ESD)	mGy
Organ dose (OD)	mGy
Dose–area product (DAP)	Gy/cm^2
Effective dose (ED)	mSv

the one most commonly used. It is the equivalent uniform whole-body dose arising from partial body irradiation (e.g., heart and chest), and is proportional to risk.

Radiation Risk

X-Rays were discovered in 1895 and the first skin cancer from radiation was diagnosed in 1902. Many early radiation workers died from leukemia or cancer without the dangers being recognized.

In general, the risk of injury to the interventional patient is small and is mainly related to the skin of the back. However, less predictable, severe consequences can also appear. The potential risks of radiation are divided under the following headings.

Stochastic Risk

"Stochastic risk" refers to the risk of low-dose radiation causing cancer or genetic abnormalities in the longer term. This is the result of irreversible DNA destruction, is totally unpredictable, and is based on probability proportional to the effective radiation (ED) dose actually received by staff. A linear dose–response relationship is assumed, and the cancer risk/radiation dose graph is extrapolated down from high-dose data to the level of spontaneous occurrence of that complication in the general population. It is assumed there is no threshold dose.

Deterministic Risk

Single large doses of radiation cause death in large numbers of cells and predictable tissue damage. The severity of damage over a certain threshold increases with the dose. Such doses are very rare in medical practice and can easily be avoided. They usually result from nuclear accidents or war. Japanese survivors of the atomic bombs were exposed to 1–4 Sv. Early leukemic deaths have largely been replaced by a continued rise in deaths from solid tumors. Knowledge of the risk associated with doses below 1 Sv is relatively sparse.

1.0–3.0 Sv:	Skin erythema, possible necrosis and skin ulceration. 5% neoplastic risk
2.0–6.0 Sv:	Nausea and vomiting and hemorrhage from intestinal mucosal damage
	Hair loss
	Skin loss
3.0–5.0 Sv:	LD50. Lethal dose to half the population

Patient Radiation Risk

Erythema may develop with doses of 2 Gy and skin burns may appear later even at a dose of 4 Gy if the fluoroscopy time is longer than 30 minutes. Risk is also dependent on the intensity and location of the exposure entrance, patient size, and fluoroscopy time. Young patients are at the highest risk of cancer and the risk gradually decreases with age. Radiation protection, the huge advance in X-ray equipment design, and training of all staff involved with X-rays has made patient radiation injury very rare. An experienced operator should be able to perform coronary angiography with a screening time of 1–2 minutes only. The usual radiation dose to the patient is about 2 mSv (Table 1.19).

However, major radiation reactions are associated with high radiation doses:

Table 1.19 Typical doses of radiation.

Typical doses of radiation (ED)	
Background natural-source radiation/year	2.2 mSv
Chest X-ray	0.01–0.02 mSv
Lateral thoracic spine X-ray	0.29 mSv
Abdominal X-ray	0.7 mSv
Coronary angiography + LV cineangiography	2 mSv
CT head	3.0 mSv
CT body	7.0 mSv
PCI	5–10 mSv

- Skin injury, e.g., temporary or permanent depilation, erythema, burns, dermal necrosis, ulceration
- Cataracts
- Bone marrow dysfunction
- Tissue atrophy
- Infertility
- Neoplastic changes, cancer

Generally, the sensitivity of a tissue to radiation is proportional to the rate of cell proliferation and inversely related to the degree of cell differentiation. Neurological tissue is thus the least sensitive and bone marrow the most sensitive to radiation damage.

Operator Radiation Risk and Dose Limits

The operator's exposure should be lower than 0.1 mSv per procedure, and in general operators should not perform more than 500 cases per year. The annual whole-body dose limit is 20 mSv for adults over 18 years. This is the dose recorded by the TLD badge under the lead apron. For women of child-bearing age, the dose should not exceed 13 mSv in any 3-month period.

The limits are:

Whole body:	20 mSv
Eye lens:	150 mSv
Skin, hands:	500 mSv

If the whole-body limit is exceeded, the operator should stop radiological work and undergo a regular medical examination.

Radiation problems are uncommon but operators may experience:

- Skin injury, mostly hands: depilation, erythema.
- Eye injury, mostly cataracts, which may occur late.
- Cancer. The most vulnerable organs are those close to the radiation (thyroid, breast, parotid, bone marrow).

Key Learning Points

- Press the foot pedal only when looking at the monitor.
- Do not use fluoroscopy when someone is standing on the left side of the table.
- Stay as far from the radiation source as possible.
- Keep the table as high as you can to feel comfortable.
- Keep the detector as close to the patient as possible.
- Learn all the tips to minimize radiation dose to patient and staff.
- Minimize cine acquisition.

2 Devices in Practice

Guiding Catheters

Essential Angioplasty, First Edition. E. von Schmilowski, R. H. Swanton.
© 2012 John Wiley & Sons, Ltd. Published 2012 by John Wiley & Sons, Ltd.

- **Catheter Support Techniques, 85**
  Passive Backup
  Active Backup
  Stabilizing Guide Position
  Difficulties with Stent Delivery
  Re-engagement of the Guide Catheter
  Mother–Child (Coaxial Double Catheter) Technique
  Guide Liner Catheter
  Wire Support Technique
  Anchor Balloon Technique

Introduction

The guiding catheter facilitates passage of multiple guide wires, balloons, stents, and other devices into a vessel and allows contrast injection. Most catheters are atraumatic, with flexible and smooth outer coating to prevent platelet adhesion and thrombus formation and a soft material at the tip to reduce the risk of vessel injury during engagement. Sufficient flexibility and torquability facilitate engagement, whereas stiffness determines backup support during device advancement. The choice of catheter is always based on personal experience, the complexity of the procedure, and the potential risk of complications.

Catheter Selection

Despite the wide range of catheter curves and shapes available, most procedures can be safely performed with a conventional Judkins type catheter. Other catheters may provide better support or allow easier device advancement, but the Judkins catheter is generally used routinely as first choice (Table 2.1).

There are no absolute rules: it may take several attempts to find a guide with the best fit.

In general, the choice of guiding catheter should be based on the following factors:
- Aortic root size
- Aortic root curve

Table 2.1 Choice of guiding catheter depending on type of lesion or vessel anatomy.

Type of Lesion/Vessel Anatomy	Guiding Catheter
Ostial	Judkins, Amplatz left
Bifurcation	Judkins, extra backup (EBU)
Severe stenosis	Amplatz, Judkins
Chronic total occlusion, tortuosities	Amplatz
Abnormal takeoff	Judkins right, multipurpose, Amplatz

- Target artery takeoff
- Length of the left main
- Vessel and lesion location and characteristics
- Devices to be used during the procedure, e.g., a larger catheter with extra backup for complex percutaneous coronary interventions (PCIs)

Catheter Size
Catheter Diameter
The outer diameter of the catheter is measured in French (F) and should correlate with size of the proximal vessel. French is an international measurement used for various medical devices and named after a French urologist who proposed the standard for urinary catheters. 1F is approximately one-third of a millimeter, and precisely equal to 0.33 mm (0.013″) (the catheter diameter is obtained by dividing the French size by 3); for example, the standard 6F catheter has an outer diameter of 2 mm. This is useful when trying to size a vessel for a balloon or stent.

It is very important to plan the technique in advance and try to predict what devices may be needed during the procedure. This will determine selection of the catheter in terms of its inner lumen and backup support. Although catheters are available in 5–10F, in daily practice catheters larger than 7F are rarely used. Generally, the smaller the better; however, larger catheters are still needed for complex PCIs or intraventricular ultrasound (IVUS)-guided procedures. In most procedures, a 100 cm, 6F Judkins type catheter is the optimal choice for a femoral approach, whereas the 5F size is suitable for radial access.

- *6F* (2.00 mm/0.070″) is a commonly used standard catheter compatible with most angioplasty procedures except for some bifurcation lesions or chronic total occlusion (CTO). It also permits radial access and allows easy and deep engagement with minimal damping. Unfortunately, the 6F guide does not offer good support and visualization, which are required in complex procedures.
- *7F* (2.33 mm/0.081″) is usually used in complex PCIs with double wiring, large stents, the potential need for two balloons for kissing inflation, a double stenting approach, double over-the-wire (OTW) catheters, and/or the need for a covered stent or debulking device. The 7F guide offers great support and better visualization and torquability, and is preferable in PCIs for multivessel disease and in patients with cardiogenic shock. The main drawback is a large puncture site, with all the implications of that, and higher risk of pressure damping with coronary intubation..
- *8F* (2.66 mm/0.91″) is always required to deliver devices (atherectomy, rotablation, IVUS, etc.).

Catheter Length
The standard catheter length is 100 cm. Shorter catheters (85–90 cm) are usually used for distal lesions, e.g., left internal mammary artery (LIMA), or

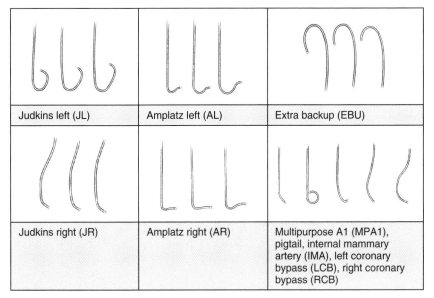

Judkins left (JL)	Amplatz left (AL)	Extra backup (EBU)
Judkins right (JR)	Amplatz right (AR)	Multipurpose A1 (MPA1), pigtail, internal mammary artery (IMA), left coronary bypass (LCB), right coronary bypass (RCB)

Figure 2.1 Commonly used guiding catheters.

retrograde CTO, whereas longer catheters (110–115 cm) are required for tall patients or in aortoiliac tortuosities.

Catheter Shape
The shape of the guiding catheter is determined by the primary and the secondary curve. The primary curve is designed to engage the ostium, whereas the secondary curve provides support. The curve selection is based on the size of aortic root and on which artery needs to be engaged. The given size of the catheter describes the distance between the primary and the secondary curve; for example, JL4 (Judkins left 4) means that the distance between the primary and the secondary curve is 4 cm.

Larger catheters are required for a dilated aorta, in complex procedures with double wiring, kissing balloons, or if a procedure requires additional devices. Small catheters (e.g., JL3.5) are used for the narrow aorta. Commonly used guiding catheters are listed in Table 2.1 and illustrated in Figure 2.1.

Left Coronary Artery Catheters
Commonly used catheters for engagement of the left coronary artery (LCA) are Judkins left (JL), Amplatz left (AL), and extra backup (EBU) (Table 2.2).

Judkins Left Shaped Catheter
These catheters are available in 3.5, 4.0, 5.0, and 6.0 cm curves, and the size of the curve to be selected depends on the size of the ascending aorta. JL4 is a standard catheter suitable for patients with a normal aorta. Patients with narrow aorta require the smaller 3.5 cm size, while those with a wide aortic

Table 2.2 Choice of guide catheter for the left coronary artery.

	Narrow Aorta	Normal Aorta	Dilated Aorta
Judkins left	JL3.5	JL4	JL5
Amplatz left	AL1	AL2	AL2/3
Extra backup	EBU3.5	EBU4	EBU4.0/4.5

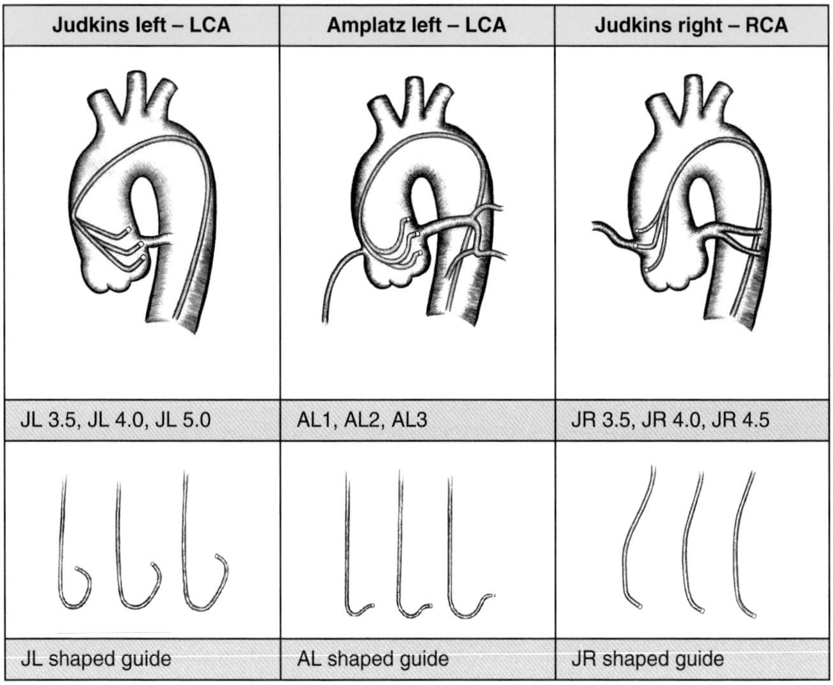

Judkins left – LCA	Amplatz left – LCA	Judkins right – RCA
JL 3.5, JL 4.0, JL 5.0	AL1, AL2, AL3	JR 3.5, JR 4.0, JR 4.5
JL shaped guide	AL shaped guide	JR shaped guide

Figure 2.2 Judkins and Amplatz shaped guide catheters.

root will need the 5.0 cm size or larger (Figure 2.2). Judkins left is easy to use and is suitable for most routine procedures.

Amplatz Left Shaped Catheter

Amplatz catheters are particularly helpful in patients with a high origin of the LCA from the aorta as well as in patients with a dilated aorta or a posterior left main takeoff. Amplatz left offers deep engagement with the coaxial alignment and strong backup in patients with a short main stem and complex circumflex lesions. When withdrawing the catheter from the LCA, remember that the Amplatz is more aggressive and tends to engage the ostium deeper than the Judkins, which may result in vessel spasm or dissection. Always withdraw the catheter slowly and carefully. AL2 is suitable for patients with a normal aorta. Patients with a narrow aorta require the smaller AL1, while patients with a wide aortic root will need AL2 or AL3 (Figure 2.2).

Table 2.3 Choice of the guide catheter for the right coronary artery.

	Narrow Aorta	Normal Aorta	Dilated Aorta
Judkins right	JR3.5	JR4	JR5
Amplatz right	AR1	AR2/3 or AL1/2 or HS	AR2/3 or AL1/2

Extra Backup Left Shaped Catheter (EBU)
The extra backup catheter is particularly helpful in complex procedures in providing stable seating for device delivery. EBU4.0 is the most commonly used size, suitable for patients with a normal aorta. For a large aorta it is best to choose EBU4–4.5 or JL5 or AL2 or AL3 for better support. The contact area with the contralateral wall of the aorta and a long secondary curve ensure great support.

Right Coronary Artery Catheters
Commonly used catheters for engagement of the right coronary artery (RCA) are Judkins right and Amplatz right (Table 2.3).

Judkins Right Shaped Catheter
These catheters are available in 3.0, 3.5, 4.0, 4.5, 5.0, and 6.0 cm. JR4 is the standard suitable for most interventions and all RCA shapes and takeoff in patients with a normal size aorta (Figure 2.2).

Amplatz Right Shaped Catheter
These catheters offer great support and are available in sizes 1, 2 and 3. AR2 is suitable for patients with a normal size aorta. If engagement with AR2 fails, switching to an Amplatz left (starting with AL1) may be helpful. AR1 is best for a narrow aorta, whereas AR3 is more suitable for a dilated aorta. Hockey Stick (HS) is a useful alternative for the large aorta.

Catheter Engagement

Catheter Management and Manipulation
There are a few basic guidelines that should help successful cannulation:
• Select a suitable size and shape catheter for the specific purpose.
• Aspirate before flushing.
• Flush before use. First flush the sheath with saline. Then flush the catheter to remove all air bubbles, and keep flushing regularly during the procedure to avoid formation of air bubbles and thrombus inside its lumen.
• Use a J wire while advancing and withdrawing the catheter. Advance a diagnostic guide catheter over the 0.035″ J wire into the ascending aorta. After the wire is withdrawn, connect the catheter to the manifold, aspirate blood to remove all bubbles, and flush it with heparinized saline.
• Advance, manipulate, and withdraw the catheter only under fluoroscopy.

- Rotate the catheter while advancing and withdrawing; don't force it.
- Draw contrast into the injecting syringe and monitor the pressure regularly during the entire procedure. If you notice pressure damping, withdraw the catheter immediately.
- Large size catheters (7F or 8F) require less force on the syringe during contrast injection.
- When the catheter crosses the aortic arch and the J wire is removed, flush the catheter again to remove any microthrombus or air bubbles.
- Catheters have thin flexible walls and are easily steerable. Advance the catheter slowly and gently. If difficulties occur and you feel resistance, a quick fluoroscopy check may be helpful. Do not advance or withdraw the catheter when you feel resistance. Determine the reason and proceed further. Forceful manipulation can cause coronary dissection or spasm, which may give the false impression of an ostial lesion.
- If you are catheterizing the RCA or grafts and engagement is difficult, try a different catheter size or type rather than manipulate extensively. Avoid wedging the tip against the vessel wall as this may result in ischemia, dissection, or vessel closure.
- Standard guide catheters have closed tips without side holes, and pressure damping occurs with ostial lesions.
- Although catheters with side holes are not routinely used, they can provide good local perfusion and are recommended with small vessels. They also allow measurement of aortic pressure. They are not recommended in ostial lesion procedures. One of the first signs of the presence of an ostial lesion is pressure damping during catheter engagement. This will not occur with a side-hole guide.

Pressure Damping

Engagement of the coronary artery must not interfere with arterial inflow. Flattening or ventriculization of the aortic pressure wave, sometimes seen on the monitor, indicates that during cannulation the catheter tip has occluded forward blood flow. As a consequence, injection of even a relatively small volume of contrast may provoke an arrhythmia or myocardial ischemia and in some cases dissection. Although this situation is more frequently associated with engagement of the ostium of the RCA (with the catheter tip reaching the conus branch), reduction of the guiding catheter pressure may also occur with cannulation of the left main.

There are several reasons for pressure damping (see Figure 2.3):

- Severe ostial lesion either in the left main or in the RCA.
- Artery spasm caused by cannulation of the catheter tip being too deep or too high, particularly during RCA engagement.
- Engagement of a small artery, e.g., conus branch, during cannulation of the RCA.
- Too large a catheter size (F) blocking the ostium of the coronary artery.
- Presence of air bubbles or thrombus in the catheter.

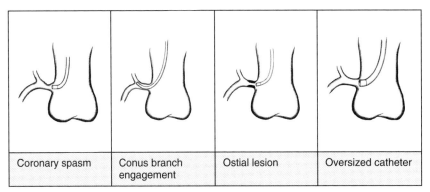

Coronary spasm	Conus branch engagement	Ostial lesion	Oversized catheter

Figure 2.3 Common reasons causing pressure damping.

• Kinking of the catheter from excessive torque.
• When you detect pressure damping, withdraw the catheter immediately. In cases of coronary spasm, the presence of an ostial lesion, or with small branch engagement, the pressure should immediately return to normal. If this maneuver fails and the pressure remains flat, check with fluoroscopy for catheter kinking. If there is any doubt, change the guiding catheter.
• When normal pressure is restored, consider possible reasons for pressure damping. Inject small amounts of contrast to assess the situation. In a case of a severe ostial lesion, skip the less relevant projections and obtain only the most important ones. Inject 200 μg glyceryl trinitrate (GTN) intracoronarily to reverse possible spasm, or change the catheter to engage the ostium of the artery properly.
• If arterial pressure remains flat there is a possibility of air injection, the presence of thrombus, or vessel dissection. Check the ECG oxygen saturation and the patient's condition. Resuscitation measures may be necessary, including intra-aortic balloon pumping.

Left Coronary Artery Engagement

Left main cannulation is usually relatively simple and hardly ever requires any manipulation (Figure 2.4). However, in some patients a slight anticlockwise rotation may be needed to ensure proper alignment of the catheter tip.

The following technical tips can be of help in engaging the left main safely:
• Start with the left anterior oblique (LAO) 50° projection.
• If you notice that the catheter has not reached the required position, or reversed contrast flow appears, change the catheter for a smaller or larger size rather than keep manipulating. Extensive manipulation always carries the potential risk of left main dissection.
• In case of difficulties with engagement, a deep breath in or out by the patient may be helpful.
• Always be aware of possible left main anomalies or varieties of the left main takeoff (pp. 41–51).

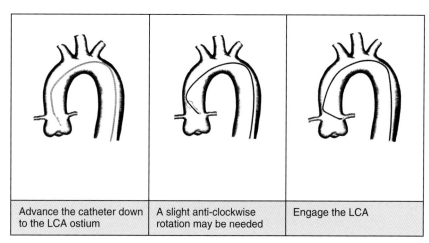

Advance the catheter down to the LCA ostium	A slight anti-clockwise rotation may be needed	Engage the LCA

Figure 2.4 Left coronary artery cannulation.

• Keep an eye on pressure damping, which usually occurs due to high catheter engagement, severe left main stenosis, or spasm.
• In an ostial LAD lesion it is better to choose a Judkins type catheter with a short tip, obtaining a more coaxial position in the ostium. Excessive manipulation and deep engagement should be avoided (see "Ostial lesions", p. 241).
• In some cases, e.g., short left main or separate ostia, selective engagement of either the LAD or the left circumflex artery (LCx) may be required.
• If the left main is too short to cannulate and results in selective advancement of the catheter into either the LAD or the LCx, position the catheter in the LAD first and choose projections most suitable for the best LAD visualization. Then change the catheter for a larger size, e.g., JR5, engage the LCx, and carry on with optimal LCx views.

Right Coronary Artery Engagement

Engagement of the RCA is more demanding than that of the left main and always requires catheter manipulation (Figure 2.5). LAO 50° projection is optimal. To engage the RCA use a JR4 catheter, advance the catheter down to the aortic valve, keep pulling back slowly, and rotate clockwise at the same time. Proceed slowly and inject a small amount of contrast if necessary to mark the track. As the catheter rotates towards the RCA ostium, release the torque.

In case of difficulties with engagement possible reasons are:
• Severe ostial lesion.
• Severe tortuosities.
• Anomalous origin of the RCA. The origin of the RCA may be more superior and more leftward than normal, or it may arise close to the left main. In case of anomalies a rapid injection close to the ostium will help mark the vessel

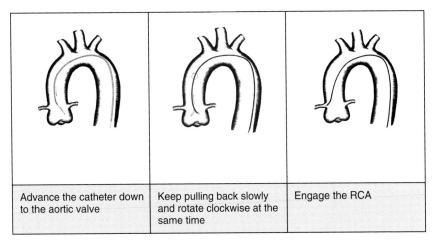

Advance the catheter down to the aortic valve	Keep pulling back slowly and rotate clockwise at the same time	Engage the RCA

Figure 2.5 Right coronary artery cannulation.

track. The JR4 should be replaced with an AL1 or AL2 catheter and this should be advanced close to the left main. Slight clockwise rotation with test injection may help find the origin of the RCA, which should be located between the left main origin and the usual site for a right coronary ostium.

If the RCA ostium still cannot be found, perform an aortic root injection in the LAO projection.

Coronary Artery Takeoffs
Left Coronary Artery Takeoff
The LCA takeoff is defined as the angle between the aorta and the ostium of the left main and it is described as superior, posterior, right, acute, or obtuse. Different catheters may be required to engage the left main successfully; however, the Amplatz left is the first choice (Table 2.4, Figure 2.6).

Right Coronary Artery Takeoff
There are various types of RCA origin. Standard Judkins right is usually suitable for all types of RCA takeoff; however, it does not ensure good backup support and cannulation requires more time and effort. If difficulties arise, a multipurpose catheter can be a good alternative (Table 2.5, Figure 2.7). In case of anterior takeoff, use a Judkins left and rotate it slightly clockwise. This will provide a fairly stable platform and good backup.

Transradial Angiography
Although there a wide spectrum of specific transradial catheters are available, such as Kimny, Ikari, or Barbeau, femoral guide catheters are very adaptable to a transradial approach, and standard Judkins left or right, Amplatz, or EBU for extra support can be used successfully in most cases. Good backup and

Table 2.4 Choice of guide catheter depending on left coronary artery takeoff.

LCA takeoff	Catheter
LCA superior	Amplatz left, Judkins left 3.5/4
LCA posterior	Amplatz left, Judkins left 4/EBU

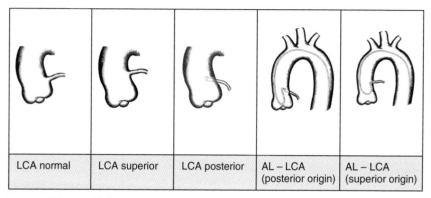

| LCA normal | LCA superior | LCA posterior | AL – LCA (posterior origin) | AL – LCA (superior origin) |

Figure 2.6 Types of left coronary artery takeoff and choice of guide catheter.

Table 2.5 Choice of guide catheter depending on right coronary artery takeoff.

RCA takeoff	Catheter
RCA anterior	Judkins right, Amplatz, Amplatz left, Judkins left
RCA superior	Judkins right, Amplatz left, Judkins left, EBU right, Shepherd's crook
RCA inferior	Judkins right, multipurpose MPA1
Shepherd's crook	Shepherd's crook, Hockey Stick (HS), LIMA

coaxial alignment with the target vessel are essential. In some situations specific transradial catheters are very helpful, not only in providing excellent support, but also in allowing treatment of both left and right coronary arteries with a single guide. Whatever catheter is chosen, one has to remember that the radial artery is very spasmogenic and engagement should be done with great care and limited manipulation. All catheter exchanges should be performed over the J wire. If any resistance is encountered during catheter passage, a quick check under fluoroscopy is helpful in identifying the reason. It is usually due to spasm, a loop, or entering a side branch. One of most common problems during cannulation is when the J wire advances into the descending rather than the ascending aorta. This may be caused by tortuosities of the brachiocephalic artery or by aortic unfolding. In order to

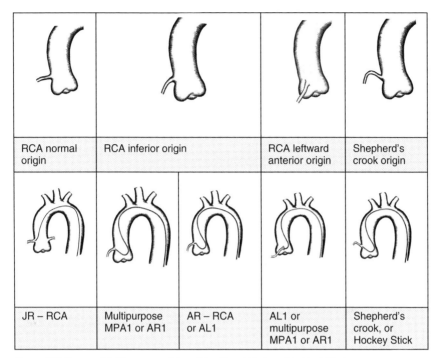

RCA normal origin	RCA inferior origin		RCA leftward anterior origin	Shepherd's crook origin
JR – RCA	Multipurpose MPA1 or AR1	AR – RCA or AL1	AL1 or multipurpose MPA1 or AR1	Shepherd's crook, or Hockey Stick

Figure 2.7 Types of right coronary artery takeoff and choice of guide catheter.

redirect the wire, advance both the wire and the catheter purposely into the descending aorta and withdraw the wire into the guide catheter. Then withdraw the catheter into aortic arch and rotate it anticlockwise, pointing its tip toward the ascending aorta. Ask the patient to take in a deep breath and advance the wire again, At this point the catheter can be negotiated into the ascending aorta.

Right Radial Approach
Radial cannulation techniques for both the right and the left coronary artery are similar to the femoral approach. In general, the catheter for the radial approach should be one size (0.5 cm) smaller than that for the femoral approach with a similar aortic root. For example, if for a femoral approach you would choose JL4, for the radial approach use a JL3.5. When using the right radial approach, be careful pulling the catheter back into the left coronary artery. During this maneuver a catheter tends to engage the ostium deeply, which may cause spasm or dissection.

Left Coronary Artery Engagement
Judkins Left Catheter Proceed in LAO 50° projection. The standard choice is a JL3.5. Pull the arm straight and extend it slightly towards the head. Advance the J wire into the ascending aorta, then advance the catheter below the left

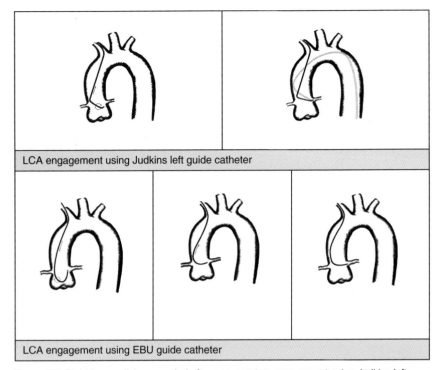

LCA engagement using Judkins left guide catheter

LCA engagement using EBU guide catheter

Figure 2.8 Right transradial approach. Left coronary artery engagement using Judkins left guide catheter and EBU guide catheter.

coronary origin and pull the J wire out. Go down to the aortic valve (slightly deeper than in the femoral approach), withdraw the catheter a fraction to the level of the RCA orifice, and rotate it anticlockwise. This usually does not need any further manipulation and the catheter should engage, providing stable passive backup. If the catheter does not reach the orifice, however, inject a small amount of contrast to mark the vessel origin. Slowly withdraw the catheter, rotate it gently, and advance again (Figure 2.8). Deep inspiration by the patient may help facilitate engagement.

Extra Backup Catheter When you use an EBU catheter, advance it down to the aortic valve to form a U loop shape and rotate it slightly clockwise. Withdraw the catheter gently until the contact area is long, ensuring good backup, and the catheter will form an L loop. Then engage the origin of the left main (Figure 2.8). In case of difficulties, a little anticlockwise rotation may be helpful.

Right Coronary Artery Engagement
LAO 50° projection is also recommended for RCA cannulation. Although the optimal choice is a Judkins right, this provides less stability from the right

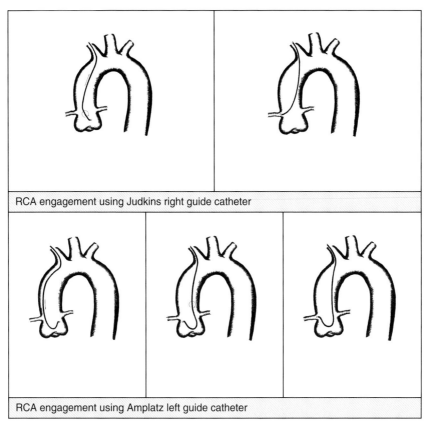

RCA engagement using Judkins right guide catheter

RCA engagement using Amplatz left guide catheter

Figure 2.9 Right transradial approach. Right coronary artery engagement using Judkins right guide catheter and Amplatz left guide catheter.

radial approach, and in some cases a catheter with greater reach may be needed, particularly when dealing with ostial lesions. If strong backup is required, an Amplatz left (start with AL1 for a normal aorta) is a great option.

Judkins Right The standard choice is JR3.5. Advance the catheter down to the aortic valve with the tip pointing to the left main. Simultaneously rotate the catheter clockwise and slowly withdraw it (Figure 2.9). When proceeding with an angioplasty, advancing guide wires and balloons through a JR catheter will ensure deeper engagement and will secure good backup.

Amplatz Left This is an alternative to the Judkins right catheter. Choose Amplatz left 1 or 2 depending on the size of the aorta. Advance the catheter down to the aortic valve and rotate it clockwise while advancing (Figure 2.9). You should reach the orifice relatively easily, but deep engagement with this type of catheter is not possible.

Left Radial Approach

The optimal projection for cannulation from the left radial access is also the standard LAO 50° view.

This approach is usually more challenging. The anatomy of the subclavian artery and the angle between the subclavian artery and the aortic arch determine success. It is easier to obtain passive backup and to engage the RCA than the LCA. During engagement the catheter adheres to the inner side of the ascending aorta. This means that the catheter is bent somewhere in the middle of the aorta, and if the subclavian artery is vertical and the aorta is horizontal, even a small JL3.5 appears to be too large to engage the LCA. In this case you will need to rotate the catheter clockwise, inject a small amount of contrast to check the vessel position, and advance the catheter pointing towards the ostium. Notice, however, that in this case you are unlikely to get contralateral aortic backup. The LCA can also be engaged by gently withdrawing the catheter until it reaches the ostium of the LCA. Likewise, in this case the catheter may not gain support from the opposite wall of the aorta. If engagement with Judkins left fails, try an EBU catheter or an Amplatz.

Bypass Graft Angiography

A few practical points should be considered when dealing with bypass grafts:
- Review previous coronary angiogram before the procedure.
- Focus on the number of anastomosed grafts, anatomy, and location.
- Keep in mind that in some cases a sequential graft (jump graft) may supply two arteries.
- Metallic clips or sternal wires may help to visualize the track of a graft.

Vein Graft Angiography

Generally, vein graft procedures are associated with a higher dose of contrast, increased radiation exposure, and longer procedural time. There are no limitations regarding vascular access. Either femoral or radial arteries can be used for graft cannulation, but left radial or femoral access is easier for visualization of a LIMA graft.

Plan your strategy in advance and remember a few rules to proceed safely:
- Cannulation itself carries a higher risk of thromboembolism and aortic injury. This is due to the presence of atherosclerotic plaques, particularly in old vein grafts or as a result of extensive catheter manipulations in the aorta.
- In most patients angiography of native vessels should be performed first, followed by mammary artery graft and vein grafts. This sequence helps to visualize distal vein graft insertion sites and localize bypasses before cannulation.
- Check which internal mammary artery has been used as graft previously. If the LIMA, select the left arm to ensure access to the left mammary artery and to the vein grafts. For right internal mammary artery (RIMA) engagement, choose the right arm.

Guide Catheter Selection
The majority of grafts should be engaged using bypass-dedicated guide catheters, i.e., right coronary bypass (RCB) catheter for right coronary graft and left coronary bypass (LCB) catheter for left grafts. Some operators prefer to start with a Judkins right 4 (JR4) for all grafts, but achieving a stable position in the graft ostium may be difficult, in which case opacification will be poor and back-up inadequate. In addition to the bypass-dedicated guide catheters, the Amplatz right and left catheters are often used. From the practical point of view, in the case of sharp inferior takeoff in the right coronary vein graft the best choice is a multipurpose catheter with a shallow angulation (MPA1). In the case of anterior takeoff of the RCA or in a dilated aorta, the first choice is Amplatz right (AR1) and then Amplatz left (AL1 to AL3).

Saphenous Vein Graft to the Right Coronary Artery
A bypass to the RCA should be located slightly above the origin of the RCA (right takeoff from the aorta) (Figure 2.10). The optimal visualization can be obtained from the LAO 40° projection. Use a JR4 or RCB catheter and try to position the catheter tip slightly higher than the expected vein graft orifice. Rotate the catheter clockwise and advance it down to the aorta (Figure 2.11). Watch for pressure damping, as this can indicate presence of an ostial lesion, and injection into the vein graft with a severe ostial lesion increases the risk of arrhythmias. Other catheters such as the Amplatz, multipurpose, or hockey stick catheter can also be useful.

Saphenous Vein Graft to the Left Coronary Artery
Vein bypass grafts to the LCA have an anterior takeoff and are located on the anterior wall of the ascending aorta, slightly higher and to the left of the RCA

Grafts from the Aorta	Bypass Location	Catheter Selection	Bypass Position
Graft to the right coronary artery or to the distal left circumflex	The lateral wall of the aorta above the right sinus of Valsalva	RCB, JR4 multipurpose, AL1/2	
Graft to the left anterior descending artery	More anterior location to the right coronary artery	JR4 LCB, AL1/2, multipurpose	
Graft to the diagonal branches	The anterior wall of the aorta above the left sinus of Valsalva		
Graft to the obtuse marginal branches	More anterior location to the left anterior descending artery		

Figure 2.10 Guide catheter selection based on bypass location in vein graft angiography. LCB, left coronary bypass; RCB, right coronary bypass.

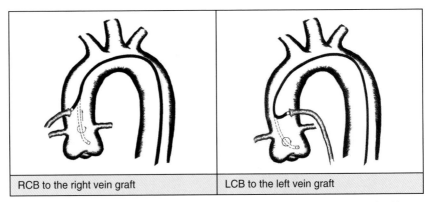

| RCB to the right vein graft | LCB to the left vein graft |

Figure 2.11 Vein graft engagement with right (RCB) and left (LCB) bypass-dedicated guide catheters.

(Figure 2.10). The ostium of the LAD graft is usually the lowest and the closest to the aortic valve. Diagonal and circumflex grafts are located slightly above. The ostium of the circumflex graft usually has the highest takeoff from the aorta. The best choice of catheter to engage the graft to the marginal branches is the Amplatz left, mostly because of its good backup.

When engaging a graft avoid extensive manipulation. The LAD graft is relatively easy to cannulate using an LCB catheter (Figure 2.11). This can be done either after the right vein graft cannulation by pulling the catheter back or, alternatively, by placing the catheter slightly above the LAD vein graft orifice with clockwise rotation. The same technique applies to the circumflex graft, which is located slightly higher than the LAD vein graft. Potential difficulties are usually associated with different takeoffs, and in these cases the catheter should be probed across the aorta at a different level. Sometimes a strong contrast injection is useful to identify the atypical takeoff or occlusion of a missing graft. Different catheters such as the multipurpose or Amplatz left can also be very helpful.

Arterial Graft Angiography
Anatomy of the Arch of the Aorta
Three main arteries arise from the ascending aorta:
• The brachiocephalic (innominate) artery, which has two main branches – the right common carotid artery and the right subclavian artery. The right subclavian gives rise to the right vertebral and the right internal mammary arteries.
• The left common carotid artery, which divides into the external and internal carotid arteries.
• The left subclavian artery, to the left arm which gives rise to the left vertebral artery and the left internal mammary artery.

Both the left and the right internal mammary arteries arise most commonly from the inferior aspect of the first part of the subclavian artery (Figure 2.12).

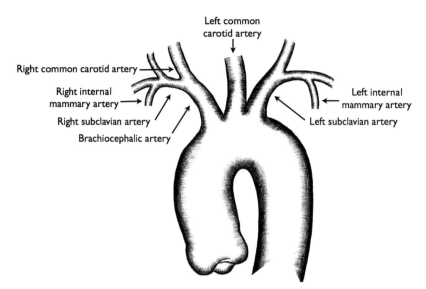

Figure 2.12 Anatomy of the arch of the aorta.

Arterial Graft Engagement

Cannulation of arterial grafts is often more demanding than vein graft cannulation. Difficulties usually arise due to variants in the anatomy and shape of the aortic arch and origin of the internal mammary artery. Sometimes the subclavian artery is severely stenotic or tortuous, particularly in older patients with coexisting peripheral vascular disease.

Left Internal Mammary Artery Graft

The best choice of catheter to engage the LIMA is a dedicated internal mammary artery catheter (IMC). This catheter provides coaxial seating in the ostium of the mammary artery with support from the subclavian artery. However, a JR4 catheter can also be an option.

A few points may be useful for successful LIMA engagement (Figure 2.13): Using the femoral approach:

• Select the LAO 50° projection for accessing the left subclavian artery from the aorta. When the catheter is beyond the LIMA use the RAO 40° projection.

• Some operators prefer the PA projection for LIMA engagement. Advance the catheter into the arch of the aorta and reach the origin of the left subclavian artery.

• When you reach the ostium of the subclavian artery, gentle clockwise rotation of the catheter will help the catheter tip enter the subclavian artery origin. Avoid vigorous manipulation, as this carries a risk of dissection, injury, or embolism.

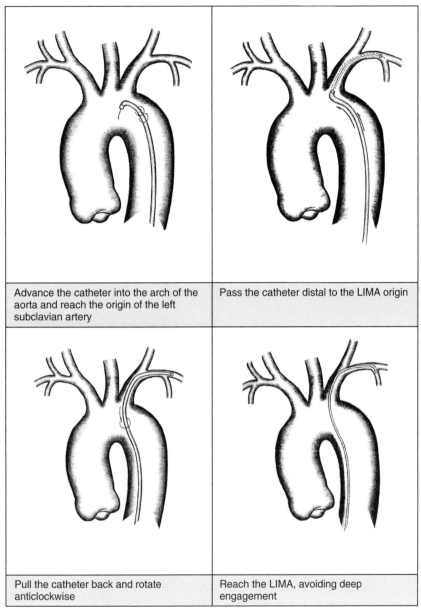

Advance the catheter into the arch of the aorta and reach the origin of the left subclavian artery	Pass the catheter distal to the LIMA origin
Pull the catheter back and rotate anticlockwise	Reach the LIMA, avoiding deep engagement

Figure 2.13 Left internal mammary artery engagement.

• Once the left subclavian artery is engaged, advance the guide wire well down the artery, and then advance the catheter beyond the origin of the LIMA. Withdraw the guide wire.
• Slowly pull back the LIMA catheter and rotate it slightly anti-clockwise.
• Avoid deep cannulation and watch for pressure damping.
• In case of failure to engage the LIMA, inject a small amount of contrast and check the catheter position under fluoroscopy. If the catheter is close to the origin but it is difficult to reach the origin, a deep inspiration by the patient or changing the arm position may be helpful. If the LIMA cannot be cannulated but you are close to the LIMA ostium it may still be possible to wire it.
• If the subclavian engagement is difficult or impossible to achieve from a femoral approach, the left radial may be an alternative.

Right Internal Mammary Artery Graft
The best catheter to enter the RIMA graft is the Judkins right. Although engagement of the RIMA is technically similar to that of the LIMA, difficulties may arise in patients with a dilated aortic root and abnormally steep takeoff of the RIMA. Sometimes access from the right arm may be necessary.
   If you use femoral access, proceed as follows (Figure 2.14):
• Advance the catheter into the arch of the aorta.
• Once you reach the brachiocephalic trunk, rotate the catheter anticlockwise to change the position of the guide tip and advance the guide into the subclavian artery.
• Proceed further as described above for LIMA graft cannulation.

Vein Grafts Engagement from the Radial Approach
The best choice of guiding catheter for this purpose is JR4, Multipurpose or bypass graft catheters. If cannulation using these catheters fails or if the backup is not adequate, Amplatz left may be of help. Left and right internal mammary grafts can be successfully engaged from the left and the right transradial approach using either Judkins right or Internal mammary catheters.

Catheter Support Techniques
Catheter backup is very important to ensure a stable catheter position. The support area is located opposite the ostium on the contralateral wall of the aorta, providing stability for advancing and exchanging wires, balloons, and stents through the lesion. Backup depends on catheter shape, size, tip, lateral wall support, and coaxial alignment. Extra backup (EBU) catheters have a long secondary curve and the contact area with the opposite aortic wall is greater than with the Judkins catheter (Figure 2.15).

Passive Backup
Passive backup is achieved when the catheter engages easily in the origin of the vessel without any additional manipulation and is stable in the ostium (Figure 2.16). This type of support provides a very stable sitting position, but a long catheter tip is preferable (6F minimum). The Amplatz type catheter

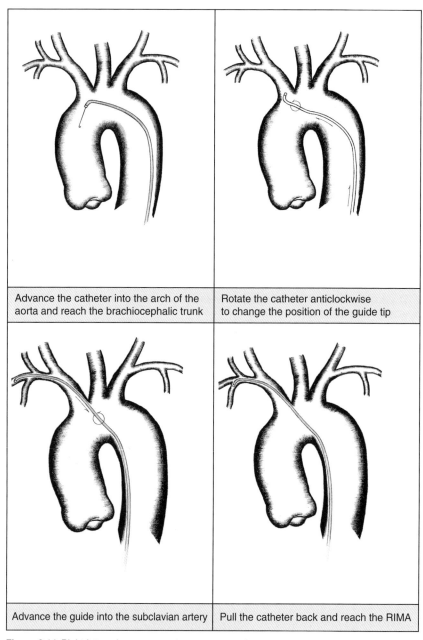

Advance the catheter into the arch of the aorta and reach the brachiocephalic trunk	Rotate the catheter anticlockwise to change the position of the guide tip
Advance the guide into the subclavian artery	Pull the catheter back and reach the RIMA

Figure 2.14 Right internal mammary artery engagement.

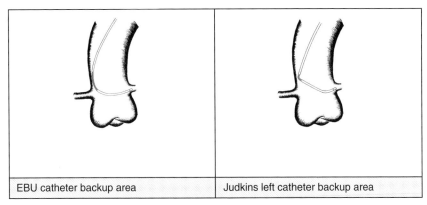

| EBU catheter backup area | Judkins left catheter backup area |

Figure 2.15 Backup support area for EBU and Judkins guide catheters.

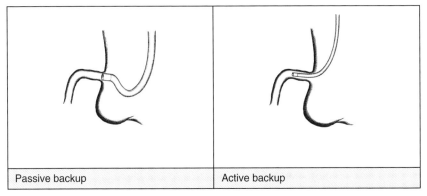

| Passive backup | Active backup |

Figure 2.16 Passive and active backup.

provides good passive backup. Note that the 5F catheter is too small and will not provide passive backup support.

Active Backup

Active backup always requires further catheter manipulation to secure deeper engagement and firmer seating (Figure 2.16). This is crucial, particularly in complex procedures, as deep engagement facilitates delivery of balloons or other devices across the lesion.

Active backup is easier with small catheters (size 6F or even smaller). It is important to try and keep the catheter tip coaxial when deeply engaged to avoid catheter-induced proximal dissection. While stable active backup and deep seating into the LAD requires simultaneous anticlockwise rotation and slow advancing of the catheter, clockwise rotation is needed for engagement of the RCA.

Sometimes it is difficult to keep the guiding catheter in the origin of the vessel. The catheter may disengage from the ostium, losing both catheter and guide wire position. If this happens, the procedure has to be restarted from the beginning and the lesion recrossed. This may influence the outcome of the entire procedure.

Stabilizing Guide Position
If the guiding catheter position is unstable and the guide backs out, the following options may be helpful:
• Deeper engagement with support from the aortic valve allows sufficient support to advance the balloon. The danger is that the guide will prolapse into the left ventricle, pulling the wire and balloon out of the artery.
• Strive to keep the guide wire as far down the relevant vessel as possible, as this will help provide guiding catheter support.
• Use a stiffer wire.
• Use a lower-profile balloon.
• If you use a standard JL4, change guide catheter to, e.g., AL1 or AL2 – but this will require recrossing the lesion with the wire.

Difficulties with Stent Delivery
If difficulties with stent delivery occur and the stent does not cross the lesion, causing guide disengagement, consider the following options:
• Improve guide support.
• Repeat predilatation with a larger balloon at high pressure (up to 20 atm) and/or a larger-diameter balloon.
• Use stiffer wire.
• Use a buddy wire.
• Use a different, more deliverable stent.
• Use the anchor balloon technique.
• Withdraw the catheter slightly to a more neutral position outside the ostium of the artery, as soon as a device has been delivered successfully. This allows maximum forward coronary flow.

Re-engagement of the Guide Catheter
If the wire is looped in the aorta and the guide is disengaged, try to re-engage the artery without losing the wire position (Figure 2.17):
• Do not pull on the wire.
• Withdraw the guide until the wire loop is straightened.
• Fix the wire and advance the guide to re-engage the vessel.

Mother–Child (Coaxial Double Catheter) Technique
This technique provides great seating and excellent catheter backup support, which is very helpful in dealing with the following situations:
• Aorto-ostial lesions
• Severe tortuosities located proximal to the target lesion

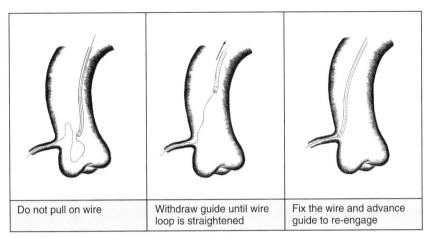

| Do not pull on wire | Withdraw guide until wire loop is straightened | Fix the wire and advance guide to re-engage |

Figure 2.17 Re-engagement of the guide catheter.

- Dilated aorta
- Abnormal coronary artery takeoff

The mother–child system is usually needed if previous cannulation attempts have been unsuccessful. Although this technique provides very good support, it also carries the risk of air embolization or dissection. This may happen particularly during cannulation with the "child" catheter, when the child catheter is wedged against the artery wall. Always check the blood back flow after stent deployment, and keep monitoring distal coronary pressure.

The mother–child technique step by step (Figure 2.18):

- Use a standard large 6F or 7F Judkins or Amplatz guiding catheter (the "mother").
- Advance a long smaller 5F or 6F multipurpose or Amplatz diagnostic catheter (the "child") inside the large diagnostic catheter. The inner catheter diameter should be approximately one French size smaller than the standard large one, e.g., mother 6F and child 5F.
- Connect the smaller catheter to the pressure and contrast injection. This allows tip pressure monitoring during contrast injection.
- Advance a wire and cross the lesion.
- Intubate the child catheter deeply into the vessel and proceed with balloon and stent.
- Alternatively, advance a second (buddy) wire to the distal vessel to achieve better backup and withdraw the child diagnostic catheter.

Guide Liner Catheter

This is a simplified version of the mother–child technique. A coaxial guide extension allows deep seating and extra backup support with the possibility of a rapid exchange. The guide size is approximately one French size smaller than the guide catheter so it can be delivered through standard guide catheter.

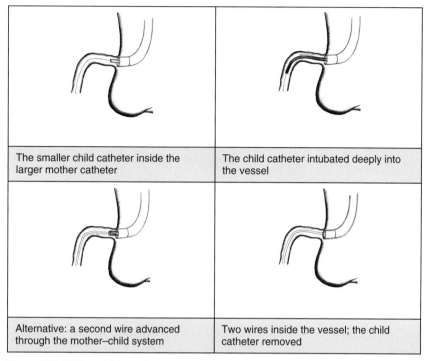

The smaller child catheter inside the larger mother catheter	The child catheter intubated deeply into the vessel
Alternative: a second wire advanced through the mother–child system	Two wires inside the vessel; the child catheter removed

Figure 2.18 Mother–child technique.

The rapid exchange allows deployment through a Y adapter without limiting the length of devices.

Wire Support Technique
Buddy Wire: Proximal and Distal Wire Support Technique
This is a simple and quick support technique which is particularly helpful when you use a standard 6F catheter. To achieve a stable catheter position, advance a second, stiffer wire into the side branch proximal to the treated main branch lesion (Figure 2.19, upper left) or, alternatively, distal to the treated main branch lesion (Figure 2.19, upper right).

The buddy wire is basically an additional (second) guide wire that gives more backup to the guiding catheter and more support to the balloon or stent. It is very useful in complex, challenging lesions such as tortuosities (the wire helps straighten the vessel), calcifications, distal lesions, and in-stent restenosis. It can also facilitate positioning of distal protection devices and help manage coronary anomalies.

The buddy wire technique step by step:
- Choose a side branch that is easy to cross.
- Advance the first wire into the target vessel.

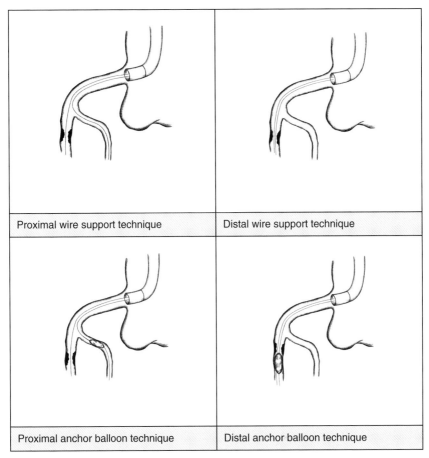

| Proximal wire support technique | Distal wire support technique |
| Proximal anchor balloon technique | Distal anchor balloon technique |

Figure 2.19 Guiding catheter wire and anchor balloon support techniques.

- Fix the guide catheter.
- Advance the second, stiffer wire into the side branch and keep it there while proceeding.

Anchor Balloon Technique
Proximal and Distal Anchor Balloon Support
If the buddy wire does not provide sufficient support, use a small 1.5 mm balloon and deploy it at low pressure (2–4 atm) in the proximal side branch (Figure 2.19, lower left) or distal to the treated lesion (Figure 2.19, lower right).

Proxis Anchor Balloon Support
The Proxis catheter is commonly used as a proximal embolic protection device for saphenous vein graft angioplasty. The tip of this device is relatively

atraumatic, allowing deeper and stable engagement. Furthermore, this can also be used as a backup support particularly for selective engagement of the ostium in ostial lesions.

Key Learning Points

- Predict what devices may be needed during PCI before selection of a guide catheter.
- Use a J wire while advancing and withdrawing the catheter.
- Advance, manipulate, and withdraw the catheter only under fluoroscopy.
- During cannulation, be aware of potential pressure damping.
- Use support techniques to ensure a stable catheter position.

Guide Wires

Introduction

Over the last few years there has been a huge development in wire technology. A wide spectrum of wires is now available which are both vessel- and lesion-specific.

Essentially, a wire should be safe, flexible, and provide good support. The choice of a wire is always personal, based on the operator's experience. When starting, it is sensible to use one's favorite workhorse wire, and then expand the range when dealing with a more complex lesion. In most procedures one wire is enough. However, if one fails to enter the artery or cross the lesion, or if additional support is required, then a different or sometimes a second wire is needed.

The average size of wire is 0.014″ diameter, and, generally, the smaller wire, the more flexible it is. Stiffer or larger wires, e.g., 0.16″, provide more support and torque control and are particularly useful in tortuous vessels or when the guide support is inadequate. On the other hand, stiff wires are more aggressive and are more likely to cause spasm or dissection. They tend to straighten out the tortuous segments and at the same time change vessel geometry.

A few caveats will help in wire selection and overcoming difficulties during wire manipulation:

• Choose a wire on the basis of lesion characteristics and vessel anatomy.
• Shape the tip of the wire precisely, according to the shape of the vessel.
• When recrossing a vessel through stent struts during a bifurcation procedure, shape the wire into a wide J and rotate it during insertion. If you feel resistance, withdraw the wire gently as you have probably placed the wire behind the struts.
• Remember that the tip should move easily without creating loops and without bending.
• When the tip bends, do not push it but withdraw it, slowly rotate it, and advance again.
• Never force the wire in attempting to cross the lesion.
• Try to avoid excessive rotation.
• In a tortuous lesion use a steerable, tracking, support wire with tip control (BMW, Whisper).
• Rotate the wire while advancing balloons or stents. Rotation improves steerability and facilitates advancement.
• If dealing with a heavily calcified, tight lesion or CTO, always start with a soft floppy wire as some seemingly tough lesions are softer than expected. However, a more aggressive, CTO-dedicated wire will probably be needed.
• After successfully crossing a chronically occluded lesion, check the wire position with angiography and make sure that the distal wire is in the true lumen. This is absolutely essential as balloon inflation in the subintimal space may perforate the vessel.

Wire Selection

Selecting an appropriate wire helps achieve a successful result, saves time, and reduces contrast dose. The properties of a wire are determined by its structure:

• Flexibility: Ability to bend with direct force (Table 2.6)
• Trackability: Ability to bend around tortuosities, aligning with vessel anatomy
• Torquability: Allows control of the distal tip of the wire by rotation of the proximal tip
• Steerability: Allows delivery of the wire down the vessel
• Lubricity: Ability to attract or repulse liquids
• Support: Ability to support the passage of various devices (Table 2.6)
• Visibility: Radio-opacity under fluoroscopy

Wire Components

The three main components of a wire are its core, coating, and distal tip (Figure 2.20).

Table 2.6 Choice of guide wire based on flexibility, device support, and type of coating.

Flexibility	Device Support	Coating
Floppy: Choice Floppy Hi-Torque Floppy	Light support: Choice Floppy Hi-Torque Whisper Hi-Torque Balance	Hydrophilic Choice PT Floppy Asahi Fielder
Intermediate: Choice Intermediate Hi-Torque Intermediate Standard: Choice Standard	Moderate support: Hi-Torque Whisper Hi-Torque BMW Extra support (tortuosities, calcifications) Choice Extra Support Choice PT Extra Support	Hydrophobic Hi-Torque Whisper Pilot

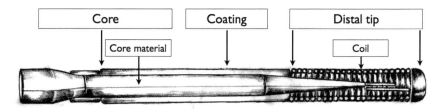

Figure 2.20 Wire components.

Core

The core is the innermost and stiffest part of the wire, which determines wire stability, support, flexibility, and steerability, all depending on the material used.

Core Material Stainless steel is strong and provides very good support and torquability. Nitinol is very elastic with good flexibility, steering, and great shape retention in tortuous lesions.

Core Diameter The diameter of the core determines flexibility, support, and torquability. Thinner wires (smaller diameter) are more flexible, whereas thicker wires (larger diameter) are more supportive and torquable (Figure 2.21).

Core Taper The taper determines the torquability of the wire. A shorter taper provides greater support and force, but is more likely to prolapse. A longer taper provides less support but increases the chance of successful tracking (Figure 2.22).

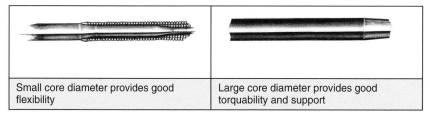

Small core diameter provides good flexibility	Large core diameter provides good torquability and support

Figure 2.21 Wire characteristics: Core diameter.

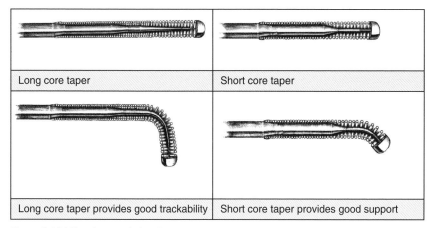

Long core taper	Short core taper
Long core taper provides good trackability	Short core taper provides good support

Figure 2.22 Wire characteristics: Core taper.

Coating

The coating is the outer covering on the core, which affects the lubricity, trackability, and deliverability of the wire. The coating facilitates the movement of the wire and helps overcome tortuosities (see Table 2.6).

Hydrophilic Coating this provides greater lubricity as it attracts water and becomes slippery on with contact with liquids. This helps reduce friction with the vessel wall and improves trackability. Wires with hydrophilic coating are commonly used in very tortuous or calcified lesions and in bifurcations to help crossing into a side branch through stent struts. They should be advanced carefully to avoid risk of subintimal tracking and vessel injury, e.g., perforation or dissection. The hydrophilic wire may recoil or migrate forward during a procedure. This movement may even cause tip perforation. Great care is also needed changing balloons or stents as wiping the hydrophilic wire may result in its inadvertently being pulled out of the vessel. A very tight grip on the wire is needed to prevent this, and regular screening checks of the wire position during balloon exchange. Try and avoid jailing a hydrophilic wire behind a stent as there is a slight risk of wire fracture on its withdrawal.

Hydrophobic Coating this repels water but the wire has better positive feed-back and tip control. These silicone coated wires feel more stable inside the vessel, are easier to control and do not tend to recoil or migrate. They can be jailed more safely behind stents.

Distal Tip

The distal end of a wire can have either a one-segment core, which provides good steerability and tip control, or a two-segment core, which is very soft, flexible, and easy to shape but more likely to prolapse. The wire tip can be covered with coils or with polymer. Coil and cover affect support, trackability, and visibility. Tip style affects steering, which is determined by stiffness, tip shape, and lubricity

Types of Wires

Workhorse and Extra Support Wires

A workhorse wire is used routinely initially, the choice depending on the operator's experience. This wire should be safe rather than stiff, e.g., BMW, Choice PT Floppy, Pilot. Workhorse wires may be hydrophilic or hydrophobic and should provide good torque transmission. Extra support wires allow delivery of devices easily, but are harder to steer, whereas flexible wires are easy to steer but not so supportive with device delivery. It is important to find a balance between flexibility and stiffness as well as torque control and support (see Table 2.6).

Stiff and Soft Wires

Stiff wires are commonly used in older, well-established, and severely calci-fied lesions. The stiffer the tip, the better the pushability and the higher the chance of crossing a tight lesion, but at the cost of a higher risk of spasm or perforation.

Wire Manipulation

The wire should be advanced into the vessel slowly and gently. The tip should be shaped to match the takeoff or the curve of the vessel. The wire should move easily without creating loops and without bending or kinking.

Shaping a Wire

Shaping a wire facilitates manipulation (Figure 2.23). The shape should match the vessel anatomy (angulation, tortuosity, bifurcation angle) and the type of lesion (proximal/distal, long/short). A wire can be shaped primarily and secondarily to match a vessel shape. In tortuous vessels both the primary and the secondary bend should be about 45°. In most vessels a J curve facilitates wire steerability. In crossing a circumflex marginal lesion an S-shaped bend may be necessary.

All wires are flexible and the tip is easy to shape. The tip of a wire can be shaped by bending the tip between the fingers over a needle, guide-wire introducer, scissors, or mosquito forceps. Shaping should be performed gently

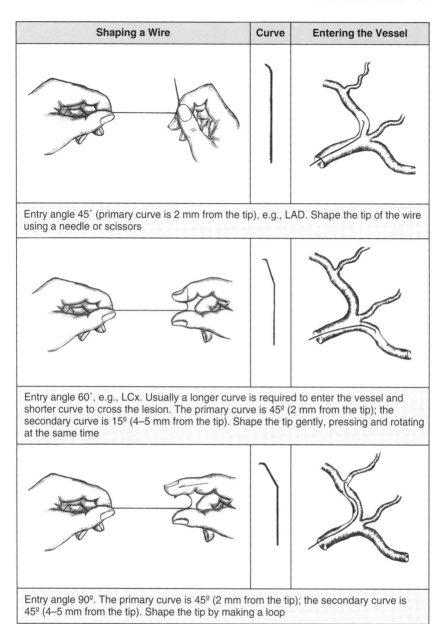

Shaping a Wire	Curve	Entering the Vessel
Entry angle 45° (primary curve is 2 mm from the tip), e.g., LAD. Shape the tip of the wire using a needle or scissors		
Entry angle 60°, e.g., LCx. Usually a longer curve is required to enter the vessel and shorter curve to cross the lesion. The primary curve is 45° (2 mm from the tip); the secondary curve is 15° (4–5 mm from the tip). Shape the tip gently, pressing and rotating at the same time		
Entry angle 90°. The primary curve is 45° (2 mm from the tip); the secondary curve is 45° (4–5 mm from the tip). Shape the tip by making a loop		

Figure 2.23 Shaping a wire.

to avoid damaging the structure of the wire. If the wire becomes kinked in this maneuver it must be discarded as the core will have fractured.

Wire Steering

When resistance is felt and the tip of the wire starts bending, do not push it, but withdraw and slowly rotate it clockwise and anticlockwise. Then advance

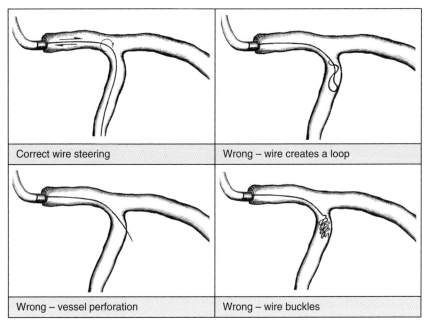

Correct wire steering	Wrong – wire creates a loop
Wrong – vessel perforation	Wrong – wire buckles

Figure 2.24 Wire steering.

again. Never force the wire in trying to cross the lesion, and try to avoid rotating it 360° (risk of tip fracture or wire twists). Extensive manipulation may damage the plaque, causing thrombus formation, occlusion, spasm, perforation, or dissection (Figure 2.24).

Difficulties with Manipulation

Sometimes a wire does not seem to enter an artery or cross the lesion and keeps prolapsing into unwanted smaller branches. Here are a few tips to overcome this problem:

• *Optimal visualization.* If there are difficulties entering a vessel or crossing a lesion, first change the projection and check the wire position in at least two orthogonal views. For example, if trying to enter the LAD, the RAO cranial view is usually used. If the wire is moving towards the circumflex, try the spider view to see the LAD entry from a different angle. Contrast injection is helpful.

• *Support techniques.* If the vessel is tortuous it is often difficult to manipulate a wire smoothly. Support techniques such as the anchor balloon technique provide great backup for the guide catheter, but can also support a wire passage and improve wire steerability. A second wire (buddy wire) can also be used, which will stabilize the whole system. Alternatively, switch to a stiffer, more aggressive wire to improve torque control. This, however, carries a higher risk of vessel perforation. Another possibility is to use a balloon in the vessel well short of the lesion, keeping it uninflated.

• *Prolapsing.* In some situations a wire tends to prolapse during the entry into the target vessel, for example at the LAD/LCx bifurcation. This is usually caused by a short core taper (a wire with a short tip which provides good support, but at a cost of poorer trackability). In such a case it is sensible to switch to a stiffer, long-tapered wire that can enter the vessel deeper.

• *Making a loop.* In cases of severe branch-ostial lesions, particularly with a short stump, a purposely created loop may help entry into the vessel. Advance the wire deeper into the main branch, past the side branch, and try to create a loop in the main branch. Then pull the wire slightly back so that the tip of the wire enters the side branch automatically, dropping down into it from the opposite direction. Remember that a loop must not be created unintentionally from excessive manipulation.

• *Deep inhalation.* This may help the entry into the target vessel. Deep inhalation straightens and narrows the angle between coronary arteries, allowing easier wire passage.

Key Learning Points

• Familiarize yourself with available wires and select one workhorse wire for most procedures.
• Shape the tip precisely, matching the shape of the vessel.
• Avoid excessive manipulation and never try to force the wire across the lesion.
• Stiff, aggressive wires provide good support but carry a higher risk of vessel injury.
• Find a balance between flexibility and stiffness as well as torque control and support.

Balloons

Introduction

Essentially, balloon angioplasty results in acute lumen gain. The mechanisms differ depending on the lesion characteristics. Whereas in a heavily calcified lesion balloon inflation is associated with plaque fracture and dissection, in a fibrotic lesion the gain is due more to plaque compression and vessel stretch.

Balloon-Only Angioplasty

Although balloon-only angioplasty (POBA: "plain old balloon angioplasty") has been shown to improve early outcomes, long-term results remain a problem, and even a successful balloon angioplasty has many limitations:
- Significant residual stenosis
- Frequent plaque shift: a special problem at the carina (see "Bifurcation lesions", p. 204)
- Vessel dissection
- Balloon slippage during inflation
- High restenosis rate (up to 50%)
- Vessel recoil (from its elastic properties)

In many cases, however, balloon angioplasty remains the only available treatment option. Balloon intervention is still the most common strategy in patients with in-stent restenosis, small vessel disease, and complex tortuous vessels as well as in bifurcation lesions, where provisional side branch stenting is the currently recommended treatment strategy (see "Bifurcation lesions", p. 217).

General Considerations

Important technical tips to be considered during balloon procedures include the following:
- A stable guide catheter position with good backup and deep engagement are essential, particularly in tight complex and tortuous lesions.
- A deep inspiration by the patient will help straighten a tortuous segment and may be helpful.
- Predilate a lesion if necessary. In complex PCIs, predilatation should be performed routinely.

• In pre- and postdilatation, balloon length should always be shorter than the final stent length.
• The balloon should be positioned in the center of the stent and must not extend outside the stent.
• After inflation, make sure that the balloon is deflated completely. It is wise to have a quick check on fluoroscopy.
• Withdraw the balloon slowly until it is back in the guide. Make sure that the balloon has regained its wrapped state upon deflation. If in doubt after a fluoroscopy check, remove it completely from the guide.
• Always postdilate using a noncompliant balloon.

Standard Balloons

In general, compliant and semicompliant balloons are used for predilatation and POBA in normal, not complex lesions. Noncompliant balloons are used for postdilatation and POBA in tough, calcified lesions. Essentially, the more compliant a balloon is, the more limited is the pressure range.

Compliant Balloon

This is a flexible balloon which increases its diameter with increasing inflation pressure. One compliant balloon can be used several times for various vessels during the same procedure as the inflation pressure determines the diameter. Since higher pressure results in a larger diameter, there is always a risk of overstretching, and care must be taken to check the balloon diameter at each pressure from the chart on the balloon package. If a lesion is long, it is wise to perform a two-step dilatation: dilating the distal segment first at lower pressure, followed by the proximal part at a higher pressure, to avoid the risk of dissecting the distal segment (Figures 2.25 and 2.26 and Table 2.7).

Noncompliant Balloon

This type of balloon is stiffer than a standard compliant balloon and is always used for stent post-dilatation ensuring optimal stent expansion and apposition. A noncompliant balloon tolerates 50%-higher inflation pressures than a compliant balloon and has a constant relationship between changes in applied pressure and the changes in observed volume. This allows use of greater force without the risk of overstretching other parts of the treated segment particularly the distal segment. A noncompliant balloon can reach and maintain the required diameter despite very high pressure inflation. The diameter is predictable and usually constant over its whole length. This is particularly relevant in long or calcified lesions (Figure 2.25).

Semicompliant Balloon

Semicompliant balloon is relatively stiff and can maintain its size even in high inflation pressure. Not commonly used in daily practice.

Parameters	Compliant balloon	Noncompliant balloon
Stiffness	Flexible	Stiffer
Risk of overstretching	Higher	Lower
Toleration of inflation pressure	Smaller	Larger up to 50%
Diameter at high pressure	Unpredictable	Predictable
Precision	Low	High
Forces	Smaller and dispersed	Greater and focused

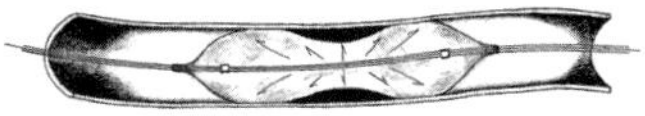

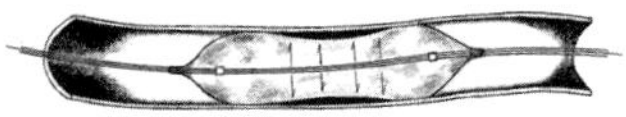

Figure 2.25 Differences between a compliant and noncompliant balloon.

Type of balloon	Balloon design
Compliant balloon	
Cutting balloon	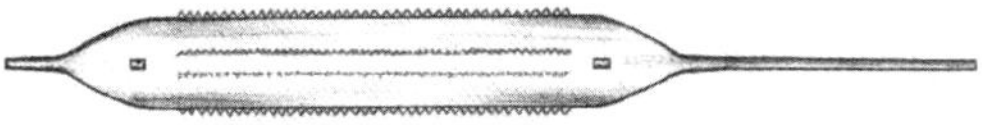
Over-the-wire catheter	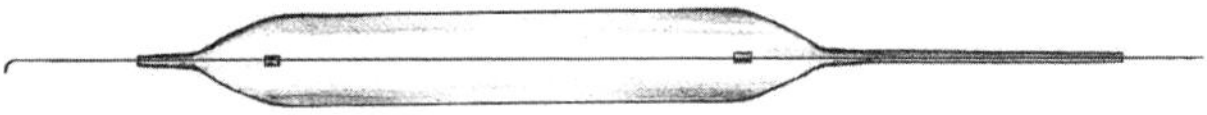
Rapid exchange	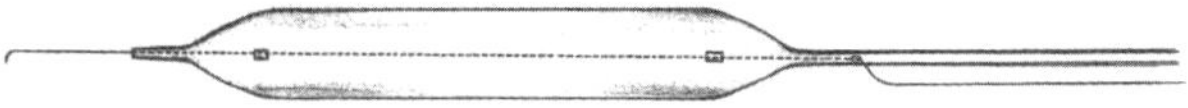

Figure 2.26 Types of coronary balloons.

Table 2.7 Differences between a compliant balloon and a cutting balloon.

Parameters	Compliant balloon	Cutting balloon
Arterial wall damage	Higher	Lower
Media	Multiple rips and tears	No disruption
Endothelium	Disrupted	Minor disruption
Inflation pressure	8–20 atm	6–8 atm
Inflation time	Longer	Shorter
Inflation number	Multiple	Single

Specific Balloons

Balloons made for specific purposes are often needed for complex lesions. Currently available balloons are made from polyurethane materials with either a hydrophilic or hydrophobic coating and a silicone base.

Cutting Balloon

The cutting balloon is a noncompliant balloon dedicated to lesions resistant to high-pressure balloon inflation. The inflation pressure is low (4–8 atm) and the vessel is dilated with less force. The cutting balloon consists of three or four atherotomes attached to the sides of the balloon. During inflation the atherotomes score the plaque by severing the fibrotic part of the vessel, which results in more organized plaque disruption and greater luminal gain than in standard high-pressure balloon expansion. This type of balloon is often used in:

- Ostial lesions
- Restenotic lesions
- In-stent restenotic lesions
- Small vessels and short lesions

The cutting balloon is not recommended, however, in highly tortuous vessels and severely calcified lesions because of the higher risk of vessel perforation. Where there are difficulties in advancing the device through moderate tortuosities or calcification, a buddy wire with a standard balloon inflation may help overcome this (Figure 2.26 and Table 2.7).

Over-the-Wire Balloon

The over-the-wire (OTW) balloon is a balloon catheter with a guide wire positioned inside. The OTW balloon is usually 145–155 cm long with 300 cm wire in the lumen. A guide wire can move through the entire length of the catheter and exits at the hub rather than from a side hole. Both guide wire and balloon can move independently. Two operators are required to change the wire (Figure 2.26).

Rapid-Exchange Balloon

The so-called rapid-exchange (Rx) balloon is very helpful for a quick exchange. It consists of a balloon catheter and a guide wire which enters the balloon at its distal tip and can be moved separately from the balloon catheter. The Rx is 180 cm long with 195 cm guide wire inside the lumen. A single operator can manage it by fixing the wire and advancing the balloon simultaneously (Figure 2.26).

Balloon Size

Balloon Diameter

A rule of thumb for optimal balloon selection is to compare the vessel diameter with the diameter of the guiding catheter, which is usually 2 mm (assuming the use of a 6F guide). It is helpful to remember quarter sizes of available balloons and balloon compliance. IVUS measurements may help in balloon size selection. If in doubt, it is always safer to start with a balloon 0.5 mm smaller than the initial estimate and progress to a larger balloon if necessary.

Balloon Length

Several rules help in the selection of an ideal balloon length. They are different for predilatation and postdilatation.

Predilatation and Postdilatation

Predilatation

This is an important part of lesion preparation that determines stent sizing and positioning. It helps assess lesion compliance and improves coronary flow before stent implantation.

Predilatation can be performed with a compliant, semicompliant, or noncompliant balloon, depending on the type of lesion. If a compliant balloon will not expand adequately switching to a small-size noncompliant balloon inflated at high pressure or a cutting balloon should be considered. If both balloons fail to dilate the lesion, debulking may be necessary with rotablation.

Predilatation of a short focal lesion should be performed with a short balloon fully covering the lesion. To avoid dilating and damaging normal vessel at each end of the lesion, the balloon should not be longer than the lesion itself. Predilatation of a long, diffuse lesion, however, should be performed with a long balloon which is longer than the lesion rather than with two short balloons. This may mean using a 30 mm balloon for diffuse disease. Although choosing one long balloon always carries a potential risk of over-inflation of the distal segment and underinflation of the proximal segment, the risk of vessel dissection is lower and the long balloon is generally a very safe device.

A few caveats with predilatation:
- Always predilate long tortuous or complex lesions.
- Always predilate calcified lesions.
- Avoid predilatation in grafts if possible (see p. 275).

- Avoid predilatation in primary PCI if possible (see p. 140).
- Never deploy a stent in a vessel which cannot be predilated adequately.
- Consider debulking a lesion which cannot be adequately dilated prior to stenting.

Postdilatation
Postdilatation should be performed with a short noncompliant balloon (shorter than the stent) to avoid vessel injury beyond the stent. Balloon markers should be placed symmetrically within the ends of the stent (if two markers) and centrally within the stent (if a single marker). The balloon should be inflated at high pressure to optimize stent apposition.

Crossing the Lesion
This depends on the design of the balloon and its profile (pushability and crossability), guide catheter backup, and preparation of the lesion. In most cases, with the lesion well prepared, the balloon slides into the vessel across the lesion smoothly so that additional maneuvers are not needed.

Calcified Lesion
In heavily calcified lesions the balloon may not cross the lesion, causing difficulties such as catheter disengagement (backing out). In such cases the catheter will require better support, more stable backup, or deeper seating. It may be possible to engage the catheter deeper or to use one of the guide support techniques (see p. 85) or to switch to a different guiding catheter, e.g., EBU. If these techniques fail, you can switch to a smaller or shorter balloon with an extra-support wire. Using the tapping technique on the balloon catheter may help. A small balloon deployed proximal to a very tight lesion will create a channel and may facilitate crossing.

Tortuous Vessel
Crossing a lesion may also be challenging in very tortuous vessels. In this situation, the simplest way is to ask the patient to take a deep breath and then to try to advance a balloon. Another solution is to use a second wire (buddy wire), or alternatively to withdraw the balloon and switch to a stiffer wire. Both techniques may facilitate the passage by straightening the vessel. Guiding catheter stability is also very important and support techniques should be used to provide optimal backup.

Balloon Positioning
Marker bands (single or dual) in the shaft of the balloon determine the balloon location during its positioning. In predilatation the balloon should cover the lesion completely, while during postdilatation a noncompliant balloon shorter than the stent should be positioned in the center of the stent (Figure 2.27).

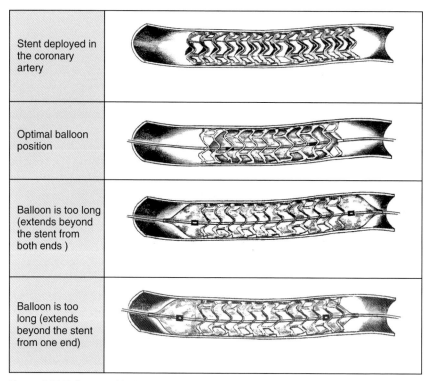

Stent deployed in the coronary artery	
Optimal balloon position	
Balloon is too long (extends beyond the stent from both ends)	
Balloon is too long (extends beyond the stent from one end)	

Figure 2.27 Balloon positioning within a coronary stent during postdilatation.

Balloon Inflation

An inflation device is used to inflate and deflate balloon catheters (Figure 2.28). The device consists of a syringe, a pressure gauge calibrated from 0 to 30 atm to monitor the inflation pressure, a piston handle, and a tube to connect the device to the balloon catheter. When unlocked, the piston handle is ready for aspiration. The syringe should be filled with mixture of contrast and saline (in the proportion 1:1 or 1:2), and all bubbles from the syringe and connecting tube must be removed. The tube should be connected to the Luer lock of the balloon catheter. The inflator is then ready to use:

• Pull the piston handle fully back and lock it in "aspiration" position to achieve negative pressure and maintain a vacuum in the balloon before inflation.

• To inflate, unlock the piston handle to reach a neutral position (0 atm).

• It is important to keep the inflation device pointing downwards to avoid getting bubbles in the connecting tube.

• Keep turning the grip. The balloon should be inflated quickly to reach the required pressure. Some operators prefer a slow inflation to stretch the vessel gradually, but this has not been proved to be of benefit.

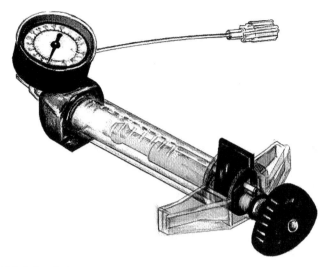

Figure 2.28 Inflation device.

• The balloon or stent is now inflated. Hold for a while and observe the result on the screen.
• First inflation is usually approx. 30 seconds (see below). It may be shorter if the balloon suddenly expands from the dog-bone shape, or longer if the balloon fails to expand adequately.
• Balloon inflation may cause angina, and the patient should be warned of this possibility.
• To deflate the balloon, pull the piston handle fully back, reaching negative pressure, and lock it.
• After successful inflation, make sure the balloon has been deflated completely. A quick check under fluoroscopy before withdrawal is recommended. In some very rare cases a balloon may fail to deflate with the inflation device. This may occur due to balloon entanglement or, more often, to balloon or guide wire entrapment within a very tight or calcified lesion.
• For postdilatation inside a stent, the balloon can be deflated once the required diameter has been achieved. Long postdilatation inflations should not be necessary.

Inflation Pressure
Inflating to an optimal pressure is essential in achieving a good result. Balloon pressure charts on the package label always indicate two pressures, which have been tested by manufacturers both in a rig and in vivo (Table 2.8):
• Nominal pressure (e.g., 9 atm): The pressure at which the balloon reaches its specified diameter.

Table 2.8 Definitions of inflation pressure.

Inflation pressure	Definition
Nominal pressure	Pressure at which the balloon can reach its nominal diameter (as stated on the label)
Rated burst pressure	Pressure at which and below which the balloon will not burst (based on in vivo tests)
Working range	Pressure range between nominal pressure and rated burst pressure

- Rated pressure (e.g., 16 atm): The pressure at or above which the balloon may burst. The balloon should not burst below this pressure but may burst at any pressure higher than this pressure.
- The range between the nominal and rated pressure is the working range of the balloon.
- The size of the balloon in this working range should be checked on the manufacturer's chart and will depend on balloon compliance.

It may be possible to exceed the rated pressure with tough lesions, but this increases the risk of balloon rupture, and balloon performance varies above the rated pressure.

Balloon Rupture

Balloon rupture within the working range is rare, but it may occur with a heavily calcified lesion or from multiple inflations and deflations, particularly in calcified plaques. Balloons burst either circumferentially into two halves or longitudinally along the length of the balloon. If this occurs there is a sudden decrease in the inflation pressure on the gauge, and contrast dispersion around the balloon is visible on angiography. Blood may be aspirated down the inflation lumen. It is important to withdraw the ruptured balloon slowly and to check the vessel in case of dissection or perforation.

It is very important to maintain wire position with a balloon rupture as vessel dissection or even perforation is a possibility, and urgent stenting may be necessary.

Inflation Time

How long should the balloon remain inflated?

Successful predilatation is marked by the expansion of the balloon, which changes suddenly from a dog-bone shape to a cylindrical sausage shape as the fibrous plaque of the lesion is cracked. This may be associated with a sudden slight drop in pressure on the inflation pressure gauge as the balloon suddenly expands.

The balloon should be kept at maximum pressure for at least 15 seconds. If the balloon will not inflate fully even at high pressure – suggesting a very tough or calcified stenosis – then longer inflations or switching to a high-pressure, noncompliant balloon may be necessary. Thirty seconds is long enough for predilatation and stent deployment in most lesions. Be prepared for longer inflations in very tough lesions, assuming the hemodynamics are stable.

Short inflations should cause minimal or no angina, but longer inflations may cause chest pain and the patient should be warned of this possibility. Adequate sedation and analgesia are important. Diamorphine aliquots of 2.5 mg IV may be necessary in some cases.

For postdilatation the aim is simply to ensure good all-round stent strut apposition. The stent is postdilated with a short, noncompliant balloon positioned in the center of the stent and deployed at high pressure for 5–10 seconds only. Long inflations at this stage are unnecessary. IVUS can be used to check satisfactory apposition if there is doubt and the dilatation repeated if necessary.

Balloon Entrapment

There are several strategies to free an entrapped balloon.
• First, try to inflate and deflate the balloon alternately using the inflation device. Alternatively, replace the inflation device with a syringe and try to deflate the balloon directly from the inflation port.
• Secondly, gently retract and advance the balloon backward and forward with slight rotational movements. Simply pulling it back vigorously may work, but risks damaging the vessel.
• Thirdly try the buddy balloon technique. Advance another balloon parallel to the entrapped one to stretch the vessel and free the balloon. Good catheter support will be needed to deal with two balloons. A second, stiffer wire may also be helpful to straighten the vessel.
• A risky solution is to inflate the balloon at a very high pressure to rupture it. This will inevitably cause dissection or possible perforation and may considerably complicate the procedure.
• Finally, if all above strategies fail, surgical removal is the only remaining option.

Key Learning Points

• Predilatation is an important part of lesion preparation.
• Calcified lesions may cause balloon rupture.
• Do not deploy a stent in an inadequately prepared lesion.
• Postdilatation with a noncompliant balloon at high pressure improves stent expansion.
• The postdilatation balloon should be positioned in the center of the stent, and should be shorter than the stent.
• Use specific balloons where appropriate.

Stents

Introduction

Since the introduction of the Palmaz-Schatz stent in 1994, stent technology has evolved tremendously. Increasing numbers of coronary interventions now include safe treatment of complex coronary lesions, unprotected left main stem stenosis, and high-risk patients. Recent meta-analysis from more than 30 trials has demonstrated that PCI with both on- and off-label use of drug-eluting stents reduces symptoms, ischemia, rates of restenosis, and target vessel revascularization. It has been clearly shown that drug-eluting stents do not increase death and myocardial infarction compared with bare metal stents.

The primary goal of stent implantation is to achieve an optimal luminal area without damaging the artery, ensure rapid endothelialization, and prevent chronic inflammation. The ideal stent should have thin struts, be easily introduced with a low crossing profile, and have good scaffolding without a polymer coating to minimize vessel damage and chronic inflammation. It should also eliminate the need for long-term dual antiplatelet therapy and be compatible with noninvasive follow-up such as CT or MRI.

Table 2.9 Changing characteristics of stents over time with improving stent technology.

Bare Metal Stent	Drug-Eluting Stent	Bioabsorbable Stent
Vascular injury	Tissue pharmacodynamics	Device absorption
Neointimal response	Delayed vascular healing	Vascular remodeling

Continuous improvements in stent technology provide safety and efficacy to angioplasty procedures as well as easier and safer stent implantation. Whereas the first bare metal stents caused vascular injury and neointimal response, the new-generation stents are fully absorbable, leaving behind healthy vessel (Table 2.9).

Stent Implantation

Predilatation and Postdilatation
Balloon predilatation helps facilitate the positioning of a stent, particularly in tight or calcified lesions or if stent sizing is a problem. An accurate assessment of the vessel size, especially distal to the lesion, is very important as an undersized stent increases the risk of future in-stent restenosis. After placement of a stent, a shorter noncompliant balloon should be used to postdilate the lesion at higher pressure. Stent implantation without previous balloon predilatation is direct stenting.

Stent Length and Diameter
Stent length should be determined by the length of the lesion, measured from one normal reference vessel to the next normal reference vessel (the distance between disease-free areas). If in doubt, a longer stent should always be chosen to make sure that the lesion is covered completely.

The practical way to choose the *stent diameter* is to compare the diameter of the treated vessel with the diameter of the guiding catheter (which is 2 mm for a 6F guide). The most common mistake is sizing a stent with reference to the proximal vessel diameter. Murray's principle states that the proximal vessel diameter ×0.67 is equal to the sum of the main branch and the side branch. Therefore, particularly in a long lesion with a significant disproportion between proximal and distal diameters, the stent size should match the diameter of the distal vessel. This rule applies to most coronary vessels.

Stent Positioning
Accurate stent positioning is particularly difficult in treatment of ostial lesions and saphenous vein grafts. Sometimes stent positioning may be disturbed by respiratory or cardiac motion. In the case of extensive respiratory motion, a deep inspiration and breath-hold or shallow breathing can be helpful. If cardiac motion is a problem, gentle stent balloon inflation at very low pressure (2 atm) will help to fix the stent in the intended position before it is fully deployed.

It is also helpful to study the stent before introducing it to check the relationship of the end of the stent to the balloon marker. With some designs the stent overlies the marker and in others there is a gap of several millimeters between stent and marker. This is important for accurate stent placement.

Stent Deployment

A stent is delivered by the balloon inside it. "Delivery" refers to the way the stent is introduced and transported to the lesion, whereas stent "deployment" refers to the expansion within the vessel wall. Optimal stent deployment is essential; this increases drug delivery and reduces the risk of stent thrombosis and in-stent restenosis and the need for target lesion revascularization.

The duration of stent balloon inflation is also very important. It is known that a short inflation time limits complete stent expansion and is associated with greater immediate elastic recoil. Furthermore, studies have shown that increasing the inflation time from 10 to 60 seconds results in a significant increase in minimal luminal area. If a stent seems to be undersized at angiography, a longer inflation time up to 60 seconds at high pressure is recommended.

Stent Underexpansion and Apposition

Suboptimal stent deployment is often associated with either physical properties of the vessel wall, underestimation of the original vessel diameter with undersizing of the stent size, type of lesion (severe calcification, tortuosity, bifurcation, ostial lesion), inadequate balloon compliance, or low-pressure inflation (<10 atm). Predilatation, adequate angiographic visualization, or the use of IVUS help optimize stent deployment.

Incomplete stent apposition means a separation of at least one stent strut from the vessel wall (with evidence of blood present behind the struts).

Safety and Efficacy

"Safety" refers to the potential risk of stent thrombosis, whereas "efficacy" refers to the restenosis rate and suppression of neointimal hyperplasia. These two properties should be considered together. The safety and efficacy of drug-eluting stents are determined by radial strength, durability, the delivery system (compatible balloon), trackability, visibility, thrombogenic effect, and strut thickness.

Bare Metal Stents

Although bare metal stents reduce the need for repeat revascularization compared to balloon angioplasty, their use is limited in the drug-eluting stent era.

In practice bare metal stents are still used if the patient has planned non-cardiac surgery or has difficulty in maintaining long-term dual antiplatelet therapy (usually due to high risk of bleeding or resistance to aspirin or clopidogrel). Bare metal stents can also be used for simple lesions in big vessels, in low-risk patients, and in vein grafts. They are used less in primary PCI for acute myocardial infarction with increasing evidence in favour of drug-

Table 2.10 Differences between bare metal stents and drug-eluting stents.

	Bare Metal Stents	Drug-Eluting Stents
Compliance with DAPT	Poor compliance, short term	Good compliance, long term
DAPT duration	1 month	1 year
Inflammatory	Few days	Few days to weeks
Tissue formation	Weeks	Months
Neointima formation	1–2 weeks	Several months
Complete healing process	2–4 weeks	Several months

DAPT, dual antiplatelet therapy.

eluting stents in these patients. In pregnancy, however, bare metal stents should be used.

Drug-Eluting Stents

The main differences between bare metal stents and drug-eluting stents (DES) relate to the vascular wall injury and healing pattern, e.g., the process of protein absorption is very short after bare metal stent implantation, but it takes months after DES use. Likewise, the vascular repair process with bare metal stents is relatively short, taking hours or days, whereas DES release their antimitotic drugs slowly over a few weeks (see Table 2.10).

DES have dramatically reduced the rate of in-stent restenosis and the need for subsequent target vessel revascularization compared to bare metal stents. However, delayed vascular healing with DES resulting from the vessel response to the polymer and the drug, as well as lack of complete re-endothelialization, has increased the risk of stent thrombosis. Although very rare, this remains a problem. Moreover, patients who receive DES always require prolonged dual antiplatelet therapy for a minimum of 1 year. Efficacy in diabetic patients is poorer due to an impaired nitric oxide pathway.

Platform, Drug, and Polymer

DES consist of a platform, an agent (antimitotic drug), and a polymer. The platform is the metallic scaffolding. The polymer is a surface coating responsible for biocompatibility and the degradation profile. Drug release into the vessel wall controls the inflammatory reaction immediately after stent deployment and the proliferation of smooth muscle long after implantation. The agent elutes either from the stent matrix (platform) or from the polymer coating. The polymer is designed to deliver a drug over a specific time. Unfortunately, many polymers have quite undesirable features and are recognizable as a foreign body, causing various allergic reactions, inflammation, aneurysm formation, or delayed healing. Durable, stable polymers are used in early-generation stents (Taxus stent). Some new-generation stents have bioabsorbable polymers which are fully metabolized and highly biocompatible. The polymer resorbs fully within a few months and does not induce any inflammatory reactions. Very new polymer-free stents show promising results and may become an alternative to standard polymeric stents.

On- and Off-Label Indications

On-label indications for DES implantation are limited to symptomatic patients with single de novo lesions shorter than 30 mm and 2.5–3.5 mm in diameter. These have been evaluated in many clinical trials.

Off-label use of DES refers to patients with in-stent restenosis, graft lesions, long lesions (>30 mm), small-diameter vessels (<2.5 mm), or large-diameter vessels (>3.5 mm). Although real-life experience shows worse short-term outcomes (mostly ischemic complications) with off-label use of DES than with standard on-label use, off-label use of DES is very common. Unfavorable outcomes are most likely to be associated with the patient's clinical profile, lesion characteristics, and more advanced coronary disease rather than with specific shortcomings of the devices themselves. Most patients receiving DES need complex PCIs and present with diffuse disease, left main stenosis, a bifurcation lesion, chronic total occlusion, or already existing restenosis. Nevertheless, even with off-label use, DES are more effective than bare metal stents, and the overall in-hospital and 12 month major cardiac adverse events rates remain low. Indications for use of DES are listed in Table 2.11.

Drug-Eluting Stent Selection

Although all available DES have been proven safe and efficacious, various factors determine the optimal stent choice. Patient selection should be based on a careful assessment of the medical history and overall clinical presentation: severity of symptoms, vessel and lesion characteristics (anti-restenotic needs), compliance with dual antiplatelet therapy, and cost effectiveness.

Table 2.11 Indications for the use of drug-eluting stents.

On-label use	Off-label use	Situations where drug-eluting stents should be avoided
Vessel diameter 2.5–3.5 mm	Vessel diameter <2.5 mm	Contraindications to DAPT
Lesion length ≤30 mm	Lesion length >30 mm	Patient unlikely to comply with DAPT
De novo lesion	In-stent restenosis	Medical treatment or bypass surgery are preferable treatment options
	Acute myocardial infarction	
	Left main lesion	
	Bifurcation lesion	
	Chronic total occlusion lesion	Excellent final result may be expected without drug-eluting stent
	Saphenous vein graft lesion	
	Multivessel disease	

DAPT, dual antiplatelet therapy.

Table 2.12 Relative priorities of safety and efficacy in stent selection for various indications.

Prioritize safety	Prioritize efficacy
Emergency PCI	Long lesions
Primary PCI	Diabetic patients
Bleeding risk	Small vessels
Forthcoming elective surgery	High restenosis risk
Elderly patients	Grafts
Doubts regarding antiplatelet therapy compliance	Ostial lesion
Bifurcation lesion	Left main coronary artery stenosis
Comorbidities	Multivessel disease

PCI, percutaneous coronary intervention.

Safety and efficacy should be well balanced. Safety is always a priority in emergency procedures, in high-risk patients with acute coronary syndrome, in the elderly, who may have difficulties with the long-term dual antiplatelet therapy, in patients with a high risk of bleeding, and in those who may need elective surgery in the near future or have comorbidities or a poor socioeconomic status. Safety is also a priority with bifurcation lesions and large vessels. Efficacy should be considered the priority in patients with diabetes, a high risk of restenosis, small vessels and long lesions, grafts, ostial lesion, thrombotic lesion, multivessel disease, or left main stenosis. These priorities in stent selection are summarized in Table 2.12.

Stent Thrombosis
Although very late stent thrombosis is less of an issue with the new generation of drug-eluting stents, it carries catastrophic implications. In the ENDEAVOR IV study, analysis showed a reduction of 1.5% in the rate of stent thrombosis for a zotarolimus-eluting stent compared with a paclitaxel-eluting stent, and the LESSON-1 trial demonstrated a 0.5% stent thrombosis rate for an everolimus-eluting stent vs 1.6% for a sirolimus-eluting stent. The most common predictors of stent thrombosis are noncompliance with dual antiplatelet therapy, smoking, diabetes, impaired renal function, and low ejection fraction (see p. 303). Effective dual antiplatelet therapy is essential to minimize the risk of stent thrombosis.

Dual Antiplatelet Therapy
Dual antiplatelet therapy after DES implantation is extremely important. Mounting evidence shows that prolonged antiplatelet therapy reduces the risk of stent thrombosis, death, and myocardial infarction. The exact duration of treatment remains controversial and has not been established,

but it is thought to be a minimum of 1 year following DES deployment (see p. 113).

New-Generation Durable-Polymer Drug-Eluting Stents

The new generation of DES show an improved efficacy and safety profile, a lower rate of myocardial infarction, and a lower risk of very late stent thrombosis compared with the early-generation durable-polymer DES. However, mortality remains similar and they still show some disadvantages. The major consideration is the presence of a permanent foreign body within the vessel, which causes chronic inflammation, delays re-endothelialization, and increases the risk of stent thrombosis and restenosis. All patients require long-term dual antiplatelet therapy.

• The Xience V stent has shown good results in many clinical trials. A soft tip allows good pushability and reduced vessel injury. A higher rated burst pressure permits higher pressure deployment.

• The recently introduced Promus Element platinum–chromium everolimus-eluting stent system offers great radial strength, conformability (expanded stent flexibility), and visibility. This stent is particularly useful in long and tortuous lesions and shows good early results (PLATINUM trial). An example of Promus Element conformability is shown in Figure 2.29.

Bioabsorbable Drug-Eluting Stent Platforms

This new stent technology is based on bioabsorption – a process in which both the polymer and the stent matrix are gradually absorbed. They lose their chemical structure by hydrolytic, enzymatic or oxidative reactions. Although in practice the terms "bioabsorbtion," "bioresorption," and "biodegradation" are used interchangeably, they do in fact have different meanings. While "biodegradation" refers to the process in which stents lose their desirable chemical structure, "bioresorption" suggests that the polymer is changed by the process.

After a stent has delivered a drug, it would appear to be no longer needed. Worse, it may even be harmful. Bioabsorbable stents are fully metabolized after drug delivery and are naturally absorbed without leaving any permanent metallic implant. After absorption has taken place, the vessel is completely healed and normal. These stents are particularly beneficial for patients with metal allergies.

Lack of a permanent metallic implant carries various implications. First, the stented segment is able to respond to ischemia as its vasomotor and endothelial function is regained and returns to normal. Potentially, there is no risk of late stent thrombosis, or at least the risk is minimized as there is no foreign body in the artery wall and subsequently no inflammation. Also, coronary artery bypass surgery will prove easier for the surgeon, should it prove necessary, as there will be no possible metallic stent at the desired anastomotic site. Finally, bioabsorbable stents are compatible with CT

Table 2.13 Advantages of bioabsorbable stents.

No permanent scaffolding
Fully metabolized
Fully absorbed
No chronic inflammation
Decreased risk of stent thrombosis
Easier reintervention
No metal at site of possible future CABG anastomosis
No image interference with CT and MRI (noninvasive follow-up)

and MRI, which allows noninvasive follow up without image interference from the metallic stent. Advantages of bioabsorbable stents are listed in Table 2.13.

Bioabsorbable stent design is based on a fully bioabsorbable polymer (poly-L-lactic acid, PLLA), which enters the metabolic cycle and dissolves into water and carbon dioxide within a few months. The polymer is safe and is commonly used in orthopedic plates, sutures, screws, etc.

A variety of bioabsorbable polymer-based stents have been developed:

• The Igaki–Tamai was one of the first polymeric stents with a PLLA platform, self-expanded with zig-zag hoops.

• "Limus family" stents with a PLLA coating have a lower drug dose and higher spatial distribution, with thinner struts and better vessel coverage and delivery.

• Biolimus A9, which shows promising early results from the LEADERS trial. BioMatrix is a biolimus eluting stent with biodegradable polymer. This has immunosuppressive and anti-inflammatory properties and the coating fully absorbs within 6 months. In comparison with the sirolimus eluting Cypher stent, it showed superior strut coverage and superior outcomes in the STEMI trial with a similar rate of stent thrombosis (less than 0.5%).

• BioMime, a sirolimus-eluting stent with a cobalt–chromium platform and very thin struts, has a unique open and closed cell design ensuring good radial strength and flexibility. It provides almost full endothelialization within 2 weeks.

• The Jactax paclitaxel-eluting stent with ultrathin bioerodable abluminal polymer delivers only a small dose of paclitaxel. It releases the drug in 60 days and fully resorbs within 4 months.

• The Elixir fully bioabsorbable myolimus-eluting stent, with cobalt alloy platform, thin coating, and thin struts, promises better vessel coverage, better flexibility, and improved deliverability. Bioabsorbable polymer-based limus-releasing DES demonstrate as good safety and efficacy as early-generation durable-polymer-based DES with a similar late catch-up phenomenon.

• BVS, an everolimus-eluting stent with platform and struts made from PLLA, is balloon-expandable with the MultiLink Vision delivery system.

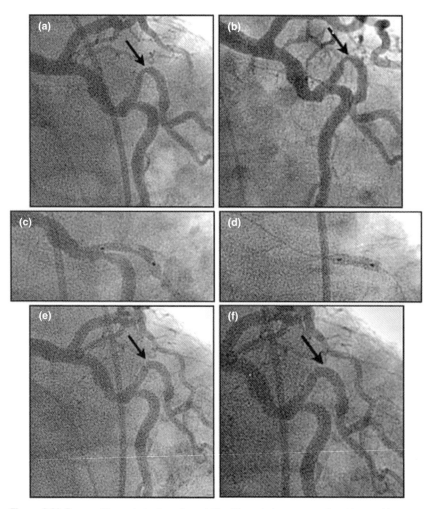

Figure 2.29 Promus Element stent conformability. Stenosis is seen on a bend in an obtuse marginal artery (**a,b**). Wire and a deployed stent straighten the artery (**c**). Postdilatation at 24 atm with a 2.75 × 9 mm noncompliant balloon (**d**). The 2.75 × 12 mm Promus Element stent conforms to the vessel contour without straightening the artery (**e**). Final result (**f**).

Excellent results have been shown with this stent, which is largely absorbed within 2 years, leaving restored vasomotion.

Less Successful Bioabsorbable Stents

Stents such as the REVA, BTI (fully absorbable salicylic acid stent), or bioabsorbable magnesium alloy stents showed initial unfavorable results in first in-man studies and more investigations are needed to optimize outcomes. The

REVA is a balloon-expandable drug-eluting stent with tyrosine delivered on a polycarbonate platform. Results from the RESORB trial have demonstrated higher than expected target lesion revascularization between 4 and 6 months after implantation, probably due to the polymer design. BTI–sirolimus with salicylic acid polymer and anti-inflammatory and antiplatelet properties also showed unfavorable results, probably due to insufficient drug dose and too fast drug release. A higher dose of drug with slower release might optimize the outcome (under investigation). A bioabsorbable magnesium alloy stent with magnesium platform and slow degradation has also shown a high restenosis rate and target lesion revascularization of almost 50%.

Polymer-Free Drug-Eluting Stent Platforms

Although polymer-free and porous-eluting stents are still under development, they may prove a great advantage in the future. A lack of polymer or polymer-free drug release could potentially reduce polymer-related late adverse events caused by a polymer coating.

Polymer-free stents may ensure good neointimal healing, improve surface integrity, restore the process of endothelialization, and subsequently reduce the risk of thrombus formation. It is also possible that they shorten the required duration of dual antiplatelet therapy. Essentially, the idea is to create a bioactive agent which impregnates the surface of the stent and dissolves in a nonpolymeric biodegradable carrier on the stent surface. The second important factor in this technology is an abluminal coating (i.e., outer surface of the stent only) which holds drug and allows the stent to deliver the drug directly into the vessel wall from its reservoir.

Polymer-free stents include the following:
• The BioFreedom stent, a Biolimus A9 eluting stent, which also completely eliminates polymer and allows more rapid drug clearance to enhance vascular healing.
• CID Optima, a polymer-free stent that releases a drug from a reservoir straight into the vessel wall.
• Amazonia Pax, a chromium–cobalt alloy platform with open cell design and very thin struts, based on the same pattern as the CID Optima.
• Another new concept in stent design is the ISAR-TEST2, which contains a dual drug system, delivering both a drug (sirolimus) and an anti-restenotic agent, probucol, which has shown good results in reducing restenosis rates.

Drug-Eluting Balloons

Drug-eluting balloons (DEBs) may become an attractive alternative to DES, particularly in selected patients in whom the use of DES is limited, e.g., those with small vessels, long lesions, left main stenting, in-stent restenosis, or diabetes.

The concept of drug-coated balloon technology is completely different to that of coated stents. Whereas DES deliver the drug over days or weeks, DEBs provide immediate and short-lasting drug release straight after balloon expansion, ensuring great contact between the drug and the vessel wall. The idea is to design a balloon which will replace a stent and ensure precise drug delivery, reduce the rate of restenosis, and shorten the process of vascular healing with minimal local negative effect.

The first-generation DEBs provide passive, uncontrolled drug elution into the intima of the artery by balloon expansion and do not have an intrinsic delivery system. The antimitotic drug can achieve a therapeutic level and the balloon polymer is able to keep the drug in place. The drawback is that it does not allow its proper transfer. There is also the potential risk of various toxic reactions and a possible need for multiple inflations. A further concern is the possible risk of distal embolization or tissue damage.

DEBs such as the zotarolimus-eluting balloon, nanoparticle polymer-free sirolimus balloon, or Paccocath, a paclitaxel-coated balloon, are still being investigated. Although outcomes from the PEPCAD V bifurcation study with a paclitaxel-eluting balloon plus bare metal stent implantation in bifurcation lesions show a higher risk of late stent thrombosis, results from the PEPCAD program will tell us whether DEBs are safe with the potential to be a realistic alternative to DES in selected patients.

Trials
SPIRIT IV
In this study almost 4000 patients were randomized to receive an everolimus-eluting stent or a paclitaxel-eluting stent. The trial also examined the differences in performance of the two stents in diabetic patients. The results demonstrated enhanced safety and efficacy of the everolimus-eluting stent compared to the paclitaxel stent without routine angiographic follow-up.

The primary end point of the trial was target lesion failure at one year, a composite measure of cardiac death, target vessel myocardial infarctionor ischemia-driven target lesion revascularization. Major secondary end points of the trial were target lesion revascularization at 1 year, and a composite of cardiac death or target vessel myocardial infarction at 1 year. For the everolimus stent, target lesion failure at 1 year was 4.2%, and for the paclitaxel-eluting stent, target lesion failure was 6.8%, a significant 38% reduction for the everolimus stent. At one-year, ischemia-driven target lesion revascularization was 2.5% for the everolimus stent and 4.6% for the paclitaxel stent, a significant 45% reduction. The composite rates of cardiac death or target vessel myocardial infarction at 1 year were not statistically different for the two stents. The rates of stent thrombosis, however, were significantly reduced with the everolimus stent compared to the paclitaxel-eluting stent (0.3% vs. 1.1% respectively). In the diabetic patient subgroup, the study found a comparable rate of target lesion failure with both stents, whereas in patients without diabetes, the everolimus stent reduced target lesion failure by 53% compared to the paclitaxel-eluting stent.

LEADERS

In this study 1707 patients with chronic stable coronary artery disease or acute coronary syndromes were randomized to treatment with either biolimus-eluting (n = 857) or sirolimus-eluting (n = 850) stents. At 9 months and 1 year the biolimus- and the sirolimus-eluting stents seemed equivalent in respect of major adverse cardiac events (MACE rate). However, biolimus appeared to be associated with a higher rate of binary in-stent restenosis in long lesions and target lesion revascularization. Results showed that a biolimus stent made from a biodegradable polymer represents a safe and effective alternative to a sirolimus-eluting stent made from a durable polymer in patients with chronic stable coronary artery disease or acute coronary syndromes.

ISAR-TEST 4

This real-world study randomized 2603 patients with stable coronary artery disease or acute coronary syndrome who underwent stenting with DES in de novo lesions, receiving either a biodegradable polymer sirolimus-eluting stent or a permanent polymer DES (a sirolimus-eluting Cypher or an everolimus-eluting Xience stent). The biodegradable polymer stent consisted of a stainless steel, microporous, thin-strut platform coated on site with a mixture of rapamycin, biodegradable polymer, and a biocompatible resin. A biodegradable polymer DES has been hypothesized to help overcome the delayed arterial healing and inflammatory response induced by the permanent polymer of conventional DES. Two-year outcomes were similar for the two groups. TVR was 11.7% in the permanent polymer stent, and 11.0% in the biodegradable stent, and stent thrombosis 1.7% and 1.1% respectively.

ABSORB

In this open-label study 101 patients with a single de novo lesion were enrolled for treatment with the poly-L-lactic acid backbone and poly-D,L-lactic acid everolimus-eluting bioabsorbable polymer BVS stent. The rate of MACE was 4.4% and there were no reports of thromboses. The study showed the feasibility of implantation of the bioabsorbable everolimus-eluting stent with an acceptable in-stent late luminal loss (0.19 mm) and a low stent area obstruction.

SORT OUT II

In this study 2098 patients with ST-elevation myocardial infarction (STEMI), non-STEMI, unstable angina, and stable angina were randomized to receive a paclitaxel- or sirolimus-eluting stent. In the comparison between the paclitaxel and sirolimus stents, there were no significant differences in the rate of clinically driven MACE at 9-month follow-up.

Key Learning Points

• Stent length should be determined by the length of the lesion measured from one normal reference vessel to the next normal reference vessel.

• Predilatation should be performed with a compliant balloon, postdilatation with a noncompliant balloon.

• Safety refers to the potential risk of stent thrombosis, whereas efficacy relates to the restenosis rate and suppression of neointimal hyperplasia.

• Biodegradation is the process in which stents lose their desirable chemical structure by hydrolytic, enzymatic, or oxidative reactions.

• Bioabsorbable stents are fully metabolized after drug delivery and are naturally absorbed without leaving a permanent metallic implant.

• Spasm, perforation, restenosis and stent thrombosis are the most common complications of stent implantation.

• Drug-eluting balloons may become an alternative to drug-eluting stents in some circumstances

---

Closure Devices

Introduction

Although manual compression is still used after diagnostic angiography, closure devices are an attractive alternative, particularly in fully anticoagulated patients after PCI in whom a femoral or radial puncture was performed without problems. There is no evidence that closure devices are superior to manual compression in terms of complication rates; however, there are many advantages that make them popular.

Femoral Hemostasis

Closure devices provide an immediate arterial seal and allow sheath removal regardless of anticoagulation therapy. Time to hemostasis and ambulation is shorter, increasing the number of day-case procedures. However, manual compression takes time as the activated clotting time (ACT) should be well below 150 seconds. Closure devices are also safe and comfortable for the patient and easy to use, with a proven low rate of failure.

A few points to help in the successful deployment of a closure device:

• Before placement, check the groin (for possible swelling or hematoma) and inform the patient that the closure device will be deployed.

- If there is a hematoma, manual compression and a Femostop device should be used.
- Perform routine femoral angiography at the end of the procedure with contrast injection through the femoral sheath. Vascular anatomy is checked to detect potential risk factors for retroperitoneal hemorrhage, such as sheath insertion above the inferior epigastric artery, or for femoral arterial disease. Ensure at angiography that the femoral artery is a minimum of 4 mm in diameter and there is no bifurcation within 1 cm of the arterial entry site. The best view for assessment is RAO 20°.

For the AngioSeal device:
- Keep tension on the suture during deployment.
- Avoid tamping too forcefully.
- If there is no resistance during tamping, hemostasis will be inadequate.
- Continued bleeding is probably due to inadequate deployment and tamping of the collagen plug.
- Rarely, if there is a suspicion that collagen has been deployed intra-arterially, duplex ultrasound can be helpful.
- Check the femoral and foot pulses.
- If the femoral pulse is absent, exclude possible thrombotic obstruction with ultrasound and consult a vascular surgeon.
- Make sure that the Femostop device is available and familiarize yourself with this device before the procedure.

In addition there are some issues that must be considered before device deployment. These will increase the risk of using a femoral closure device:
- Intermittent claudication. Avoid femoral access on that side.
- Heavily calcified femoral artery. This increases the risk of vessel closure or local bleeding.
- Several previous catheter procedures with scar tissue or previous surgery on the femoral artery.
- Multiple punctures of the femoral artery (this may increase the risk of bleeding).
- Small vessel (<5 mm) diameter.
- Sheath larger than 8F, which will cause a larger puncture hole and difficulties with deployment.
- Nerve irritation caused by the sheath.
- Bifurcation puncture.
- Patients on warfarin, ongoing thrombolysis, or glycoprotein inhibitor infusion will have an increased bleeding risk, and may need an additional Femostop device.

Selection of Closure Device

The choice of hemostasis device should be based on safety, patient comfort, cost, and operator experience. A variety of closure devices are currently available.

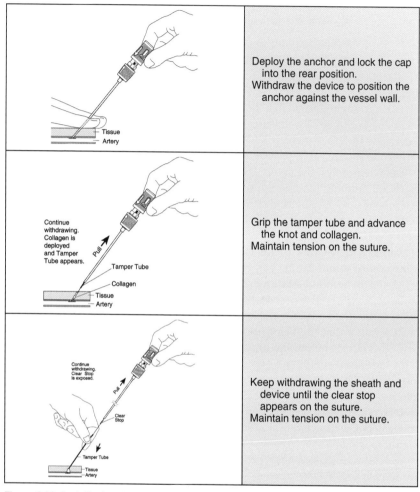

Figure 2.30 AngioSeal anchored plug closure device. (Angio-Seal™ is a trademark of St. Jude Medical, Inc. or its related companies. Reprinted with permission of St. Jude Medical™, ©2011 All rights reserved.)

Collagen-Based Anchored Plug Devices

These devices (e.g., AngioSeal) are very easy to use and are popular in many catheter labs. The AngioSeal is composed of an absorbable collagen sponge and an absorbable polymer anchor/footplate that are connected by an absorbable self-tightening suture. The device seals the arterial hole between the anchor and the collagen sponge by pulling up the footplate from inside the artery and tamping the sponge on the outside (Figure 2.30). The sponge and footplate are fully absorbable within 60–90 days.

Collagen-Based Unanchored Plug Devices

Devices such as the VasoSeal or Duett are no longer on the market because of high failure and increased complication rates. However, recently intro-

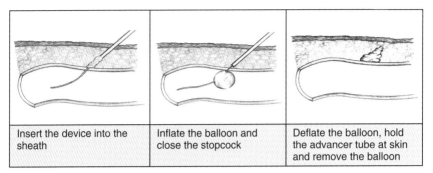

| Insert the device into the sheath | Inflate the balloon and close the stopcock | Deflate the balloon, hold the advancer tube at skin and remove the balloon |

Figure 2.31 Mynx unanchored plug closure device.

duced femoral closure devices are based on the same technology and seem more successful. Sealing biopolymer agents are deployed through the vascular sheath. ExoSeal is a third-generation device which provides painless deployment delivering polyglycolic acid (PGA). Within 3 months the plug enters the metabolic cycle and is degraded into water and carbon dioxide. The Mynx device is another unanchored plug device that provides immediate sealing with a water-soluble sealant located in the balloon. After balloon deflation and device removal, the sealant is left on the surface of the arterial puncture, ensuring natural healing (Figure 2.31). Mynx is made from a polyethylene glycol polymer which dissolves in 1 month.

Stitch-Based Devices
These are vascular suture devices (e.g., PerClose) that also require an aseptic procedure and are more demanding technically. The advantage is that they can be used in patients with vascular disease. the disadvantage is very occasional suture failure or local discomfort for the patient.

Staple-Based Devices
These devices are very easy to use even in patients with vascular disease, e.g., StarClose. A metal clip is delivered onto the surface of the vessel to close the artery (Figure 2.32). The great advantage is that there is no material left inside the vessel. This is indicated for patients in whom a small 5F or 6F sheath is used.

Mechanical Compression
The mechanical compression device Femostop (Figure 2.33) is effective and very popular in many catheter labs. These devices ensure adequate hemostasis causing minimal discomfort to the patient and are particularly useful in cases of:

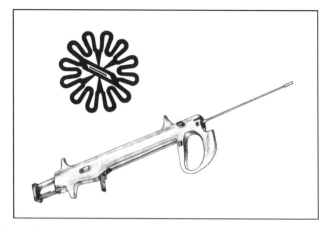

Figure 2.32 StarClose staple-based clip closure device.

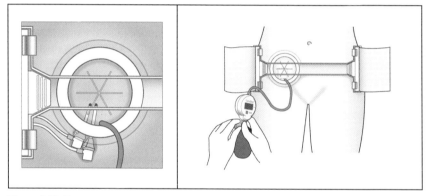

Figure 2.33 Femostop mechanical compression. (FemoStop™ is a trademark of St. Jude Medical, Inc. or its related companies. Reprinted with permission of St. Jude Medical™, ©2011 All rights reserved.)

- Low femoral puncture
- Use of catheter larger than 6F
- Developing hematoma
- Continuing bleeding on manual compression
- Patients on warfarin or glycoprotein inhibitor infusion

Manual Compression

This is the easiest and the cheapest method with good results, particularly in patients in whom small size catheters (standard 6F) are used. However, it is less comfortable for the patient and is time-consuming. Moreover, if heparin has been given, the ACT must be checked and be below 150 seconds before sheath removal. Otherwise the patient has to return to the unit with the sheath still in the groin, stay longer, and remain immobilized before the ACT is

Table 2.14 Differences between manual compression and closure devices.

Manual compression	Closure devices
Patient discomfort	Patient comfort
Sheath can be removed after ACT check	Sheath can be removed immediately after the procedure
Long time to ambulation	Short time to ambulation
Complications associated with prolonged compression	Immediate sealing, no compression

rechecked prior to sheath removal. Differences between manual compression and closure devices are summarized in Table 2.14.

Complications of Closure Devices (see pp. 289–293)

Vascular devices minimize the risk of complications associated with hemostasis and are very rare. However, the following complications may occur:
- Incomplete or failed closure
- Hematoma
- Pseudoaneurysm
- Embolization
- Loss of distal pulse
- Femoral artery occlusion

If placement of a closure device fails and difficulties with hemostasis occur, manual compression or a Femostop device is usually effective. A pseudoaneurysm may present late as a very painful swelling over the puncture site (a hematoma is uncomfortable but not usually very painful). The pseudoaneurysm is confirmed with ultrasound and can often be closed by compression with the ultrasound probe directly on the neck of the aneurysm. Alternatively, a local thrombin injection into the aneurysm is effective. A surgical consultation is needed for the lost femoral pulse, and an embolectomy may be necessary for the ischemic leg.

Radial Hemostasis

The simplest way to achieve hemostasis after diagnostic angiography from the radial artery is manual compression. After PCI, patients are anticoagulated and radial compression can be obtain using either the Hemoband or the Terumo TR radial band (Figure 2.34).

Radial hemostatic devices are safe and comfortable for the patient. The TR band is a dual system based on two separate balloons. A larger balloon compresses the entire puncture site whereas a smaller balloon gives is angled for point compression. The band is transparent and provides full visibility of the access site, allowing monitoring of the puncture site. The great benefit is that the band provides selective hemostasis at the puncture site, avoiding compression of the nerve and the ulnar artery.

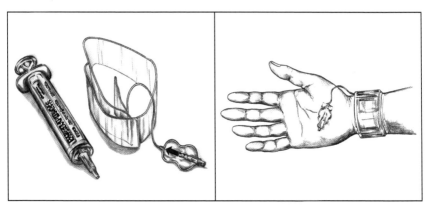

Figure 2.34 Terumo TR radial band for radial artery compression. (Reproduced with permission from Terumo Medical Corporation. All rights reserved. All brand names are trademarks or registered trademarks of Terumo.)

Key Learning Points

- Before placement, check the groin (swelling, hematoma).
- Perform routine femoral angiography at the end of the procedure.
- Use closure devices with caution in patients with peripheral vascular diseases.
- In case of a complication, consult a vascular surgeon.
- Closure devices have not proved to be superior to manual compression.

3 The Interventional Patient

Elective PCI for Stable Coronary Artery Disease

Introduction

Elective percutaneous coronary intervention (PCI) is recommended when medical treatment fails to control angina satisfactorily, particularly when non-invasive stress tests show ischemic areas of myocardium. In patients with stable angina, PCI compared with medical treatment reduces symptoms and ischemia, prevents future events, and provides a better quality of life.

The largest study to date comparing PCI with medical treatment is the COURAGE trial (2007). COURAGE demonstrated that angioplasty with bare metal stenting reduced angina and the need for medications and improved quality of life compared with medical treatment in symptomatic patients. Drug-eluting stents however were only used in 3% of patients. This study also showed that PCI does not increase the long-term risk of death or myocardial infarction. The COURAGE Nuclear Substudy suggested that, compared with medical treatment alone, PCI plus medical therapy resulted in greater improvement in the extent of ischemia on myocardial perfusion scanning at 6–18 months. Before deciding whether to proceed with PCI or not, it is important to make sure that the patient has real ischemia with at least a moderate perfusion defect and a chance of improvement.

Essential Angioplasty, First Edition. E. von Schmilowski, R. H. Swanton.
© 2012 John Wiley & Sons, Ltd. Published 2012 by John Wiley & Sons, Ltd.

However, not all modalities were tested adequately and in consequence the study suggested that PCI added to optimal medical therapy did not reduce risk of death, myocardial infarction, or other major cardiovascular events.

It should be noted that outcomes were determined by the end point of all-cause death and myocardial infarction. Patients were a highly selected, low-risk patient group, often with incomplete, suboptimal angioplasty, a low rate of procedural success and minimal use of drug-eluting stents. The trial was also underpowered with regard to all-cause death or myocardial infarction. Although more than 35,000 patients were screened for the study, only 3000 were eligible and less than 2500 included. Many patients with severe disease who could have benefited from PCI were excluded from the trial. One-third of patients in the group selected for medical treatment crossed over to PCI. This trial has not found favor with interventionists and its results have not had a major influence on current coronary artery disease management.

Previous studies (ACME, RITA-2) had already confirmed that there was no evidence that revascularization in low-risk patients with stable angina improved survival or rate of myocardial infarction. Therefore, in these patients medical therapy is recommended.

Selection of Patients for PCI or CABG

If medical therapy has been ineffective or poorly tolerated, interventional treatment must be considered. Proper indications and clinical assessment are essential. Patient selection should be based on severity of symptoms and the presence of ischemia, comorbidities, and age. An interventional strategy is contraindicated only in the absence of symptoms or lack of evidence of ischemia, confirmed on noninvasive stress tests.

With the indications above in single-vessel disease, PCI is always recommended. Likewise, two or three relatively short lesions with a low SYNTAX score and the probability of complete revascularization increase the chances for successful PCI. Angioplasty has been proven to reduce symptoms and improve exercise tolerance. Results from 15 trials show that in multivessel disease PCI provides similar prognostic and symptomatic benefit to coronary artery bypass grafting (CABG), and there is no difference in death and myocardial infarction rates between these two strategies, although redo revascularization rates are higher in the PCI groups.

Therefore, surgery should be considered only in highly selected patients who are good candidates for complex revascularization. CABG is of more benefit in these highly complex symptomatic patients, particularly those with:
• Severe ischemia with diffuse, multivessel (three-vessel) disease with SYNTAX score > 33
• Chronic total occlusion (CTO) supplying a large part of viable myocardium
• Significantly impaired left ventricular function with three-vessel disease

- Additional valve disease requiring surgery
- Diabetic patients particularly with left anterior descending (LAD) artery involvement requiring a left internal mammary artery (LIMA) graft.

Surgery offers complete revascularization and may be a safeguard against disease progression in the future. This is due to the risk of plaque rupture and progression of disease in nonstenotic segments (occurring in arterial segments already bypassed). Careful patient selection is essential as surgery carries an increased risk of complications in patients (e.g. stroke) with significant comorbidities or in the elderly.

Elective PCI Step by Step
Inform the patient and obtain written consent.

Before the Procedure
Assess the risk and take a brief medical history. In particular check for the following:
- Results from previous angiography or revascularization (PCI/surgery). Number and site of previous grafts
- Diabetes
- Renal function (creatinine, glomerular filtration rate)
- Stroke
- Bleeding disorders
- Peripheral vascular disease
- Comorbidities
- Recent surgery
- Allergies (including allergy to contrast). Patients with previous known contrast allergies should receive prophylactic treatment 24 hours before angiography (see pp. 288–289).
- Current medical treatment: patient on antiplatelet therapy or warfarin? on metformin?
  - Warfarin should be discontinued for at least 48 hours before angiography to ensure INR <1.8
  - Metformin should be discontinued before angiography and resume 48 hours after procedure if renal function is normal
  In addition:
- Perform a physical examination including peripheral pulses. Check for carotid bruits, previous groin surgery, abdominal aortic pulsation.
- ECG.
- Establish satisfactory venous access.
- Perform Allen's test if considering radial access.
- Check routine blood tests: including full blood check and platelet count, glucose, renal function, electrolytes, INR (if on warfarin), and also blood group, and save serum.
- Patients with higher risk for thromboembolization should receive full heparinization.

• Manage chest pain if it occurs before or during the procedure. This is important. Oral nitrates are often inadequate. IV nitrates may be necessary and IV diamorphine 2.5–5.0 mg may be needed.
• The operator must obtain written consent. If the patient is unconscious, this should be obtained from the next of kin if possible.

In the Catheter Laboratory

• Ensure satisfactory hemodynamic monitoring, pulse oximetry, availability of intra-aortic balloon pump (IABP), defibrillator, and temporary pacing.
• Keep a close eye on the patient's blood pressure, heart rate, and O_2 saturation throughout the procedure.
• Cardiac chest pain may also occur with coronary artery spasm, side branch occlusion, vessel dissection, or distal embolization.
• Remember the possibility of noncoronary chest pain: aortic dissection, pericarditis, esophagitis, esophageal tear (Mallory–Weiss), peptic ulceration.
• Prepare more than one site when choosing vascular access, assess the risk of bleeding: e.g., peptic ulcer history, platelet count, systemic hypertension.
• Give adequate antiplatelet and antithrombotic therapy (see Chapter 4).
• Quickly assess overall coronary status in two projections. Identify the culprit lesion(s).
• Use intracoronary glyceryl trinitrate to assess vessel size.
• Consider possible complications. Is there surgical back-up?
• Ensure adequate vascular hemostasis.

After the Procedure

• Inform the patient and family what has been done.
• Write a report of the procedure (brief medical history, indications for PCI, procedure details including type and size of balloons and stents used, closure devices if any, and further recommendations)
• Inform the patient of the importance and duration of dual antiplatelet therapy and possible consequences of early discontinuation.
• Check an ECG after procedure.
• Check the access site.
• Check blood tests (renal function, biomarkers, glucose, electrolytes).

Key Learning Points

• Elective PCI is recommended when medical treatment fails to control angina adequately.
• Bypass surgery should be considered in highly selected patients who are good candidates for complex revascularization.

PCI in Acute Coronary Syndromes

Introduction

Acute coronary syndromes are caused by rupture of an atherosclerotic plaque in the artery wall. The ruptured plaque increases platelet adhesion and activation, and by releasing inflammatory mediators leads to platelet aggregation. These reactions are responsible for coronary thrombus formation occluding the vessel partially or completely. Early and transient occlusion presents clinically as unstable angina, while prolonged occlusion results in non-ST or ST-segment-elevation myocardial infarction (NSTEMI, STEMI) with myocardial damage (Figure 3.1).

The spectrum of acute coronary syndromes is wide and the diagnosis is based on symptoms, changes in ECG, cardiac enzymes, and other cardiac biomarkers. In all patients with a medical history suggestive of acute coronary syndrome, physical examination, full blood screen, and ECG are necessary to

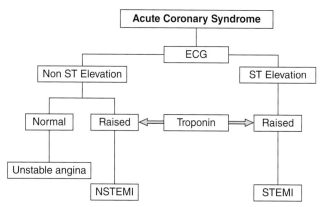

Figure 3.1 The spectrum of acute coronary syndromes. NSTEMI, non ST elevation myocardial infarction; STEMI, ST elevation myocardial infarction.

determine the diagnosis. Patients with atypical chest pain or with an uncertain diagnosis should be observed in a short stay unit, until full evaluation is complete and the diagnosis confirmed. If the initial ECG is normal but the history suspicious, the ECG should be repeated at 1 hour and subsequent intervals as necessary. If acute coronary syndrome is confirmed, urgent hospital admission is necessary.

Risk Assessment

In patients with confirmed unstable angina or NSTEMI, a risk assessment will determine further treatment options. TIMI risk score or modified GRACE score may be helpful (see website www.wiley.com/go/essentialangioplasty. com). Patients with a low risk score should have a stress test. This may be either a treadmill test, a dobutamine stress echocardiogram, or a stress myocardial perfusion scan. They are treated medically in the first instance and followed up in the outpatient clinic.

In high-risk patients (GRACE score >140) an invasive strategy is required. Factors associated with an increased risk of in-hospital mortality include advanced age, congestive heart failure, peripheral or cerebrovascular disease, elevated serum creatinine, impaired left ventricular ejection fraction, cardiogenic shock, treatment of acute myocardial infarction, urgent or emergency status, prior CABG, or need for intra-aortic balloon pump. Risk factors in patients undergoing PCI are shown in Figure 3.2.

PCI for Acute ST-Elevation Myocardial Infarction (Primary PCI)

Introduction

The main goal of primary PCI is to restore flow in the infarct-related artery to achieve full and sustained epicardial and microvascular flow and minimize risk of complications.

Several meta-analyses have confirmed the benefit of primary PCI over thrombolysis for acute myocardial infarction. Primary PCI reduces the dura-

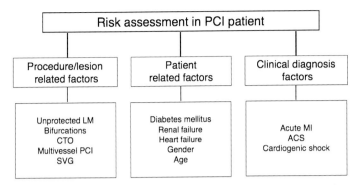

Figure 3.2 Risk assessment in the interventional patient. ACS, acute coronary syndrome; CTO, chronic total occlusion; LM, left main; PCI, percutaneous coronary intervention; SVG, saphenous vein graft.

tion of hospital admission and readmission, recurrent angina, reinfarction, and mortality. The interventional approach also provides more complete reperfusion with limitation of the infarct area with improved left ventricular function, and lowers the risk of major complications including stroke. Primary PCI is preferred particularly in high-risk patients, those in shock, and those with contraindications to fibrinolytic therapy.

Although primary PCI is the preferred treatment option, the choice of reperfusion therapy depends on the following factors:

- *Time from onset of symptoms.* This is a very important factor as prompt pharmacological thrombolysis within 2 hours of symptom onset can abort a myocardial infarction. Reperfusion rates after thrombolytics are critically time-dependent, with no significant benefit after a 6 hour delay from symptom onset. The call-to-needle time must be less than 60 minutes, and the hospital-door-to-needle time less than 30 minutes if a primary PCI service is unavailable.
- *Risk of the acute myocardial infarction itself* (see risk factors below). In general, the higher the mortality risk from the infarct, the more PCI is preferred.
- *Bleeding risk.* The higher the risk of bleeding, the more PCI is preferred.
- *Door-to-balloon time.* Time is muscle, and the shorter the door-to-balloon time, the better. This is the ultimate goal of a good primary PCI service (see below). Time delay is as important in primary PCI as in thrombolytic therapy. The DANAMI 2 trial showed that, provided pain-to-balloon time was less than 3 hours, primary PCI was superior to thrombolysis. The PRAGUE 2 trial suggested that both therapies carried the same mortality up to 3 hours, but after this time primary PCI was superior. Primary PCI inevitably carries an initial delay (PCI-related delay), but provided this delay is less than 1 hour PCI remains superior. Door-to-balloon time must be less than 1 hour and primary PCI should be performed within 90 minutes of first medical contact if possible.

- *Availability of a primary PCI service.* In remote areas a primary PCI service may not be an option, necessitating pre-hospital thrombolysis.
- *Operator and center experience.* All PCI centers should aim to run a 24/7 service, which requires an absolute minimum of six experienced interventional cardiologists on a rota.

Regional Wall Motion Abnormalities

Shortly after the onset of chest pain and long before evidence of ECG changes, myocardial ischemia produces regional wall motion abnormalities (RWMA). The wavefront concept of myocardial infarction states that infarction increases in a transmural wavefront, starting from the endocardium and moving out to the epicardium. The longer the duration of arterial occlusion, the more severe is the ischemia. Occlusion lasting longer than 1 hour leads to subendocardial necrosis and subsequently increases the transmural extent of the infarct (transmurality), until infarct size covers the entire area at risk. Based on this concept the infarct-related artery (IRA) should be opened as quickly as possible to limit the duration of ischemia in the occluded area and protect viable myocardium in the area at risk. Infarct size is also dependent on hemodynamic factors such as blood pressure and heart rate, and residual flow in the area at risk is determined by the potential presence of collaterals and antegrade flow in the IRA.

Area at Risk and Infarct Size

In patients with an acute myocardial infarction, early reperfusion benefits left ventricular function and remodeling and also reduces the severity of RWMA and infarct size. Angiographic studies with cardiac magnetic resonance (CMR) assessment show that in cases of complete transmural myocardial infarction treated by reperfusion therapy, the anatomical area at risk visible at angiography is very similar to the infarct size. The infarct-endocardial surface area is similar to the anatomical myocardium area at risk. In consequence, combining measurements of anatomical area at risk estimated at angiography and infarct size as assessed by CMR may determine the myocardial salvage achievable by reperfusion therapy. The area at risk can also be estimated by the percentage of left ventricular endocardial surface area affected by the infarct on CMR.

In cases with long periods of ischemia causing a transmural infarction, the infarct size visible on CMR is exactly the same as the risk area assessed by both scores. In patients with a prompt reperfusion strategy and subendocardial infarction, the infarct size is smaller than the risk area.

Myocardial Salvage and Infarct Transmurality

There is a relation between myocardial salvage and infarct transmurality. Patients with developed collateral flow or those who underwent early reperfusion present lower infarct transmurality and consequently increased myocardial salvage, which is defined as the difference between the infarct size and the initial area at risk. The presence of collateral flow does not decrease the lateral boundaries of the infarct ,which are established after the first hour of symptom onset. Collaterals, however, have been shown to reduce the infarct transmurality score.

Prehospital Procedure and Cath Lab Access

All patients with STEMI should be taken directly to a PCI center if possible. Trained paramedics in the ambulance interpret the ECG, give a loading dose of clopidogrel 600 mg, aspirin 500 mg IV bolus or oral soluble aspirin 300 mg, heparin 5000 U IV bolus or bivalirudin 0.75 mg/kg bolus, and warn the cardiothoracic center of their arrival. Telemetry of difficult ECGs to a local cardiologist may help. It is important that the local ambulance service and the hospital reception team are coordinated to allow direct transfer of the patient on arrival in the hospital to the catheter laboratory. Admission via the Emergency Department has been shown to prolong the delay and increase mortality. Ideally a 24/7 service should be available with the on-call team including an experienced coronary interventionist. Written criteria and agreements for transferred patients should be ready, and one or more primary PCI beds must be available in the hospital at all times. Primary PCI should be considered in all patients with STEMI, particularly high-risk patients in cardiogenic shock (who are less than 18 hours from symptoms and less than 75 years old), and those in whom fibrinolytic therapy is contraindicated or who have already received thrombolytics.

On Arrival in the Cath Lab

- Does the history of chest pain suggest a myocardial infarction?
- Any previous history of previous myocardial infarction, CABG, or PCI?
- Any history of cocaine abuse, or recent chemotherapy (spasm)?
- Does the ECG show more than 2 mm ST elevation (convex upwards) in more than one lead?
- Does the ECG show more than 2 mm ST depression in leads V1–V3 (posterior myocardial infarction)?
- Does the ECG show left bundle branch block (LBBB)?
- Any physical signs?
- What is the left ventricular ejection fraction (LVEF)? Clinical assessment and echocardiography if possible.

Examination

It is very important to examine the patient quickly on the catheter table before proceeding with the primary PCI procedure. Other conditions mimicking a myocardial infarction must be considered.

- All pulses present and equal (aortic dissection)?
- Aortic regurgitation (aortic dissection)?

- Pericardial rub?
- Epigastric tenderness or abdominal mass?
- Third heart sound (S3) and basal rales in left ventricular failure?
- Pansystolic murmurs of a ventricular septal defect or mitral regurgitation?
- Raised jugular vein pressure, right ventricular heave, and hypoxia in pulmonary embolism mimicking an inferior infarct?
- History of vomiting with some hematemesis (Mallory–Weiss esophageal tear)?

Management

- Operator must obtain patient consent.
- A loading dose of thienopyridines should be given as soon as possible before or at the time of PCI. If these agents have not been administrated before, give clopidogrel 300–600 mg or prasugrel 60 mg, plus soluble aspirin 300 mg (if not given by the paramedics), beta-blockers (not in heart failure or in cardiogenic shock), and heparin or bivalirudin. Compared to a 300 mg loading dose of clopidogrel, a 600 mg dose acts more rapidly and is more potent within the first 48 hours. Prasugrel is even more potent than clopidogrel and with its faster onset of action preferable in primary PCI. Prasugrel is not recommended in patients with a history of previous stroke or transient ischemic attack (see Chapter 4).
- Ensure IV line access. Start infusion of 500 ml normal saline unless the patient is in pulmonary edema.
- Start finger-tip O_2 oximetry and give O_2 if saturation is below 95%. If the patient is cold, or shocked finger-tip oximetry will be unreliable. In this situation start O_2 anyway and check arterial blood gases.
- Monitor blood pressure noninvasively until direct arterial pressure monitoring is available.
- Perform routine blood tests, plus troponin and creatine kinase measurement. Group and save serum.
- Check sufficient analgesia has been given.
- Defibrillator pads are attached to the patient's chest at the start of any primary PCI procedure and prior to any high-risk case. The electrodes should be widely separated. Neither should be directly over the sternum (bone has high impedance to electric current). The best positions are right upper chest anteriorly and the other electrode on the patient's back.
- 12 ECG leads attached.
- Intensive glucose control with insulin once primary PCI procedure has been completed to achieve and maintain glucose below 180 mg/dl, avoiding hypoglycemia.

An anesthetist should be in the lab if the patient is in cardiogenic shock (systolic BP <90 mmHg), hypoxic (oximetry saturations <90% on O_2), if resuscitation from a cardiac arrest has already occurred, or if the patient is clearly unstable hemodynamically.

Diagnostic Angiography
• The femoral route is preferable with possible need for additional pacing or IABP insertion, and speed of access.
• Right femoral vein 6F sheath. Pacing wire to right ventricular apex in patients with inferior or posterior infarcts or atropine-resistant bradycardia.
• Left femoral artery sheath (for IABP) if patient unstable or in cardiogenic shock. Establish intra-aortic balloon pumping and right ventricular pacing in a shocked patient before starting the primary PCI procedure. IABP should be used in patients with persistent hypotension, cardiogenic shock, in case of recurrent ischemia with hemodynamic instability, poor left ventricular function or a large area of myocardium at risk.
• Unfractionated heparin 70 U/kg (in addition to possible previous heparin given in the ambulance).
• Start with the diagnostic Judkins catheter to check the nonculprit vessel first (assessed from the ECG), switching to the guiding catheter for the diagnostic angiogram of the culprit vessel. This saves time.
• Use a limited number of projections (2–3 for left coronary artery and 1–2 for right coronary artery). One shot of the nonculprit vessel may be enough if it is clearly normal.
• Has the patient potential surgical anatomy? E.g., left main stenosis with collaterals to IRA?
• Perform left ventriculography after PCI if necessary.

When Not to Proceed with PCI
Primary PCI should not be performed in the following situations:
• If infarct vessel shows TIMI 3 flow and high-risk morphology
• If there is proximal multivessel disease with TIMI 3 flow and the patient without chest pain
• If the infarct vessel supplies a small amount of myocardium
• If stenosis in the infarct vessel is less than 70% with TIMI 3 flow
• If there are mechanical complications such as aortic dissection, unless the main stem is threatened by the dissection.

Primary PCI Procedure
Guide Wire Selection
Insert a 0.014″ guide wire across an acute occlusion with balloon back-up if necessary. Advance this wire to the distal coronary segment. Use a second wire if necessary to protect any large adjacent vessel. Do not predilate.

TIMI Flow, Thrombus Burden and Thrombus Aspiration
These should be assessed as follows.
  TIMI 0–1 flow: perform *thrombus aspiration* (see also pp. 150–158). Intracoronary thrombus increases the risk of no reflow, distal embolization, abrupt closure, and major adverse cardiac events (MACE). Thrombus should be removed either mechanically or pharmacologically in order to improve the

safety of primary PCI. Thrombectomy improves perfusion and should be performed as the first therapeutic procedure, before any balloon dilatation. Several catheters are available (e.g., Export, Diver, Pronto, Thrombuster catheters) with simple monorail design. Thrombus aspiration at this stage helps avoid thrombus propagation down the culprit vessel following balloon dilatation, and also migration of thrombus down a side branch or large adjacent vessel when the balloon catheter is removed. The aspiration catheter should be passed if possible to the distal part of the vessel as thrombus may propagate distally. Usually this maneuver is highly successful, with both red and white thrombus seen in the aspirate. Several passes of the aspiration catheter should be made. Angiography should then show the distal vessel and the length of the lesion causing the original occlusion. In young patients where the thrombus is often the main lesion, thrombus aspiration alone may be enough to create an excellent result. Thrombus aspiration has been shown to improve clinical outcomes at 1 year in the TAPAS trial.

If *TIMI 2–3* has not been achieved, small balloon predilatation should be performed before stenting. After initial balloon dilatation, watch for possible reperfusion arrhythmias. (This is usually a benign, self-terminating idioventricular rhythm.) As fresh thrombus is still inevitably present, try to minimize the amount of predilatation used.

If *TIMI 2-3* flow has been restored or the thrombus burden is small, perform direct stenting. The thrombotic burden of total occlusions varies but is usually small.

If the thrombus burden is large, perform thrombectomy and then direct stenting. A large thrombus burden carries a higher risk of stent thrombosis.

Vasodilators

Once flow is established, vessel diameter may change significantly. Vasodilators should be given to assess the vessel properly. Give intracoronary nitroglycerin 100 μg or adenosine 1000–2000 μg in 60 μg increments if no-reflow (see p. 294).

Adjunctive Therapy During Primary PCI

Major bleeding is a powerful predictor of mortality in patients undergoing primary PCI for STEMI. In high-risk patients treatment with bivalirudin rather than a combination of heparin and glycoprotein inhibitors (GPIs) results in a significant reduction in bleeding, thrombocytopenia, and transfusions, and consequently lower mortality in primary PCI.

To limit risk of PCI-related bleeding:

• Consider radial access if the patient is hemodynamically stable.

• Give proton pump inhibitors to patients with a history of peptic ulceration or gastrointestinal bleeding.

• Be careful with doses of antithrombotics, particularly in elderly patients and patients with low body weight and impaired renal function.

• Use direct thrombin inhibitors (bivalirudin) for high-risk patients.

Glycoprotein IIb/IIIa inhibitors (GPIs) Before giving abciximab, ask the patient if there is any history of a bleeding tendency and ask specifically about peptic ulceration, gastrointestinal bleeding, epistaxes, or bleeding hemorrhoids. Abciximab should be avoided in any of these circumstances. In addition, if there has been difficulty with femoral artery access requiring multiple punctures and a possible hematoma, its use should be reconsidered.

In selected patients abciximab may now be administered intravenously once the wire is across the stenosis/occlusion and demonstrated on angiography to be in the true lumen. If the guide wire is not correctly positioned, there is always the small risk of hemopericardium due to possible wire perforation of the vessel wall caused by further attempts to position the wire correctly. Patients should receive the bolus dose in the lab, and start the 12 hour infusion when back on the cardiac care ward. Abciximab dose: bolus dose 0.25 mg/kg IV immediately, followed by 12 hour infusion at 10 μg/min in a total of 50 ml normal saline. In patients who have received high-dose clopidogrel the use of a GPI does not appear, however, to improve clinical outcomes significantly.

Heparin In patients who received heparin previously, an additional bolus may be needed to maintain a therapeutic ACT (>250 seconds). The dose depends on prior GPI administration. Alternatively, bivalirudin can be given in the cath lab.

Bivalirudin Bivalirudin is useful as an antithrombotic agent in primary PCI either with previous heparin treatment or without it.

Atropine In patients with proximal RCA lesions a Bezold–Jarisch reflex may occur, causing bradycardia and hypotension. Vagal reactions are also common, especially in younger patients or those with continuing pain. Atropine should be given 0.6–1.2 mg up to a maximum of 2.4 mg together with normal saline. If the patient does not improve with this, switch quickly to right ventricular pacing.

Treat Only the Culprit Lesion

A commonly asked question is: should other nonculprit significant lesions be stented at the same procedure once the culprit lesion has been dealt with? This is the subject of an ongoing trial (CVLPRIT). The theoretical advantages are a more complete revascularization at one sitting. However, myocardial infarction induces a prothrombotic state (fresh thrombus releases thrombin) and there is an increased risk of stent thrombosis in either vessel. In selected patients some operators prefer to stent the culprit lesion and all additional significant lesions. Other operators prefer to do these non culprit lesions at a separate procedure. The only exception to this is in patients with cardiogenic shock. In these cases attempts are made to stent all severe stenoses at the initial procedure.

In summary: No data is available yet to guide strategy which must remain at the operator's discretion. Treat all significant lesions in cardiogenic shock.

Drug-Eluting Stents

Drug-eluting stents (DES) are now used routinely. Bare metal stents were initially recommended because of the slightly lower stent thrombosis risk, but the TYPHOON trial has shown better outcomes with DES, with significant reduction in restenosis and need for repeat revascularization. Do not undersize the stent. Postdilate where necessary. Thrombotic lesions are usually soft and do not need routine postdilatation.

Patients receiving DES must be compliant with long-term dual antiplatelet therapy.

Consider using bare metal stents if:
• Patient is unlikely to comply with dual antiplatelet therapy.
• Patient is likely to need surgery within the next year.
• Patient is already on warfarin.
• Patient has a bad peptic ulcer history or is using regular daily analgesics (e.g., for arthritis).

Keeping Out of Trouble During the PCI Procedure Itself

• Don't be too ambitious in high-risk cases. Dealing with the severest culprit lesion may be enough to relieve the patient's symptoms (see above, "Treat Only the Culprit Lesion").
• Call for an anesthetist early if the hemodynamics are unstable or if the patient is continuing to get severe angina.
• Have you overlooked something? Is there an occluded vessel or a dissection you have not noticed? Review the diagnostic pictures quickly and compare with the most recent films.
• Use the IABP early if hemodynamics are unstable.
• Have further discussions with a cardiac surgeon if possible. Although it is unlikely a patient will be accepted following a complicated or failed primary PCI procedure, patients may be salvaged by surgery, and it is important that in these critical cases a joint discussion is held.

Figure 3.3 shows an example of primary PCI.

Postangioplasty Care

• *Bed rest.* Following a primary PCI the patient remains on complete bed rest for at least 12 hours while on the abciximab infusion. Mobilization too early will increase the risk of a femoral artery hematoma or false aneurysm.
• *Bloods* are taken at 12 and 24 hours for peak creatine kinase and troponin to estimate infarct size. Renal function is checked and the platelet count monitored. Patients whose platelet count drops sharply ($<50 \times 10^3/\mu l$) after abciximab will need daily counts, may need platelet infusions if bleeding occurs, and their discharge should be delayed until the platelet count rises again.

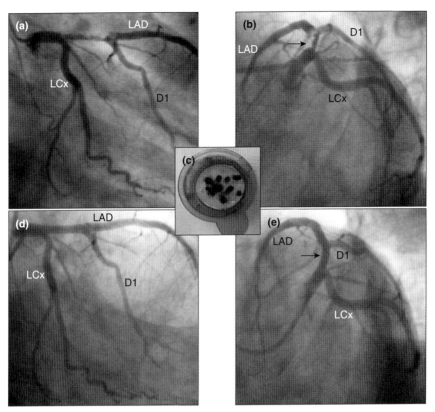

Figure 3.3 Primary PCI in acute myocardial infarction. **(a)** RAO 30. Thrombus visible in the proximal segment of the left anterior descending artery (LAD). **(b)** Thrombus visible in LAO caudal (spider view) arrowed. **(c)** Thrombus removed after multiple passes of thrombectomy device. **(d)** Angiography after stent implantation in the LAD (RAO 30 view). TIMI 3 flow. **(e)** LAO caudal (spider view) final result.

- *Echocardiography* is performed before discharge for baseline left ventricular dimensions and function.
- *Dual antiplatelet therapy.* All patients stented with either DES or bare metal stents should receive aspirin 325 mg and clopidogrel 150 mg for the first 7 days after primary PCI, then aspirin 75 mg and clopidogrel 75 mg or prasugrel 10 mg daily for at least 12 months. In patients with DES clopidogrel may be continued beyond 15 months. Prasugrel should be considered in patients at low risk of bleeding, those who are less than 75 years old, weigh more than 60 kg, and have no previous history of stroke or transient ischemic attack, no bleeding diathesis, no recent bleeding, and no recent surgery. If the risk of morbidity from bleeding is higher than the benefit from antiplatelet therapy, discontinuation should be considered. If CABG is planned in advance, clopidogrel should be discontinued at least 5 days and prasugrel at least 7 days before surgery.

• *Warfarin.* Warfarin added to aspirin and clopidogrel increases the risk of bleeding and the INR should be carefully monitored. An INR of 2.0–2.5 is recommended with an aspirin dose of 75 mg and clopidogrel 75 mg.
• In patients with a mechanical prosthetic valve who have had a primary PCI, aim for an INR of 2.5–3.0
• *Medications.* Patients should also receive routine ramipril 2.5 mg twice a day and low dose beta-blockade e.g., bisoprolol 1.25 mg once a day or metoprolol 25 mg twice a day, particularly for patients with a left ventricular ejection fraction below 40%. The doses of the ramipril and beta-blocker should be increased if possible on a follow-up visit.

Pharmacoinvasive Reperfusion Therapy
Patients with STEMI presenting to a hospital without the facility for primary angioplasty should either be treated with thrombolytics or transferred immediately for primary PCI.

The decision which to choose should be based on the following:
• Risk of mortality in STEMI (see below)
• Risk of fibrinolytic therapy and potential contraindications
• Duration of the symptoms (first onset)
• Time needed to transport the patient to a PCI center

Risk Stratification in STEMI
The variables listed below determine mortality risk in STEMI:
• History of previous myocardial infarction
• Age above 75 years
• Diabetes
• Resting tachycardia above 100/min
• Poor left ventricular function: left ventricular ejection fraction below 40%
• Systolic blood pressure <below 100 mmHg
• Left bundle branch block
• Congestive heart failure or cardiogenic shock
• Extent of ST-segment elevation

If primary PCI is chosen, the patient should be transferred immediately (Figure 3.4). Patients with STEMI best suited for transfer for PCI are those at higher risk, including a high bleeding risk from thrombolytics, and patients who present to the hospital more than 4 hours after first onset of symptoms. The decision should also take into account the transport time to the PCI center.

Patients with STEMI best suited for fibrinolytic therapy are those at lower risk who present early after symptom onset (<2 hours) with a low bleeding risk. If fibrinolytics are chosen, patients should receive the agent and the myocardial infarction risk should be assessed based on the criteria above.
• High-risk patients who have received fibrinolytic therapy as primary reperfusion should be transferred to a PCI center as soon as possible for diagnostic angiography and possible PCI. They should receive heparin, aspirin, and clopidogrel or prasugrel in the ambulance.

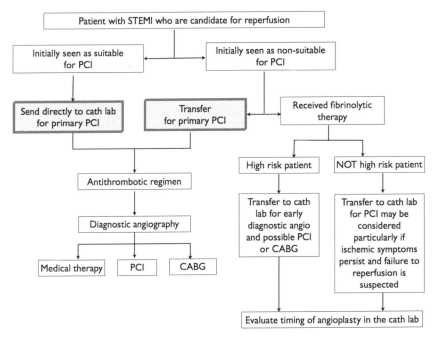

Figure 3.4 Transfer for PCI in patients with STEMI.

Table 3.1 Absolute and relative contraindications to fibrinolytics in patients with STEMI.

Absolute Contraindications	Relative Contraindications
Any prior intracranial hemorrhage	Severe uncontrolled hypertension
Known structural cerebral vascular lesion	Traumatic or prolonged CPR >10 minutes
Known malignant intracranial neoplasm	Major surgery within the past 3 weeks
Ischemic stroke within the past 3 months	Recent internal bleeding within the past 2–4 weeks
Suspected aortic dissection	Noncompressible vascular puncture
Active bleeding or bleeding diathesis	Prior exposure to streptokinase (>5 days) or prior allergic reaction
	Pregnancy
Significant head or facial trauma within the past 3 months	
	Active peptic ulcer
	Current use of anticoagulants

CPR, cardiopulmonary resuscitation.

• Patients who are not at high risk and have received a thrombolytic already may also be considered for transfer to a PCI hospital as soon as possible, particularly if symptoms persist and failed reperfusion is likely.

Absolute and relative contraindications to fibrinolytics in patients with STEMI are listed in Table 3.1.

PCI After Failed Thrombolysis (Formerly Called Rescue PCI)
Failure of thrombolytic therapy to relieve pain or reduce the ST-segment elevation by more than 50% after 90 minutes of administration is failed thrombolysis. In failed reperfusion all high-risk patients treated primarily with a thrombolytic, abciximab, heparin, and aspirin have better outcomes when transferred immediately for PCI rather than continuing medical therapy without intervention (CARESS-IN-AMI trial). Repeating the thrombolytic is of no value (REACT trial). These patients should be transferred quickly to a PCI center, and it must be assumed thrombolysis has failed. Do not wait to determine whether reperfusion was successful or not.

Early PCI After Successful Thrombolysis (Formerly Called Facilitated PCI)
An early invasive strategy and nonemergency PCI within 3–24 hours of successful fibrinolysis after full-dose lytics may be harmful. PCI after successful fibrinolysis should be performed only in patients who develop recurrent myocardial infarction, severe myocardial ischemia during recovery from STEMI, cardiogenic shock, or hemodynamic instability. The lack of benefit of "facilitated PCI" was shown in the ASSENT IV and FINESSE trials. The only facilitation recommended is the use of aspirin and full-dose clopidogrel (600 mg) prior to reaching the catheter lab, and the use of abciximab once in the catheter lab (0.25 mg/kg bolus plus 0.125 µg/kg per minute infusion up to 10 µg/min for 12 hours).

In view of these negative trial data the term "facilitated" PCI is no longer used.

Delayed PCI and Late Reopening of an IRA   Patients with a totally occluded IRA studied late (>24 hours) after myocardial infarction should not have the IRA reopened if they are asymptomatic, hemodynamically stable, and have no ECG evidence of severe ischemia.

Theoretically the open artery hypothesis would support a delayed PCI strategy. Unfortunately the large OAT study completely refutes this. Reopening of an occluded artery in stable patients 3–28 days after myocardial infarction did not reduce death, reinfarction, or heart failure over a 4 year period in patients whose occluded vessel was reopened late. This surprising result occurred in spite of a high procedural success in the PCI group. In fact there was a trend to more reinfarctions in the PCI group.

Cardiogenic Shock
The condition is usually due to acute myocardial infarction with pump failure or mechanical complications; however, it can also occur in patients with myocarditis, severe cardiomyopathy, severe aortic stenosis, or insufficiency. When a large area of the left ventricle becomes necrotic and fails to pump an adequate stroke volume, cardiac output falls and both myocardial and coronary perfusion are compromised, causing tachycardia and hypotension. With time, increased left ventricular diastolic pressure further decreases coronary perfusion and increased left ventricular wall stress increases myocardial oxygen

demand. Myocardial stunning and hibernation are forms of myocardial dysfunction which may be reversible over time after successful reperfusion. Whereas myocardial stunning may occur despite restoration of normal flow, hibernating myocardium is present at rest as a result of severely reduced coronary flow and is an adaptive reaction to hypoperfusion.

Shock is present if the peak systolic pressure is below 90 mmHg and the mean aortic pressure below 70 mmHg with oliguria (<30 ml/hour) with associated signs of peripheral shutdown with cool extremities, sweating, tachycardia, pulmonary edema, hypoxia, and cerebral obfuscation.

Early echocardiography (transthoracic or transesophageal) is essential. It may show:

- Depressed contractility; focal or global hypokinesia
- Papillary muscle rupture with acute mitral regurgitation
- Postinfarction ventricular septal defect
- Pericardial tamponade
- Type A dissection (check aortic root)
- Dilated, poorly functioning right ventricle in acute massive pulmonary embolism

Cardiogenic shock is condition that requires a highly trained team including one or more anesthetists, preferably two scientific officers, and several cardiac nurses. Patients usually require intubation, ventilation, and insertion of one or more central neck lines, while the cardiologist gains access via the femoral vessels. Primary PCI should be performed in all patients aged below 75 years who develop shock within 36 hours of myocardial infarction and who are suitable for revascularization within 18 hours of the onset of shock. Patients older than 75 years should be selected individually.

A few points may be useful:

- The majority of patients who develop cardiogenic shock do so within 24 hours of a myocardial infarction.
- Usually left ventricular ejection fraction is not reduced dramatically (approximately 30%).
- In most patients, systemic vascular resistance is not severely elevated.
- Multivessel disease is often present.
- Risk of shock is higher in the elderly, in patients with anterior wall myocardial infarction, congestive heart failure Killip Class >2, systolic blood pressure below 100 mmHg and heart rate above 100 bpm).
- IABP is usually required.
- Immediate hemodynamic stabilization and rapid restoration of blood flow in the IRA are essential.

Primary PCI Procedure in Cardiogenic Shock
These patients are the very highest risk cases, and the SHOCK trial has shown improved mortality figures at 6 months with PCI. The procedure is as follows:
- Anesthetist may need to give inotropic drugs to improve hemodynamic support.

Optimize oxygenation. Intubation and full anesthesia may be needed for patients in severe pulmonary edema.
- Establish right ventricular pacing backup via right femoral vein.
- Establish intra-aortic balloon pumping via left femoral artery as soon as possible; IABP decreases mortality.
- Alternatively, an Impella pump may provide effective left ventricular support. A 13F sheath is needed to advance the pump via femoral artery access. Impella actively unloads the left ventricle with flow up to 2.5l/min and routine anticoagulation with heparin is essential.
- Echocardiography (see above).
- Limit the number of angiographic projections and volume of contrast.
- Stent the culprit lesion plus any other significant lesions in large vessels.
- Give GPI.
- If CPR is necessary, perform post-CPR ECG once the situation stabilizes. Acute coronary occlusion may still be present even if ST elevation is absent.
- The patient is likely to need ventilating overnight and balloon pumping for at least 48 hours after the procedure.
- Full heparinization is essential for the duration of the time the balloon pump is in situ. ACT >250 seconds. Thrombin time >4 × control.
- Femostop compression and suitable sedation and analgesia will be needed for balloon removal from the femoral artery. If in doubt, and the balloon pump has been in situ for several days, consider full general anesthesia and surgical removal of the balloon.
- In patients who have had a cardiac arrest outside hospital consider establishing therapeutic hypothermia for 48 hours to reduce cerebral damage.

TRIALS
HORIZONS AMI
In this study 13,600 patients with STEMI within 12 hours of onset of symptoms were treated with primary PCI. Patients were randomized to receive heparin plus GPI or bivalirudin. The two primary end points of the study were major bleeding and MACE including death, reinfarction, target vessel revascularization, and stroke within 30 days. Outcomes at 2 years demonstrated comparable rates of stent thrombosis, target vessel revascularization, and stroke in the two treatment strategies. However, treatment with bivalirudin alone compared with heparin and GPI resulted in significantly reduced 30-day rates of adverse clinical events (40% less bleeding in the bivalirudin group at 30 days).

CARESS-IN-AMI
This study randomized 600 STEMI patients less than 75 years old with more than one high-risk feature initially treated at a non-PCI center with half-dose reteplase, abciximab, heparin, and aspirin within 12 hours of symptom onset. The study was designed to evaluate the optimal treatment strategy in patients where primary PCI was not available. All patients in the first group were transferred for PCI, but the second group with standard treatment were trans-

ferred for rescue PCI if needed. The main purpose was to compare a combined pharmacoinvasive approach with the standard fibrinolysis plus selective rescue PCI approach in patients who do not qualify for primary PCI. The primary composite end point of all-cause mortality, reinfarction, and refractory myocardial infarction within 30 days occurred significantly less often in the immediate PCI group compared to the standard rescue PCI group. There were no significant differences in the rates of major bleeding at 30 days between groups. Therefore, high-risk patients with STEMI treated at non-PCI centers with an initial pharmacologic strategy have improved outcomes when transferred immediately to a PCI center rather than continuing medical therapy with transfer for rescue PCI only if there is evidence of failed reperfusion.

TRANSFER-AMI

In this study 1059 patients with STEMI were randomized for pharmacoinvasive strategy. Patients presented to non-PCI centers within 12 hours of symptom onset and with more than one high-risk feature. All patients were treated with fibrinolytic therapy and randomized to a pharmacoinvasive strategy which was either immediate transfer for PCI within 6 hours of fibrinolytic therapy or standard treatment after fibrinolytic therapy including rescue PCI as required for ongoing chest pain and less than 50% resolution of ST elevation at 60–90 minutes or hemodynamic instability.

Standard treatment patients who did not require rescue PCI remained at the initial hospital for at least 24 hours and angiography within the first 2 weeks was encouraged. All patients received standard-dose tenecteplase, aspirin, and either heparin or enoxaparin. There was no difference in bleeding between the groups. High-risk STEMI patients presenting to a hospital without PCI capability who have received fibrinolytic therapy should be transferred to a PCI center for angiography and PCI. This should be initiated immediately without waiting to determine whether reperfusion has occurred.

Key Learning Points

- Primary PCI is superior to thrombolysis in patients with STEMI.
- Thrombus aspiration is the first maneuver prior to balloon dilatation
- Use drug-eluting stents routinely unless there is a specific reason for bare metal stent.
- Early PCI after successful thrombolysis may be harmful.
- Failed thrombolysis means emergency transfer for primary PCI.
- All patients who receive thrombolysis in a non-PCI center should be transferred immediately to a PCI center, whether or not reperfusion has occurred.
- Do not give a second dose of lytic drug for failed thrombolysis.
- The term "facilitated PCI" is no longer used.
- PCI in patients with cardiogenic shock improves mortality.
- Intra-aortic balloon pump is usually required in cardiogenic shock. Ventilation is frequently required.
- Therapeutic hypothermia reduces cerebral damage in patients who have had a cardiac arrest.

PCI for a Thrombotic Lesion

Introduction

The main purpose of primary angioplasty in acute myocardial infarction is to restore normal coronary blood flow in the infarct-related artery (IRA) and regain full coronary perfusion. Sometimes, however, impaired myocardial perfusion persists despite a fully opened IRA, restoration of normal coronary TIMI 3 flow and successful angioplasty. Patients with impaired microcirculation demonstrate myocardial blush grade 0 to 2 on angiography and no resolution or incomplete resolution of ST-segment elevation on ECG. These patients have also a higher risk of early and late mortality, larger irreversible myocardial damage, limited myocardial salvage, and a higher risk of subsequent heart failure.

Suboptimal myocardial reperfusion may be secondary to various factors such as no-reflow or low-flow phenomenon, delayed reperfusion with irreversible microvascular injury, myocardial inflammation, endothelial dysfunction, and, most commonly, embolization either of the distal artery or one of the side branches or the microcirculation.

Coronary thrombus itself increases the risk of no reflow, distal embolization, and abrupt closure, and is an independent risk factor for procedural failure. Thrombus is formed following a ruptured atherosclerotic plaque and consists of platelets, red blood cells, and fibrin. Whereas a large occlusive thrombus present in STEMI is rich in platelets and loose fibrin strands, nonocclusive thrombus seen in NSTEMI consists only of red blood cells and fibrin. Embolic material consists of fragmented thrombus and plaque as well as platelet aggregates released from the lesion as a result of fibrinolytic therapy or primary PCI. Although thrombus may not be visible on angiography, it can cause microvascular dysfunction. The classification of thrombus burden is shown in Table 3.2.

There are a few important issues that should be considered:
- How can myocardial reperfusion be assessed?
- How can optimal myocardial salvage be achieved?

Table 3.2 Classification of thrombus burden.

Thrombus Grade	Angiographic Identification
G5	Total occlusion. Presence of thrombus cannot be assessed due to total occlusion
G4	Definite thrombus with the largest dimension ≥2 vessel diameters
G3	Definite thrombus with greatest linear dimension ≥0.5 but <2 vessel diameters
G2	Definite thrombus with greatest dimensions ≤0.5 of the vessel diameter
G1	Possible thrombus. Angiography shows reduced contrast density, haziness, irregular lesion shape
G0	No angiographic evidence of the presence of thrombus

- Is the use of thrombectomy devices necessary?
- What are the benefits and limitations of mechanical thrombectomy?
- Is thrombus aspiration associated with myocardial salvage?
- How can distal embolization using thrombectomy devices be avoided?
- Is predilatation necessary or it is better to perform direct stenting?
- Are antithrombotic agents required during the procedure?

Macro- and Microembolization

Macro- and microembolization of atherothrombotic material play an important role in microvascular obstruction and remain one of the major problems in patients with thrombotic lesions. Macroembolization is associated with impaired myocardial perfusion and worse clinical outcomes, and is more likely to occur in patients with a large thrombus burden. There is no particular technique for assessing thrombus burden, and for that reason selection of this subgroup of patients remains difficult.

Although there is strong evidence that macroembolization leads to worse clinical outcomes it remains unclear whether distal microembolization is a cause of impaired myocardial reperfusion in patients with a myocardial infarct.

The suggestion that microembolization may not play a major role in causing impaired myocardial reperfusion is supported by results from the EMERALD trial, which showed no benefit from distal protection despite successful removal of thrombus.

However, distal microembolization occurring during primary PCI may contribute to poor myocardial reperfusion, and in rare cases may lead to complete blockage of epicardial flow despite removal of thrombus from the IRA. Angioplasty itself causes microembolism due to increased level of myocardial cell calcium, endothelial dysfunction, vasoconstriction, and inflammation. Additional factors such as clot fragmentation, often present in STEMI, may result in a no-reflow phenomenon. This microvascular dysfunction is usually manifested by a higher troponin elevation, larger infarct size, greater likelihood of heart failure, and recurrent myocardial infarction and death.

Myocardial Perfusion

The result of reperfusion can be assessed during angioplasty using TIMI flow grades and blush grades. While TIMI flow grade describes epicardial blood flow, myocardial blush grade refers to myocardial viability in the IRA. Both scores are simple to use and very helpful as prognostic tools in patients after primary PCI.

TIMI Flow Grade

The TIMI (thrombolysis in myocardial infarction) grade describes the degree of epicardial blood flow after reperfusion therapy (Table 3.3, Figure 3.5). Good flow (TIMI 3 flow) after primary PCI is associated with a lower risk of complications and an improvement in left ventricular function. Generally, the

Table 3.3 TIMI flow grades.

TIMI Grade	Contrast Penetration
TIMI 0	No flow
TIMI 1	Minimal flow, no perfusion. Contrast passes beyond the lesion, but fails to opacify the entire coronary bed distal to the lesion for the duration of the cine sequence
TIMI 2	Partial perfusion. Contrast passes across the lesion and opacifies the coronary bed distal to the lesion. However, the entry of contrast into the vessel distal to the lesion and its clearance from the distal bed, or both, are visibly slower than in nonoccluded segments
TIMI 3	Complete perfusion. Antegrade flow into the distal segment to the lesion and clearance from the distal bed are as rapid as in nonoccluded segments

higher the TIMI grade, the lower mortality. If the artery is completely occluded and there is no flow beyond the point of occlusion, TIMI flow is 0. If there is minimal penetration across the lesion without perfusion, TIMI flow is described as grade 1. Grade TIMI 2 refers to partial perfusion with slow flow within a well-visualized artery. After successful reperfusion with completely restored perfusion rapid flow is achieved – TIMI 3 flow.

Corrected TIMI Frame Count
The corrected TIMI frame count (CTFC) has been designed to estimated TIMI flow more precisely and objectively, particularly in high-risk patients. CTFC is the time taken for contrast to enter the distal part of the artery. Frame 0 is the starting frame. In frame 1 contrast fully enters the artery, touching two borders of the proximal segment of the major coronary artery. Contrast moves forward in the following frames, reaching the distal segment of the artery in frame 21. These are shown in Figure 3.6.

Standard distal landmarks are identified for each of the main coronary arteries and are as follows (Figure 3.7):
• In the left anterior descending artery, the distal bifurcation – sometimes called the whale's tail
• In the left circumflex artery, the most distal branch of the obtuse marginal branch that includes the IRA
• In the right coronary artery, the first branch of the posterolateral (left ventricular branch) artery

In patients during primary PCI, flow rate in the IRA is important and relates to outcomes. The faster the flow, the lower the mortality. Studies have shown that mortality increases by 0.7% for every 10 frame rise. However, in patients with acute myocardial infarction, flow in the non-IRAs is also slower and can be restored to normal following successful re-opening of the IRA. There are hypotheses that this impaired flow in the noninvolved arteries may be caused

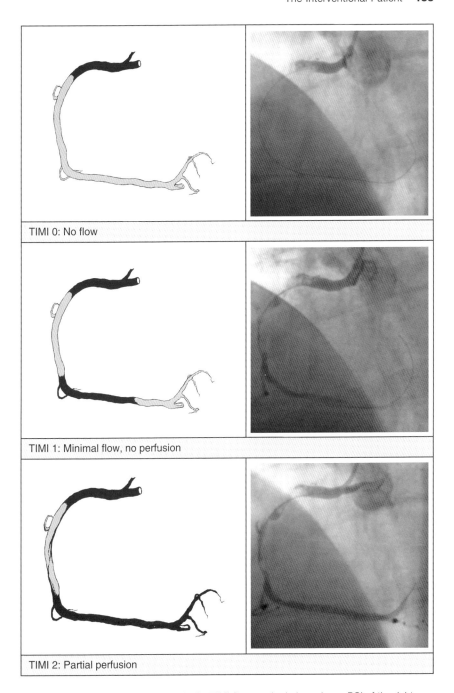

TIMI 0: No flow

TIMI 1: Minimal flow, no perfusion

TIMI 2: Partial perfusion

Figure 3.5 Progressive improvement in the TIMI flow grade during primary PCI of the right coronary artery.

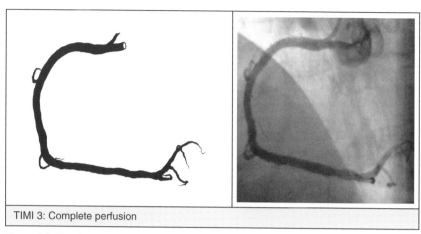

TIMI 3: Complete perfusion

Figure 3.5 (*Continued*).

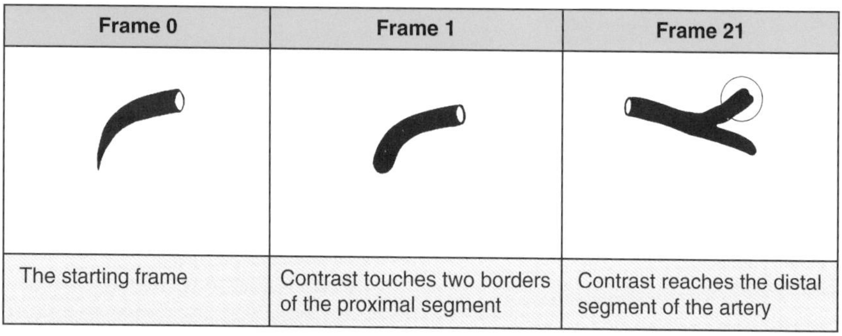

Frame 0	Frame 1	Frame 21
The starting frame	Contrast touches two borders of the proximal segment	Contrast reaches the distal segment of the artery

Figure 3.6 Corrected TIMI frame count.

Right Coronary Artery	Left Anterior Descending Artery	Left Circumflex Artery
The first branch of the posterolateral (LV branch) artery	The most distal branch of the LAD at apex	The last branch of the most distal obtuse marginal branch

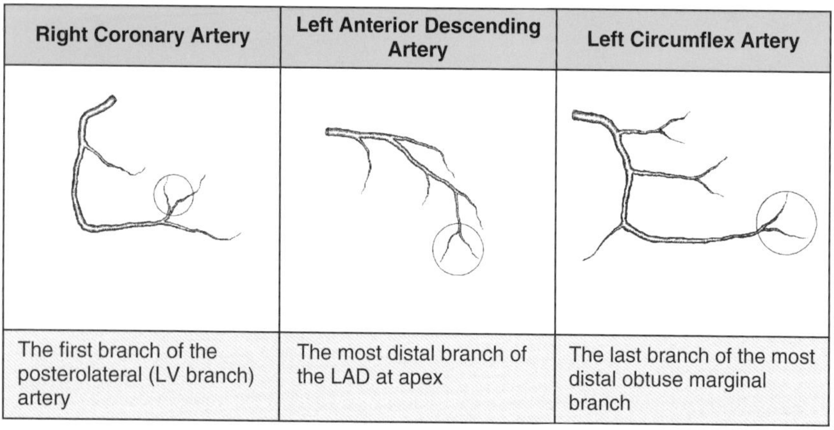

Figure 3.7 Corrected TIMI frame count (CTFC). Standard distal landmarks describing the main coronary arteries.

by necrosis in shared microvasculature or vasoconstriction in the vascular bed. Residual stenoses will also play an important role in this mechanism.

Myocardial Blush Score
Normal epicardial blood flow achieved during primary PCI in acute myocardial infarction is not always associated with restored microvascular perfusion. Myocardial perfusion can be assessed using the myocardial blush score (MBS). This is based on the presence of contrast density (described as "blush") in the distal microvasculature of the downstream myocardium after passage through the epicardial coronary artery (Figure 3.8). To assess the MBS precisely, angiographic runs should be long enough to allow careful

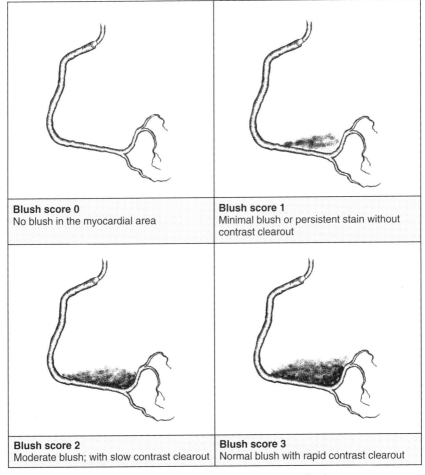

Blush score 0 No blush in the myocardial area	**Blush score 1** Minimal blush or persistent stain without contrast clearout
Blush score 2 Moderate blush; with slow contrast clearout	**Blush score 3** Normal blush with rapid contrast clearout

Figure 3.8 Myocardial blush scores. "Blush" refers to contrast opacification.

visualization of the contrast density within the infarct area. MBS also provides information about myocardial viability during angioplasty. The restoration of normal myocardial perfusion following PCI is associated with increased survival.

The presence of a blush is an independent predictor of infarct size, left ventricular function, and survival after reperfusion therapy. The lower the MBS (0 or 1), the higher the mortality and the larger the infarct size. Multivessel disease or anterior wall acute myocardial infarction are generally associated with a larger infarction and in these patients MBS 0 or 1 is more common. Minimal or no blush indicates lack of tissue perfusion in the area at risk.

• *Blush score 0* describes absence of contrast opacification in the myocardial area at risk. Contrast fails to enter the microvasculature; there is either minimal or no blush or opacification of the myocardium in the segment of the IRA, indicating a lack of perfusion.

• *Blush score 1* describes the presence of minimal contrast opacification. Contrast slowly enters but fails to exit the microvasculature; there is blush or opacification of the myocardium in the segment of the IRA that fails to clear from the microvasculature and contrast staining is still visible on the next injection (approximately 30 seconds between injections).

• *Blush score 2* refers to moderate contrast opacification. Contrast entry and exit from the microvasculature is delayed; there is blush or opacification of the myocardium in the segment of the IRA that is strongly persistent at the end of the washout phase. Contrast is still clearly visible after a couple of cardiac cycles and either does not diminish or diminishes only minimally in intensity during washout.

• *Blush score 3* represents normal contrast opacification with adequate contrast entry and exit from the microvasculature. The opacification of the myocardium clears normally and is similar to that in the non-IRA. Blush or opacification of the myocardium in the IRA clears normally. Blush that is of only mild intensity throughout the washout phase but fades minimally is also classified as grade 3.

Pharmacological Therapy

Intracoronary administration of antithrombotic agents in patients with thrombotic lesions increases PCI efficacy without increasing the risk of bleeding. A high concentration of the drug (up to 250 higher compared to parenteral administration) at the site of the thrombus may help dissolute the clot, increase receptor occupancy of GPIs, and improve microvascular function and clinical outcomes in patients with acute coronary syndrome.

• *Glycoprotein IIb/IIIa inhibitors (GPIs).* Intracoronary administration of GPIs is effective in reducing thrombus burden, improving microcirculation and epicardial blood flow in the IRA and reducing mortality. Benefits greater than parenteral administration, however, have not been proved.

• *Abciximab* inhibits platelet aggregation and deposition on the thrombus as well as platelet-induced thrombin generation. It diminishes stability of the

clot structure and makes it susceptible to fibrinolysis. Abciximab also has anti-inflammatory effects, which can improve microvascular function and reperfusion damage. Adjunctive abciximab is associated with reduction of thrombus burden during PCI.
- *Fibrinolytics.* Streptokinase and other fibrinolytics inhibit red blood cell and platelet aggregation and improve myocardial perfusion.
- *Bivalirudin.* Direct thrombin inhibitor.

Mechanical Therapy: Thrombectomy

Thrombus aspiration allows retrieval of atherothrombotic material from the occluded artery and consequently improves the final angiographic result. Thrombectomy effectively removes the vast majority of thrombus and is particularly useful in:
- Patients with a large visible thrombus burden
- TIMI 0–1 flow after crossing the lesion with a wire
- A large vessel with a large area of jeopardized myocardium
  For this reason, use of adjunctive aspiration thrombectomy has become a standard first-step procedure in primary PCI.

Although aspiration devices do not reduce myocardial damage, they prevent distal embolization and microvascular dysfunction. The TAPAS study demonstrated that thrombus aspiration during PCI in acute myocardial infarction improves microvascular perfusion and clinical outcomes at 1 year, which translates into significant reductions in cardiac death and reinfarction. Advantages and disadvantages of thrombectomy are listed in Table 3.4.

Aspiration Thrombectomy

There are several aspiration thrombectomy catheters designed to remove fresh thrombus in patients with STEMI.

Table 3.4 Advantages and disadvantages of thrombectomy.

Advantages	Disadvantages
Efficient way to remove fresh thrombus	Organized thrombus cannot be removed
High rate of restoration of coronary flow	Wall-adherent thrombus is difficult to remove
Lower risk of distal embolization in comparison with angioplasty alone	Risk of distal embolization in high-risk thrombotic lesion
Short procedural time	Lack of standard indications for the procedure
Suitable for patients with contraindications to thrombolytic therapy	Small diameter of the catheter prevents retrieval of larger thrombi
Can be performed immediately after admission	Blood loss during thrombus extraction

Manual aspiration thrombectomy devices are very simple to use. They consist of a monorail lumen for passage over a coronary wire and an aspiration lumen connected to a syringe at the proximal end for aspiration. The most commonly used are the Export and Diver CE catheters, with good results in primary PCI for STEMI.

The Diver CE catheter contains a central aspiration lumen and a soft tip with side holes for fresh thrombus or without side holes for more organized thrombus. The tip is connected with the central lumen, facilitating insertion and easy clot removal by syringe aspiration from the proximal hub. Studies with the Diver CE catheter show it is highly effective in restoring normal coronary flow in the IRA without the need for predilatation (direct stenting). There is improved ST-segment elevation resolution with less left ventricular remodeling as assessed by echocardiography. Studies using the Export catheter show similar results. Patients treated with the Export catheter have better coronary flow and myocardial reperfusion, with improved myocardial blush and ST-segment resolution and a smaller infarct size.

Rheolytic Thrombectomy
The most commonly used AngioJet device consists of a drive unit, a pump set, and a thrombectomy catheter. The dual-lumen catheter tracks over a guide wire and saline jets are directed back into the catheter, resulting in suction of thrombus through the outflow lumen into the catheter tip. The lesion should not be predilated and the device should be activated during its antegrade passage. Crossing the lesion without activation may lead to distal embolization. The use of the AngioJet device results in better coronary flow, improved ST-segment resolution, and a smaller infarct size at 1 month. The VEGAS-2 trial (Vein Graft AngioJet) has shown that rheolytic thrombectomy with the AngioJet catheter was safe and effective for thrombus removal in saphenous vein grafts and native coronary arteries. Results from the AIMI study, however, suggested that there was no benefit in terms of reduction of infarct size and there was an increased risk of major adverse cardiac events.

Distal Protection in Primary PCI
Mechanical thrombectomy devices limit the risk of distal embolization, but do not eliminate it entirely. Sometimes embolization occurs during the crossing of the lesion, or at the time of thrombectomy, or when the thrombectomy device is withdrawn.

Although distal protection devices are effective for angioplasty of saphenous vein graft lesions, they have not been shown to be effective during thrombectomy in acute myocardial infarction. Some clinical studies (EMERALD, AIMI) have failed to show positive outcomes using distal protection with thrombectomy. This may be due to limitations of the balloon/wire system. The distal protection device, whether filter or balloon, has to pass the thrombotic lesion, which itself can cause clot fragmentation and distal embolization.

Trials

TAPAS

In this study 1071 patients with STEMI were randomized for conventional PCI versus PCI with thrombus aspiration. Primary end points included myocardial blush grade, ST-segment elevation resolution, and death/reinfarction. This study demonstrated that thrombus aspiration resulted in improved myocardial perfusion. Patients who underwent thrombus aspiration in addition to primary PCI had superior outcomes for all-cause mortality, cardiac death, and nonfatal myocardial infarction compared with patients who underwent conventional PCI.

EMERALD

In this study 501 patients with acute myocardial infarction were randomized to PCI with distal protection versus PCI without distal protection. The outcomes were analyzed as a function of culprit vessel (LAD vs. non-LAD) and the use of GuardWire. Patients with an LAD infarct demonstrated significantly lower final TIMI flow grade 3, myocardial blush grade 3, and complete ST-segment resolution, had a larger infarct size and a trend towards a higher 6 month mortality. In these patients rates of reperfusion were not related to GuardWire use. In patients with non-LAD infarcts the use of GuardWire was associated with a trend towards better epicardial and microvascular reperfusion.

In conclusion, myocardial infarction in the territory of the LAD is associated with worse epicardial and microvascular reperfusion and a worse 6 month clinical outcome. The use of the GuardWire showed a trend towards better epicardial and microvascular flow in patients with a non-LAD IRA. This study demonstrated no benefit in terms of myocardial reperfusion at the tissue level, with similar rates of complete ST-segment resolution.

REMEDIA

This study randomized 100 patients with STEMI undergoing primary PCI with aspiration thrombectomy with the Diver CE catheter versus a control group. Patients treated with thrombectomy demonstrated better myocardial reperfusion with a higher blush grade (2–3) and better ST-segment resolution.

AIMI

This is the largest randomized trial to evaluate the benefit of rheolytic thrombectomy using the AngioJet with primary PCI for STEMI. The trial randomized high-risk patients with STEMI who were eligible for primary PCI. The primary end point was infarct size at 14–28 days and the secondary end points were TIMI flow post-PCI, corrected TIMI frame count (CTFC), myocardial blush, ST-segment resolution, and major adverse cardiac events (MACE) at 30 days. Results showed no differences in myocardial blush or ST-segment resolution, but TIMI flow after PCI was worse in the AngioJet arm. Moreover, infarct size was greater with rheolytic thrombectomy. MACE rates were also higher in the AngioJet group (6.7% vs. 1.7%) due to a higher mortality (4.6% vs. 0.8%). The investigators suggest that rheolytic thrombectomy does not reduce infarct size and cannot be recommended for routine use in patients with STEMI undergoing primary PCI.

Key Learning Points

- Coronary thrombus is an independent risk factor for procedural PCI failure and major adverse cardiac events.
- Reduced myocardial reperfusion may occur despite normal TIMI 3 coronary flow in the IRA being achieved.
- Embolization is associated with impaired myocardial reperfusion and worse outcomes.
- Thrombus aspiration improves final angiographic results and clinical outcomes.
- Distal protection does not reduce infarct size and does not influence clinical outcomes in primary PCI.

PCI for Non-ST-Elevation Myocardial Infarction

Introduction

Results from many studies including the TIMACS study (2009) show that in patients with NSTEMI with a high risk score, early intervention is prognostically beneficial. It has been well established that PCI within 24 hours in high-risk patients with NSTEMI (early invasive strategy) decreases the risk of death and myocardial infarction within 30 days. On the other hand, PCI delayed for more than 24 hours, TIMI grade 0-1 flow, advanced age, and higher Killip class are independent predictors of 1 month mortality (SYNERGY).

Two important guidelines:
- All high-risk patients with NSTEMI should receive prompt invasive investigation and interventional treatment as appropriate.
- All patients with confirmed NSTEMI should receive the same treatment as patients with STEMI (see procedure below step by step).

Early Invasive Strategy

"Early invasive strategy" refers to the need for diagnostic angiography with an intention to proceed with PCI if necessary. This interventional strategy is necessary in high-risk patients presenting with:

- Refractory ischemia
- Recurrent or persistent angina
- Unstable hemodynamics with clinical symptoms of heart failure and severe ventricular arrhythmias (VT/VF)

These patients should be admitted directly to the catheter lab for immediate coronary angiography and angioplasty as required. Before the procedure a loading dose of clopidogrel (600 mg) and aspirin (250 mg) should be given and additional heparin 60 U/kg (just U/kg) plus abciximab as a bolus. In cases with a high risk of bleeding, bivalirudin alone is preferable to heparin and a GPI. It has to be remembered that it takes 2 hours to achieve good antiplatelet inhibition with a loading dose of clopidogrel. Prasugrel (loading dose 60 mg) acts faster (see p. 170).

Conservative Strategy

This is a selectively invasive strategy which applies in lower-risk patients who are stable hemodynamically, are at increased risk of clinical events with an elevated troponin level, have dynamic ST/T changes on the ECG, and impaired renal function (GFR <60 ml/min per 1.73M^2).

Before the procedure, give a loading dose of clopidogrel (600 mg) and aspirin (300 mg). The patient should get to the catheter lab within 72 hours of symptom onset. In the meantime antithrombotic treatment is started:

- Bivalirudin 0.75 mg/kg or alternatively heparin (2500–5000 U IV), or
- Enoxaparin 1 mg/kg subcutaneously twice daily, or
- Fondaparinux 2.5 mg subcutaneously once a day, plus
- An upstream GPI only if necessary in those with a low risk of bleeding. For those at a high risk of bleeding, a GPI in the catheter lab may be considered.

Key Learning Points

- Diagnosis of acute coronary syndrome is based on symptoms, changes in ECG, cardiac enzymes, and other cardiac biomarkers.
- In patients with confirmed unstable angina or NSTEMI, a risk assessment will determine further treatment options.
- High-risk patients with acute coronary syndrome should be admitted directly to the catheter lab for immediate coronary angiography, followed by PCI if necessary.
- Low-risk patients who are hemodynamically stable with diagnosed acute coronary syndrome should get to the catheter lab within 72 hours of symptom onset.

The Diabetic Patient

Introduction

Diabetes and insulin resistance are independent risk factors for coronary artery disease and independent predictors for mortality in acute myocardial infarction. Seventy-five percent of patients with diabetes will die from cardiovascular disease. The prevalence of diabetes in coronary patients is increasing, and the percentage of diabetic patients undergoing PCI continues to rise also. Approximately 20% of white patients and up to 50% of South Asian patients undergoing a PCI have diabetes. Myocardial infarction may be silent in patients with diabetes.

Characteristics of the Diabetic Interventional Patient

Cardiologists play an important role in diagnosing diabetes and metabolic syndrome. Early detection of silently progressive coronary disease is essential, and routine screening for coronary disease even in asymptomatic patients is recommended especially if non-cardiac surgery is planned.

Patients with diabetes are generally older with diffuse, multivessel disease. In addition they often have a history of previous cardiac events and peripheral vascular disease affecting carotids and iliofemoral vessels (see Figure 3.9).

Factors Contributing to Vascular Disease in Diabetes

Accompanying metabolic factors such as dyslipidemia, impaired endothelial function, increased platelet activation, and a procoagulable state lead to a greater risk of major adverse cardiac events and future in-stent restenosis (see Table 3.5).

Interventional Treatment: PCI vs. Bypass Surgery

Both treatment options – PCI and CABG – are effective in diabetic patients, and both are associated with worse outcomes than in nondiabetic patients. A single revascularization strategy for patients with diabetes has not been established.

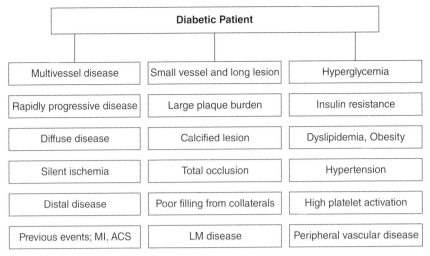

Figure 3.9 Characteristics of diabetic interventional patients.

Table 3.5 Factors contributing to vascular disease in diabetes.

Contributing Factors	Increased	Decreased
Proinflammatory state	CRP	–
	IL12	
Procoagulable state	Factor VII, X	Antithrombin III
	PAI-1	Intrinsic fibrinolysis
	Platelet aggregability	
	Thromboxane A_2	
Dyslipidemia	Triglycerides	HDL cholesterol
	VLDL, small dense LDL	Adiponectin
Endothelial damage	Advanced glycation products	PGI2
	Endothelin release	
	Tissue factor	
	VCAM, monocyte adherence	
	Oxidized LDL	

CRP, C-reactive protein; HDL, high-density lipoprotein; IL12, interleukin 12; LDL, low-density lipoprotein; PAI, plasminogen activator inhibitor; PGI2, prostacyclin; VCAM, vascular cell adhesion molecule; VLDL, very-low-density lipoprotein.

Inevitably, angioplasty in diabetic patients is more difficult than in nondiabetic individuals. PCI requires a more aggressive strategy and, in spite of all the modern advances in interventional cardiology, still carries a higher risk of peri- and postprocedural complications. These include higher risk of contrast-induced nephropathy, thrombotic events, a greater need for repeat revascularization, and treatment of restenosis as well as increased morbidity and mortality.

Decisions about treatment of coronary disease should always be made individually, and careful patient selection is mandatory. The time factor and discussion with a cardiac surgeon are also very important. One recent study (BARI 2) showed that high-risk patients benefit from prompt surgical revascularization. The earlier BARI 1 trial showed that the benefit of cardiac surgery over PCI was due to the LIMA graft. Early bypass surgery is associated with reduced major cardiac adverse events, particularly nonfatal myocardial infarction, compared to delayed treatment or lack of treatment.

Although data from very early trials showed better outcomes in patients treated with surgery than with angioplasty (BARI, CABRI), recent advances in PCI including the use of DES and GPIs show that both interventional options result in similar long-term rates of death, myocardial infarction, and stroke. Angioplasty, however, carries a higher risk of repeat revascularization. The recent CARDia trial comparing PCI using the paclitaxel-eluting Taxus stent with CABG failed to show noninferiority of angioplasty over bypass surgery in diabetic patients at 1 year.

The BARI 2D trial failed to show an advantage of a revascularization strategy (with either PCI or CABG) over medical therapy alone. Therefore patients with diabetes must have symptoms that are uncontrolled on medical treatment before revascularization is considered.

Medical Management Before and After PCI

• *Glucose.* Normalization of the glucose level is very important. Prompt glucose-lowering treatment is required before PCI, and an insulin infusion should be started on admission. Carefully restored normoglycemia will subsequently decrease the risk of micro- and macrovascular complications. Aggressive treatment, on the other hand, carries a risk of hypoglycemia and should be avoided, particularly in patients with STEMI. These patients should maintain stable glucose levels (90–140 mg/dl); low glucose levels below 80 mg/dl should be avoided.

• *Metformin.* This should be stopped 24 hours before PCI and can be restarted 48 hours after the procedure if renal function is normal.

• *Adjunctive pharmacotherapy.* During the procedure GPIs or bivalirudin are recommended. Abciximab has been shown to reduce both 1 year mortality and target vessel revascularization in patients with diabetes (EPISTENT trial).

All patients after angioplasty should receive aggressive medical treatment targeting risk factors. Many factors such as blood glucose, blood pressure, cholesterol level, renal function, and weight should be controlled regularly to reach optimal levels:

• Glycated hemoglobin <7.0%

• LDL cholesterol level <100 mg/dl

• Blood pressure ≤130/80 mmHg

• *Dual antiplatelet therapy* after PCI with DES is crucial. Aspirin and clopidogrel proved more beneficial in this group of patients than in nondiabetic patients. Beta-blockers, statins, either ACE inhibitors or angiotensin-receptor blockers are also used.

Trials

ISAR-DIABETES

In this study 250 PCI patients with diabetes were randomized either to the Cypher sirolimus-eluting stent or the Taxus paclitaxel-eluting stent. Results at 9 months demonstrated lower rates of restenosis, target lesion revascularization, and death in patients who received the Cypher stent compared to the Taxus stent. The study showed that the Cypher stent was more effective in preventing restenosis in this high-risk group of diabetic patients than was the Taxus stent.

DIABETES

In this trial 158 PCI patients with diabetes with one or more de novo lesions were randomized for PCI either with a sirolimus-eluting stent or a bare metal stent. Compared to the bare metal stent, the sirolimus-eluting stent significantly reduced the need for repeat revascularization in these diabetic patients in a 2-year follow-up.

BARI-2D

In this study 4623 patients with coronary disease were screened and 2368 randomized to either revascularization or medical treatment. The study was designed to evaluate the efficacy of revascularization with either PCI or CABG with optimal medical therapy versus optimal medical therapy alone in patients with diabetes. There was no significant difference in rates of death and major adverse cardiac events between diabetic patients undergoing revascularization with optimal medical treatment and those who received optimal medical treatment alone.

SCAAR

In this registry 7644 consecutive patients with diabetes in Sweden were enrolled to receive PCI with either bare metal stents or DES. In this registry restenosis was halved by DES in diabetic patients with stable or unstable coronary disease with a similar risk of death or myocardial infarction in comparison with the bare metal stent group.

CARDia

This trial randomized 510 diabetic patients with multivessel disease or proximal LAD stenosis to PCI with the Taxus stent or CABG. The objective was to compare the safety and efficacy of PCI to that of CABG in patients with diabetes and symptomatic multivessel disease. Although the event rate at 1 year showed lower primary composite end points of mortality, myocardial infarction, nonfatal stroke, and secondary composite end points of death, myocardial infarction, stroke and nonfatal stroke and repeat revascularization in patients treated with bypass surgery, noninferiority criteria were not met. This study did not show noninferiority of PCI over CABG in patients with diabetes. The trial was underpowered.

Key Learning Points

• Diabetic patients are older with diffuse multivessel disease, more previous cardiac events, and peripheral vascular disease.

• Diabetes is a vascular disease with dyslipidemia and a procoagulable state.

• Both treatment options – PCI and CABG – are effective; a single revascularization strategy has not been established.

• Rates of major adverse cardiac events are higher in patients with diabetes undergoing revascularization.

• Prompt glucose-lowering treatment before PCI is essential.

• Metformin should be stopped 24 hours before PCI.

• During angioplasty, GPIs or bivalirudin are recommended.

4 | Interventional Pharmacotherapy

Essential Angioplasty, First Edition. E. von Schmilowski, R. H. Swanton.
© 2012 John Wiley & Sons, Ltd. Published 2012 by John Wiley & Sons, Ltd.

Introduction

Spontaneous or intervention-induced rupture of an atherosclerotic plaque leads to thrombus formation. This is a complex process associated with platelet activation, amplification of the coagulation cascade, release of inflammatory mediators, and platelet aggregation.

Studies have demonstrated that adequate platelet inhibition with antiplatelet agents is essential to good short-term and long-term PCI results in patients with ST-elevation myocardial infarction (STEMI) and non-STEMI (NSTEMI). However, even with optimal antiplatelet therapy, recurrent ischemia, myocardial infarction, or the need for urgent revascularization are recognized problems. Many patients have decreased levels of platelet inhibition in spite of recommended doses of aspirin and clopidogrel because of genetic factors causing relative drug resistance.

Higher and more consistent levels of platelet inhibition are associated with fewer ischemic events but at the cost of increased risk of major bleeding. This is a strong predictor of periprocedural myocardial infarction and even death. Therefore, optimal and balanced antiplatelet therapy should be selected for each individual patient based on their general condition and the potential risk of bleeding (Table 4.1). Ideal antiplatelet therapy should prevent ischemia and minimize the risk of bleeding.

Many clinical trials have confirmed that early treatment with a combination of antiplatelet drugs followed by sustained dual antiplatelet therapy benefits patients with coronary artery disease and reduces coronary events after percutaneous coronary intervention (PCI). Complex drug regimes are also possible.

There are four groups of commonly used antiplatelet agents: cyclooxygenase (COX-1) inhibitors, thienopyridine $P2Y_{12}$ inhibitors, non-thienopyridine $P2Y_{12}$ inhibitors, and glycoprotein IIb/IIIa antagonists. These are shown in Figure 4.1.

COX-1 Inhibitors

Aspirin

Aspirin is the oldest and most widely used antithrombotic agent, highly effective in the dose range 75–150 mg. Uncoated aspirin reaches the plasma peak level quickly within 30 minutes, whereas enteric coated aspirin takes over 3

Table 4.1 Doses of commonly used antiplatelet agents in interventional patients.

Antiplatelet Agent	Dose and Administration Route
Aspirin	75–325 mg before PCI, followed by 75–100 mg/day orally
Clopidogrel	300–600 mg before PCI, followed by 75 mg/day orally
Prasugrel	60 mg before PCI, followed by 10 mg/day orally

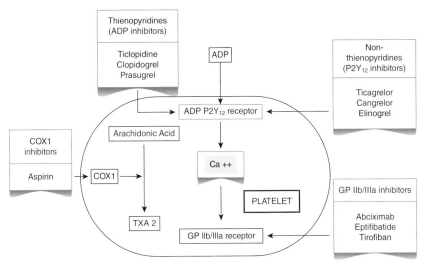

Figure 4.1 Inhibitors of platelet activation.

hours. By permanent inactivation of platelet COX-1, aspirin prevents thrombosis by inhibiting thromboxane (TXA2) synthesis and prolongs the bleeding time.

All patients undergoing PCI should receive aspirin. In case of aspirin allergy, ticlopidine, cilostazol, or prasugrel should be given as an alternative.

Thienopyridines
First-Generation Thienopyridines
Ticlopidine
This drug is rarely used now. It was shown to be inferior to clopidogrel in the CLASSICS trial and leukopenia was a possible side effect.

Second-Generation Thienopyridines
Clopidogrel
Clopidogrel is a thienopyridine antiplatelet agent with significant antiplatelet effect caused by inhibition of platelet activation mediated by ADP. This is a prodrug that must undergo two hepatic metabolic steps to reach its active form. Clopidogrel like aspirin prolongs the bleeding time without affecting the partial thromboplastin time (PTT) or activated clotting time (ACT).

Clopidogrel is an important agent used in primary and secondary prevention of coronary artery disease. Adding clopidogrel to standard medical therapy is very effective in reducing adverse vascular events in the first year after an episode of NSTEMI and improves outcomes in patients after PCI with stent implantation. Studies have demonstrated that patients with myocardial infarction treated with clopidogrel who are either active smokers or use proton pump inhibitors have a higher mortality (see below, p. 174).

Clopidogrel is most effective in the first 3 months after PCI or acute coronary syndrome (ACS). However, it is still beneficial between 3 and 12 months. The following problems may occur with clopidogrel administration:

• **Bleeding.** This is the most common complication that usually occurs during the first month of treatment. For any elective surgery in which the antiplatelet effect is not critical, clopidogrel should be discontinued 7 days before the procedure.

• **Thrombotic thrombocytopenic purpura.** This is a rare multisystem disease caused by impaired proteolysis of von Willebrand factor manifested by thrombocytopenia, unexplained fever, renal failure, neurological symptoms, and bleeding. Most cases occur within 2 weeks of starting clopidogrel therapy. Early diagnosis is critical as plasmapheresis has been shown to improve survival.

• *Resistance* (see below, p. 174).

Third-Generation Thienopyridines

Since clopidogrel is a prodrug, various factors including other medications may interact with its metabolism which increases the thrombotic risk during PCI. New-generation antiplatelet agents undergo less or no hepatic metabolism and provide a more consistent and powerful antiplatelet effect. These agents, however, act more rapidly and should be used carefully in patients with a high risk of bleeding as their potent platelet inhibition may result in severe adverse bleeding events. Recent meta-analysis of these newer agents (see below) has shown that compared with clopidogrel they reduce all-cause mortality and ischemic events in patients undergoing primary PCI for STEMI.

Prasugrel

This is a third-generation thienopyridine preventing initial platelet activation and aggregation. Prasugrel is significantly less dependent on hepatic activation, having only a single-step oxidation activation (not CYP2C19 dependent), and provides a faster onset and greater inhibition of $P2Y_{12}$-receptor-mediated platelet aggregation compared with clopidogrel. This results from a greater and more efficient generation of the active metabolite. The TRITON-TIMI 38 trial showed that, in comparison to clopidogrel, prasugrel therapy was associated with significantly reduced rates of ischemic events in patients with unstable angina, NSTEMI, or acute myocardial infarction undergoing PCI. Stent thrombosis was reduced by approximately 50% in the prasugrel group compared to the clopidogrel group. Major bleeding risk was increased in the elderly (age >75 years), patients with a history of previous stroke, or those <60 kg weight. Clopidogrel is thus preferable in the elderly, and those with a previous stroke. Prasugrel dose reduction (5 mg daily) is needed in patients <60 kg.

Prasugrel is administered orally (60 mg loading dose, 10 mg maintenance dose), with platelet inhibition time less than 1 hour. Prasugrel should be given as the first choice thienopyridine in patients undergoing primary PCI for STEMI, patients with a history of stent thrombosis, and diabetic patients.

Nonthienopyridines

Ticagrelor
This is an oral agent with reversible direct inhibition of the ADP $P2Y_{12}$ receptor, more rapid onset, and greater platelet inhibition than clopidogrel. No hepatic metabolism is required. This is a good drug in patients with ACS either with STEMI or NSTEMI. Treatment with ticagrelor significantly reduces the rate of death from vascular causes, myocardial infarction, or stroke compared with clopidogrel. Although ticagrelor has not been shown to increase overall major bleeding, the non-procedure-related bleeding rate is higher. Ticagrelor is administered orally (180 mg loading dose, then 90 mg twice daily) with platelet inhibition time 2–4 hours (PLATO trial).

Cangrelor
This is a nonthienopyridine $P2Y_{12}$ receptor antagonist which selectively and reversibly inhibits ADP-induced platelet aggregation. This ATP analog acts directly on the receptor and requires no metabolic activation. It has rapid onset and offset of action and is cleared at 1 hour after infusion (CHAMPION study). Intravenous administration: bolus dose 30 μg/kg followed by 4 μg/kg per minute for 2–4 hours; platelet inhibition time is a few minutes. It may be a useful bridge in the 5–7 days from stopping clopidogrel or prasugrel and performing CABG.

Elinogrel
This is a direct-acting reversible inhibitor of $P2Y_{12}$ receptor administered intravenously and orally: bolus dose 10–60 mg; effects within seconds (INNOVATE-PCI study). It may cause mild dyspnea.

Dual Antiplatelet Therapy

All patients should receive aspirin and clopidogrel as a loading dose before PCI, followed by continued treatment for a period of time depending on the procedure and type of stent used (see Table 4.2). The role of aspirin and clopidogrel in reducing the risk of stent thrombosis has been firmly established. Premature discontinuation of dual antiplatelet therapy, particularly after implantation of a drug-eluting stent (DES) may result in acute stent thrombosis. To avoid both the potential risk of bleeding and the consequences of premature discontinuation of dual antiplatelet therapy, the patient should be well informed about the importance of compliance with the therapy.

Risk of Bleeding

Major bleeding is an independent predictor of early and late mortality in patients with NSTEMI or STEMI and in all patients undergoing PCI. Major bleeding is defined as bleeding always requiring blood transfusion (≥2–3 units).

Table 4.2 Dual antiplatelet therapy in interventional patients.

PCI	Dual Antiplatelet Therapy
Elective	Aspirin 300 mg orally followed by 75–100 mg orally daily for life.
	Clopidogrel 300/600 mg loading dose followed by 75 mg orally daily for at least 1 year
NSTEMI	Aspirin 300 mg orally followed by 75–100 mg orally daily for life.
	Clopidogrel 600 mg loading dose followed by 75 mg orally daily for at least 1 year
STEMI	Aspirin 300 mg followed by 75 mg orally daily for life.
	Clopidogrel 600 mg loading dose followed by 75 mg orally daily for 1 month
Bare metal stent	Aspirin 75 mg daily for life.
	Clopidogrel 75 mg daily for at least 1 month (up to 12 months)
Drug-eluting stent	Aspirin 75 mg for life.
	Clopidogrel 75 mg daily for at least 12 months
High-risk patients:	Prolonged dual antiplatelet therapy beyond 6–12
Diabetes mellitus, Multivessel	months.
disease, Left main stenosis	These should be considered individually
Previous myocardial infarction	

Severe bleeding is identified when transfusion of 4 units or more is required or if any of the following occur:
- Fall in Hemoglobin ≥ 5.0 g/dl
- Hypotension requiring administration of inotropic agents
- Intraocular or intracerebral bleeding
- Need for surgical intervention

In patients with high risk of gastrointestinal bleeding, omeprazole 20 mg twice daily should be added to the standard antiplatelet therapy.

If Surgery Is Required

Recommendations on managing patients who require surgery:
- If any surgery is planned within 12 months or if the patient is unlikely to be compliant with dual antiplatelet therapy, choose a bare metal stent instead of a DES.
- If the risk of stent thrombosis is high (complex lesion, left main stenting), start tirofiban and stop it 4 hours before surgery.
- If urgent surgery is required, stop clopidogrel 7 days before surgery and continue aspirin alone. After surgery, restart aspirin and clopidogrel with a loading dose.
- In patients with ACS who are candidates for bypass surgery, ticagrelor is a promising alternative to clopidogrel (PLATO study, 2009).
- Do not replace dual antiplatelet therapy with low-molecular-weight heparin as it is ineffective.

Triple Antiplatelet Therapy

Cilostazol

Cilostazol is an antiplatelet agent with vasodilating properties. Data from recent studies suggest that adjunctive cilostazol reduces the rate of high post-clopidogrel platelet reactivity (HPPR) and intensifies platelet inhibition compared to a high maintenance dose of clopidogrel in patients undergoing PCI (ACCELL-RESISTANCE study). Moreover, in patients with acute myocardial infarction, adding 100 mg of cilostazol twice a day to dual antiplatelet therapy increases platelet inhibition more than high-dose clopidogrel (ACCELL-AMI trial).

Resistance to Antiplatelet Therapy

Low responsiveness or resistance to antiplatelet agents affects a large group of patients with coronary disease, with potential severe consequences such as myocardial infarction, stroke, or cardiac death. The standard and clinically useful definition of resistance has not been established, and we still do not have a set of management guidelines for the problem. In patients with a higher risk of stent thrombosis, platelet aggregation tests should be considered.

Aspirin Resistance

Resistance to aspirin is rare. It has been estimated that about 5% patients present with aspirin resistance (nonresponsiveness) and almost 25%(mostly women) are semiresponders. However, patients with aspirin resistance may also have a reduced response to clopidogrel.

Causes

The mechanism of aspirin resistance is complex and not fully understood, but clinical, genetic, and cellular factors are known to be associated with it. The most common reason for nonresponse to aspirin is an inadequate dose or an interaction with other nonsteroidal anti-inflammatory drugs. However, often in these cases there is a genetic polymorphism of either COX-1 or biosynthesis of thromboxane.

In all conditions associated with potential stress, such as ACS, bypass surgery, infection, or inflammation, platelet production and reactivity are very high and new platelets are continuously being released into the blood. In such circumstances, aspirin, having only a 20 minute half-life, is not capable of suppressing COX-1. Factors potentially associated with aspirin resistance are listed in Table 4.3.

Biochemical Manifestation

Resistance means that aspirin is unable to reduce platelet production of thromboxane A_2 and consequently prevent thrombosis or ischemic cardiovascular events.

Table 4.3 Factors potentially associated with aspirin resistance.

Clinical Factors	High Platelet Turnover	Genetic Factors	Bioavailability
Diabetes mellitus	Acute coronary syndrome	COX-1 mutation	Drug interaction (ibuprofen)
Obesity	Infection	COX-1 overexpression	Non- or poor compliance
Heart failure	Inflammation	GPI polymorphism	Non- or poor absorption
Previous stroke, myocardial infarction	CABG	vWF receptor polymorphism	Inadequate dose of aspirin

CABG, coronary artery bypass graft; vWF, von Willebrand factor.

The following should be considered when aspirin resistance is suspected:
- Is the patient compliant and taking aspirin regularly?
- Is the dose of aspirin adequate?
- Is the patient taking enteric coated aspirin? Avoid it!
- Is the patient taking any other nonsteroidal anti-inflammatory drugs?
- Is there any additional infection?

Sometimes simple modification of the current dose or treatment can solve the problem. Ensure that the patient is drug compliant, recommend 75–150 mg aspirin daily, and check other drugs the patient is taking to exclude any potential drug interaction.

Although there is no single standardized test available, all patients with possible aspirin resistance should have platelet function tests, including PFA-100. Skin bleeding time and thromboxane generation test (urinary thromboxane excretion) may also be helpful.

Aspirin resistance can be recognized if two or more of the following criteria have been matched:
- 0.5 mg/ml arachidonic acid-induced platelet aggregation ≥20%
- 5 μmol/l ADP-induced platelet aggregation ≥70%
- Rapid platelet function assay: acetyl salicylic acid ARU (aspirin reaction unit) ≥550

Clopidogrel Resistance

Patients who demonstrate low response to clopidogrel inevitably have a higher risk of recurrent cardiovascular events including cardiac death after PCI.

Clopidogrel resistance can be recognized when an absolute difference between baseline and post-treatment platelet aggregation is 10% or less in response to both 5 and 20 μmol/l ADP.

Table 4.4 Factors potentially associated with clopidogrel resistance.

Clinical Factors	Platelet Factor	Genetic Factors	Bioavailability
Diabetes mellitus	Low inhibition of platelet aggregation	$P2Y_{12}$ polymorphism	Drug interaction
Obesity	High platelet aggregation	$P2Y_{12}$ overexpression	Non- or poor compliance
Heart failure	High shear-induced platelet aggregation	GPI polymorphism	Non- or poor absorption
Higher-class angina	High platelet production	GPI overexpression	Dose too low

Causes

The mechanism of clopidogrel resistance is unclear. This may be associated with poor patient compliance or poor drug absorption. However, genetic, clinical, and platelet factors are also important (Table 4.4).

Some patients have shown a lack of response to clopidogrel therapy in spite of good compliance. A genetic variation in metabolism has been found. Two-step clopidogrel activation occurs via the CYP-450 cytochrome isoenzymes. Carriers of two specific alleles of CYP2C19 and CYP3A4 isoenzymes have a reduced response to clopidogrel. The TRITON-TIMI 38 trial suggested that patients with the loss of function CYP2C19 allele had an increased risk of cardiovascular events after PCI.

Biochemical Manifestation

Laboratory tests are not used routinely and there is no single test to detect clopidogrel resistance. The most reliable test for platelet inhibition with regard to the use of antiplatelet agents is the vasodilator-stimulated phosphoprotein (VASP) test. Platelet function can be monitored on flow cytometric analysis of VASP which is an intraplatelet actin regulatory protein dependent on the level of activation of the platelet $P2Y_{12}$ receptor targeted by clopidogrel. This test measures the phosphorylation status of VASP (Figure 4.2).

Clopidogrel prevents ADP from inhibiting VASP phosphorylation (VASP-P). Incomplete inhibition of the $P2Y_{12}$ receptor by clopidogrel means a fall in VASP-P after stimulation by ADP. High VASP-P indicates the presence of the active form of the $P2Y_{12}$ receptor, related to effective clopidogrel inhibition, whereas low VASP-P means inhibition of $P2Y_{12}$ receptor. Since the VASP assay directly measures the function of the $P2Y_{12}$ receptor, which is the clopidogrel target, the assay is selective for $P2Y_{12}$ inhibitors only. The VASP test should be used for selected patients at high risk of thrombotic events.

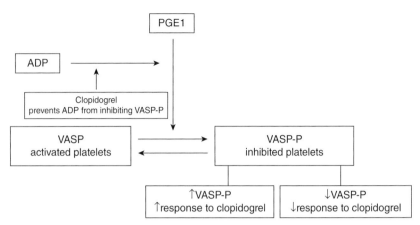

Figure 4.2 Flow cytometric analysis of vasodilator-stimulated phosphoprotein (VASP) phosphorylation (VASP-P).

Poor Responders to Clopidogrel

If patients are poor responders to clopidogrel, consider the following options:
• Increase the loading dose of clopidogrel (bolus of 600 mg clopidogrel instead of 300 mg) to ensure effective platelet inhibition over the first 24 hours after PCI.
• Give additional bolus of clopidogrel (600 mg) and check response in the VASP test if possible. Each additional bolus of clopidogrel decreases the number of patients with low response.
• Platelet aggregation tests are recommended in high-risk patients who have had left main stenting or if the stented artery was the last patent vessel.
• Clopidogrel 150 mg daily should be given if less than 50% inhibition of platelet aggregation has been demonstrated, to reduce the risk of subacute stent thrombosis.
• Switch to prasugrel or ticagrelor. This will provide more rapid onset of action, greater platelet inhibition, and less platelet response variability.
• Add another agent e.g., cilostazol.

Proton Pump Inhibitors and Clopidogrel

Proton pump inhibitors are metabolized by the CYP2C19 isoenzyme and co-treatment with omeprazole has been shown to reduce the platelet inhibitory effect of clopidogrel. A large retrospective study of 8025 patients being discharged from Veterans Affairs hospitals following ACS showed that, of the 63.9% of patients who were taking a proton pump inhibitor with clopidogrel, on multivariate analysis there was a significantly increased risk of recurrent ACS and rehospitalization (Ho et al. 2009). However, the COGENT study, which was stopped early, found no increase in cardiac events in those patients who received omeprazole in addition to clopidogrel over a 12 month period. Further studies are needed, but the need for a proton pump

Table 4.5 Indications for GPI agents in elective PCI and in patients with STEMI and NSTEMI.

PCI	GPIs
Elective PCI	Only in complex PCI, no-reflow, thrombotic lesion
NSTEMI	Only in high-risk patients
STEMI	Before or during primary PCI

inhibitor must be reconsidered in patients undergoing a primary PCI for STEMI. If one is needed pantoprazole should be used.

Glycoprotein IIb/IIIa Inhibitors

Glycoprotein IIb/IIIa inhibitors (GPIs) are effective antiplatelet agents of great benefit to patients with ACS and in elective procedures (see Table 4.5).
• They reduce mortality particularly in high-risk troponin-positive and diabetic patients.
• They are standard therapy in primary PCI for STEMI in addition to aspirin and clopidogrel (see pp. 134–161). GPI use improves TIMI flow, myocardial perfusion, and in-hospital survival. However, in patients with acute myocardial infarction undergoing primary PCI after receiving loading dose of clopidogrel (600 mg), GPIs did not show a benefit after 30 days (BRAVE-3 study).
• Bivalirudin as a single agent was found to be superior to GPIs and unfractionated heparin in primary PCI (HORIZONS-AMI trial).
• In low-risk patients a loading dose of clopidogrel (600 mg) provides a high antiplatelet effect within 2 hours of administration and the use of GPIs is unnecessary.
• In patients with NSTEMI, upstream administration of GPI agents results in reduced ischemic events, but carries a risk of major bleeding complications.
• In patients with NSTEMI who do not receive clopidogrel, GPIs should be administered before or during PCI.
• Consider the use of abciximab in patients with diabetes receiving stents. The EPISTENT trial showed this GPI reduced target vessel revascularization at 6 months and reduced mortality at 1 year in diabetic patients.
• GPIs reduce ischemic complications but increase the risk of bleeding complications from the femoral puncture site.

GPIs in Interventional Patients

GPIs should be given to the following groups of patients:
• Those undergoing elective complex procedures with thrombus visible on angiography or IVUS.
• Those who develop the no-reflow phenomenon (see p. 294).
• Those undergoing primary PCI, or with refractory unstable angina or other high-risk features (including diabetes); abciximab is the drug of choice.

Table 4.6 Doses of GPI agents in interventional patients.

GPI Agents	Dose and Administration Route
Abciximab	0.25 mg/kg bolus plus 12 hour infusion of 0.125 µg/kg per minute (max. 10 µg/min) up to 12 hours.
Eptifibatide	180 µg/kg (0.18 mg/kg) double bolus 10 minutes apart plus 18–24 hour infusion of 2 µg/kg per minute. Max infusion duration 96 hours. If renal failure (GFR < 30 ml/min), infusion should be reduced to 10 µg/kg per minute.
Tirofiban	0.4 µg/kg per minute (30 min IV infusion) plus 24 hour infusion of 0.1 µg/kg per minute. Max infusion duration 108 hours. If renal failure (GFR < 30 ml/min) infusion should be halved.

Table 4.7 Risk factors for GPI-related bleeding.

Low Risk of Bleeding	High Risk of Bleeding
Age <75 years	Age >75 years
Weight >60 kg	Weight <60 kg
No prior stroke or transient ischemic attack	Previous stroke or transient ischemic attack
No bleeding diathesis	Bleeding diathesis
No recent bleeding	Recent bleeding
No recent surgery	Recent surgery

- Those with NSTEMI and unstable angina who are at high risk based on TIMI score or elevated troponin; upstream abciximab, eptifibatide, or tirofiban should be started as soon as possible before PCI.

Abciximab, Tirofiban, and Eptifibatide

There are three GPI agents available: abciximab, tirofiban, and eptifibatide (the doses are listed in Table 4.6). The most commonly used, abciximab, provides the highest activity with the shortest half life (30 minutes) compared with eptifibatide 150 mins and tirofiban 90 mins. Abciximab has proved beneficial in reducing ischemic complications both in elective PCI and in patients with ACS (EPIC, EPILOG trials).

Major Bleeding

Although GPIs prevent ischemic complications, the risk of major bleeding remains a problem. GPIs are contraindicated in all patients with recent active internal bleeding, history of previous stroke in the last 2 years, known AV malformation or aneurysm, bleeding diathesis, use of oral anticoagulation, thrombocytopenia, major surgery, or trauma in the last 2 months or severe uncontrolled hypertension and hypertensive retinopathy. Risk factors for GPI-related bleeding are summarized in Table 4.7.

In patients with a clinical risk of bleeding (older age, low weight, previous stroke) or procedural risk of bleeding (previous PCI, long procedure, large sheath size), heparin should be added to standard GPI therapy and the sheath should be removed more than 2 hours after heparin discontinuation with the ACT below 175 seconds. The groin must be checked regularly after sheath removal. A closure device is recommended and use of the femostop device may be necessary (see Chapter 2 – closure devices).

Bleeding Prevention
A few tips to help prevent bleeding:
• Take a detailed medical history (for contraindications).
• Assess clinical and procedural risk of bleeding (see Table 4.7).
• Check platelet count if possible before procedure.
• Use a smaller sheath size for arterial access, especially in low-weight patients.
• Keep an eye on ACT (200–250 seconds); give heparin as 60–70 U/kg bolus at start of procedure and stop heparin after procedure.
• Wait for sheath removal until ACT is below 175 seconds.
• Check platelet count at the end of procedure and 24 hours after.
• Use the Femostop device in higher-risk patients (low-weight, hypertensive) prospectively before a hematoma develops.
• Check the groin for bleeding or hematoma at regular intervals.

Bleeding Management
In case of bleeding the following steps should be taken:
• Stop GPI administration.
• Use manual pressure or Femostop compression device to stop the bleeding.
• Obtain full blood count with platelets (for thrombocytopenia).
• If thrombocytopenia is confirmed and due to GPI administration, transfuse platelets and immunoglobulin.

The three commonly used GPI agents have different lengths of action. If a specific agent has been used and there is clinical bleeding or the need for emergency surgery:
• If *abciximab* has been used, stop the infusion if it is still going. Start fresh platelet transfusion as soon as possible. Remember that transfused platelets may still be bound by abciximab displaced from endogenous platelets. Although the drug has a short half life (30 mins), its effects are still detectable 7–10 days after administration due to platelet binding.
• If *tirofiban* has been used, bear in mind that the short half-life is less than 2 hours, with less than 50% platelet inhibition 4 hours after stopping the agent.
• If *eptifibatide* has been used, remember that the short half-life is 2–3 hours, with less than 50% platelet inhibition 4 hours after stopping the agent.

Thrombocytopenia

Thrombocytopenia a is rare but important complication associated with a higher incidence of severe bleeding, blood transfusion, and ischemic complications. Thrombocytopenia usually occurs within 24 hours after the procedure and is most commonly caused by abciximab. Severe thrombocytopenia (platelets $< 50 \times 10^3/\mu l$) is fortunately rare, while mild thrombocytopenia (platelets $<100 \times 10^3/\mu l$) is more common. A platelet count should be ordered routinely.

Patients who develop severe thrombocytopenia should be kept in hospital. Platelet transfusion is necessary only if bleeding complications develop. The patient may be discharged once the platelet count starts to rise and is above $50 \times 10^3/\mu l$.

Trials

CREDO

In this study 2116 patients were randomized to receive clopidogrel 300 mg plus aspirin 325 mg vs. placebo plus aspirin 325 mg prior to PCI and 28 days treatment with clopidogrel 75 mg plus aspirin 325 mg vs. clopidogrel 75 mg plus aspirin 75 mg followed by a 1 year treatment with clopidogrel 75 mg plus aspirin 325 mg vs. placebo plus aspirin 325 mg. The CREDO trial demonstrated that following a PCI procedure, maintaining dual antiplatelet therapy with aspirin and clopidogrel for up to 1 year significantly reduced the risk of adverse thrombotic events (relative risk reduction 26.9%). The time at which treatment is administered can also affect outcome, as initiating a loading dose of at least 300 mg clopidogrel is likely to be beneficial only if started more than 6 hours prior to a planned PCI procedure.

CURE

In this study 12,562 patients with ACS who had presented within 24 hours after the onset of symptoms received a loading dose of clopidogrel 300 mg followed by 75 mg daily vs. placebo plus aspirin (75–325 mg daily) for 3–12 months. The study confirmed the benefits of clopidogrel in patients with ACS without ST-segment elevation (reducing a combined end-point of Cardiovascular death, nonfatal myocardial infarction or stroke by 20%) although there was an increased risk of major bleeding among patients treated with clopidogrel.

ACCELL-AMI

This study evaluated the degree of platelet inhibition by triple antiplatelet therapy in patients with acute myocardial infarction. The effects of adjunctive cilostazol on inhibiting platelet reactivity in acute MI were studied. Ninety patients were randomized to one of three groups. On admission all patients received clopidogrel (600 mg loading dose, followed by 75 mg daily) and aspirin (300 mg loading dose and 200 mg daily for the study period). Following

PCI, they were randomly assigned to one of three groups before discharge in addition to aspirin: standard group (clopidogrel 75 mg daily), high-maintenance dose group (clopidogrel 150 mg daily), and triple therapy group (adjunctive cilostazol of 100 mg twice daily to clopidogrel 75 mg daily). Among patients with acute myocardial infarction undergoing coronary stenting, triple antiplatelet therapy resulted in a greater antiplatelet effect at 30 days compared with a high-maintenance dose of clopidogrel or standard dual antiplatelet therapy.

TRITON-TIMI 38
In this study 13,608 patients with ACS planned for PCI were randomized to receive prasugrel or clopidogrel in addition to standard therapy. The primary end point was cardiovascular death, myocardial infarction, and stroke. In patients with ACS undergoing PCI, prasugrel achieved faster and greater levels of platelet inhibition than clopidogrel, with a lower rate of ischemic events, particularly myocardial infarction and stent thrombosis, but with a higher risk of bleeding, including serious bleeding in specific patient subsets. However:
1. There was no difference in the cardiovascular death rate.
2. The trial was underpowered for a single end point.
3. Only 300 mg clopidogrel was used as the loading dose.
4. There was more major and minor bleeding in the prasugrel group, particularly in those patients who needed CABG.
5. In addition, the cost of prasugrel now considerably exceeds that of clopidogrel, which is now available as a generic prescription.

PLATO
In this trial 18,624 patients with ACS with or without ST-segment elevation were randomized to ticagrelor (180 mg loading dose, followed by 90 mg twice daily) or clopidogrel (300–600 mg loading dose, followed by 75 mg daily) for the prevention of cardiovascular events. At 12 months the primary end point of death from vascular causes, myocardial infarction, or stroke was reduced in the ticagrelor group to 9.8% compared with 11.7% in the clopidogrel group (p = 0.001). There was no significant increase in major bleeding. There was a significant reduction in death from any cause with ticagrelor (4.5% vs. 5.9% for clopidogrel), although the trial was not powered to detect a mortality difference. In addition, a significant number of patients in the clopidogrel group did not receive optimum dosing.

Although major bleeding events were similar in both groups, there was a significantly slightly higher risk of non CABG related bleeding in patients on ticagrelor (4.5% vs 3.8%).

The drug had new side effects (dyspnea, bradyarrhythmias, and a rise in serum creatinine and uric acid). This may be due to the fact that part of the molecule is similar to adenosine.

This was the largest study of a new non-thienopyridine drug compared with clopidogrel and showed the greatest benefit in mortality in STEMI patients (4.9 vs 6.0% with clopidogrel). In conclusion, ticagrelor may become an alternative to clopidogrel for patients with ACS who are candidates for PCI.

Key Learning Points

- Not all antiplatelet agents are irreversible.
- Clopidogrel is of greatest benefit within the first 3 months of treatment.
- Bleeding is the most common complication associated with antiplatelet therapy.
- In patients with procedural or postprocedural thrombotic complications on adequate doses of antiplatelet agents, always consider the possibility of drug resistance.
- GPIs are beneficial in patients with acute coronary syndromes undergoing PCI.
- The new $P2Y_{12}$ inhibitors reduce all-cause mortality and ischemic events in patients undergoing PCI for STEMI.

Antithrombotic Agents in PCI

- **Introduction, 182**
- **Unfractionated Heparin, 184**
  Activated Clotting Time: Monitoring of Anticoagulation Effect
- **Low-Molecular-Weight Heparin, 185**
- **Bivalirudin, 186**
  Switching to Bivalirudin
- **Trials, 186**
  SYNERGY
  ACUITY
  ISAR-REACT 3
  OASIS-5

Introduction

Antithrombotic agents play an important role in the treatment of patients with ACS and are essential during coronary interventional procedures (Table 4.8). The use of antithrombotic drugs is associated with improved procedural and clinical outcomes during both primary and elective procedures. Unfortunately, increased bleeding complications remain a problem and potential risks and benefits should be carefully considered in each patient.

Unfractionated heparin (UFH) binds to antithrombin III, causing rapid inactivation of free thrombin and factors XI, Xa, IX, and VIIa, causing prolon-

Table 4.8 Doses of antithrombotic agents in interventional patients.

Antithrombotic Agent	Dose and Administration Route
Unfractionated heparin (UFH)	50–100 U/kg bolus for PCI without GPI (ACT 250–300 seconds) 50–60 U/kg for PCI with GPI (ACT 200–250 seconds)
Low-molecular-weight heparin (LMWH) Enoxaparin	1 mg/kg subcutaneously twice daily or 0.3 mg/kg bolus
Bivalirudin	0.75 mg/kg bolus plus infusion of 1.75 mg/kg per hour during PCI

ACT, activated clotting time.

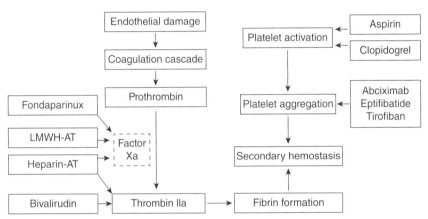

Figure 4.3 Sites of action of commonly used antithrombotic and antiplatelet agents. Heparin-AT, heparin–antithrombin III complex.

gation of the activated partial thromboplastin time (APTT) and thrombin time (TT). Low-molecular-weight heparin (LMWH) inhibits factor Xa (even when bound to platelets), preventing conversion of prothrombin to active thrombin. Neither unfractionated nor low-molecular-weight heparin can inactivate thrombin once it is bound to fibrin.

New direct thrombin inhibitors (hirudin analogs) such as bivalirudin inactivate thrombin by connecting directly to two active sites on the thrombin molecule, preventing conversion of fibrinogen to fibrin. They also inactivate fibrin-bound thrombin, unlike the heparins. They focus on the direct mediator of thrombosis without influencing other factors in the coagulation cascade. For this reason, direct thrombin inhibitors result in fewer bleeding problems compared with traditionally used UFH or LMWH.

Figure 4.3 shows the sites of action of antithrombotic and antiplatelet agents.

Table 4.9 Antithrombotic treatment in patients with STEMI and NSTEMI undergoing PCI.

PCI in ACS	Antithrombotic Agents
PCI in STEMI	Bivalirudin (0.75 mg/kg IV) or heparin (2500–5000 U IV) on arrival *and* bivalirudin (0.75 mg/kg IV plus 1.75 mg/kg per hour infusion) in the catheter lab or unfractionated heparin plus GPI
PCI in NSTEMI	Bivalirudin 0.75 mg/kg IV plus GPI only if necessary (provisional GPI) or alternatively heparin (2500–5000 U IV) plus GPI

Commonly available antithrombotic agents for PCI are the following:
• Unfractionated heparin (UFH): antithrombin III activator
• Low-molecular-weight heparin (LMWH): factor Xa inhibitor
• Bivalirudin: direct thrombin inhibitor
• Fondaparinux: antithrombin III activator, inhibits activated factor X
Standard treatment options in patients with ACS undergoing PCI:
• Patients with STEMI should receive bivalirudin or heparin on admission, followed by bivalirudin in the catheter laboratory or unfractionated heparin plus GPI.
• Patients with NSTEMI undergoing PCI should receive bivalirudin and provisional GPI, or alternatively heparin.
• Patients with STEMI and NSTEMI also need standard antiplatelet agents (aspirin 325 mg, clopidogrel 600 mg loading dose) followed by long-term dual antiplatelet therapy.
• Every patient with subacute stent thrombosis should be analyzed carefully. Inadequate platelet inhibition as well as individual variability of response to antiplatelet therapy should be considered.
Doses of antithrombotic agents in patients with STEMI and NSTEMI undergoing PCI are shown in Table 4.9.

Unfractionated Heparin
UFH is an indirect anticoagulant which binds to antithrombin to inhibit thrombin and factor Xa. Its role in patients with ACS undergoing PCI is well established. Studies have shown that UFH added to aspirin reduces the risk of acute myocardial infarction and death.

The commonly used standard dose of UFH is 50–100 U/kg bolus. If the patient also receives GPI, a lower dose of heparin (<70 U/kg) limits the risk of bleeding complications. ACT monitoring is essential to control safety and effectiveness of the anticoagulation effect. ACT should be maintained between 250 and 300 seconds if the patient does not receive additional GPI and between 200 and 300 seconds if a GPI is given.

Heparin should be used carefully. Excessive anticoagulation can cause bleeding, whereas subtherapeutic heparinization can lead to thrombus formation and coronary occlusion. Anticoagulant effect may be reversed with protamine sulfate (1 mg, reverses 100 U of heparin), with maximum dose of 50 mg (10 ml ampoule is 10 mg/ml).

UFH is contraindicated in patients with known hypersensitivity to heparin, active bleeding, severe thrombocytopenia, gastrointestinal ulcers, uncontrolled hypertension, or suspected intracranial hemorrhage.

Heparin-induced thrombocytopenia (HIT)
Heparin-induced thrombocytopenia (HIT) is a rare side effect with antibodies forming to the heparin–platelet factor 4 (PF4) complex, and thrombocytopenia developing 5–14 days after heparin administration. This may occur sooner if the patient has had heparin in the last three months. It does not occur with bivalirudin. This is a prothrombotic condition and bleeding is rare. Watch for venous (deep vein thrombosis, pulmonary embolism) and arterial thromboses (acute MI, CVA, digital ischemia). Stop heparin and switch to bivalirudin and then warfarin.

Activated Clotting Time: Monitoring of Anticoagulation Effect

The activated clotting time (ACT), which is the time required to form a clot, should be measured in the lab during the PCI procedure to assess the anticoagulation activity. Target values are:
• PCI with heparin alone: ACT 250–350 seconds
• PCI with heparin plus GPI: ACT 200–250 seconds
• If the procedure time exceeds 1 hour: ACT should be rechecked

Low-Molecular-Weight Heparin

LMWH is a safe and effective alternative to UFH for PCI procedures. It has greater bioavailability than unfractionated heparin, has fewer side effects, and does not require ACT monitoring. However, in patients with unstable angina, although LMWH is as efficient as unfractionated heparin, the risk of minor bleeding is higher.
• In primary therapy for ACS, enoxaparin should be given in dose of 1 mg/kg subcutaneously every 12 hours for 2–8 days.
• In patients more than 75 years old, the dose of enoxaparin is reduced to 0.75 mg/kg subcutaneously 12-hourly.
• In patients with impaired renal function and creatinine clearance below 30 ml/min the dose should be 1 mg/kg subcutaneously once daily (24 hours) or 0.65 mg/kg subcutaneously every 12 hours.
• In interventional patients who require GPI, the enoxaparin dose is 0.75 mg/kg IV.
• In interventional patients who do not require GPI, the enoxaparin dose is 1.0 mg/kg IV.
• If the patient has received a standard dose of LMWH and the procedure is performed within 8 hours from the last dose, no further anticoagulation is needed.
• If the patient has received a standard dose of LMWH and the procedure is performed more than 8 hours from the last dose, an additional 0.3 mg/kg IV should be given before the procedure.

Bivalirudin

Bivalirudin is a reversible direct thrombin inhibitor and a safe agent for elective procedures and primary PCI in STEMI. Its short half-life (approx. 25 minutes) contributes to the lower rates of bleeding complications. Bivalirudin is eliminated by the kidneys, and in patients with creatinine clearance below 30 ml/min an infusion dose adjustment is needed. Bivalirudin is approved for use both in patients undergoing angioplasty and also in patients with ACS not having interventional procedures.

• In patients with stable angina, bivalirudin alone or in combination with a GPI decreases 1 year mortality when compared to heparin plus GPI (REPLACE-2 trial).
• Bivalirudin is safer than UFH in patients with stable angina, ACS, and acute myocardial infarction. Bivalirudin reduces the risk of bleeding and thrombocytopenia as well as the need for transfusion compared with UFH in combination with a GPI.
• In patients with STEMI undergoing primary PCI, bivalirudin shows better outcomes than UFH plus GPI, particularly in high-risk patients. This is associated with less major bleeding and better survival (HORIZON-AMI trial).
• Bivalirudin can be used in patients with heparin-induced thrombocytopenia (it does not cause this).
• For patients undergoing PCI, the dose is 0.75 mg/kg bolus plus infusion of 1.75 mg/kg per hour during the angioplasty procedure.
• For patients with ACS not having an interventional procedure, the dose is 0.1 mg/kg followed by infusion of 0.25 mg/kg per hour.

Switching to Bivalirudin

If the patient is on UFH and the plan is to switch to bivalirudin before PCI, the best strategy is to start bivalirudin 30 minutes after the last dose of heparin. This can be done right before the PCI if the ACT is more than 225 seconds. If the patient requires PCI and the plan is to switch from LMWH to bivalirudin, the best option is to wait 8 hours after the last LMWH dose and then start bivalirudin.

Trials

SYNERGY

In this study 9977 patients with high-risk NSTEMI ACS were randomized to receive enoxaparin or UFH in order to study the influence of age on treatment outcomes with these agents. The outcomes of 30-day death, death, or myocardial infarction, and major bleeding were analyzed in relation to baseline characteristics. Elderly patients (≥75 years) had more cardiovascular risk factors and prior cardiac disease at presentation. This study showed a higher rate of severe bleeding in elderly patients treated with enoxaparin, but the overall relationships between treatment (UFH or enoxaparin) and outcomes did not vary significantly as a function of the patient's age. This study confirmed that if enoxaparin is used in patients over 75 years, dose reduction is necessary.

ACUITY

In this trial 13,819 patients with ACS undergoing cardiac catheterization within 72 hours were randomized to one of three arms: UFH or enoxaparin plus routine GPI; bivalirudin plus routine GPI; or bivalirudin alone, with GPI given only as bailout. The trial was designed to examine whether the use of bivalirudin in place of UFH or LMWH improved outcomes. In addition, it asked whether the use of bivalirudin could eliminate the need for routine use of a GPI or whether the combination of bivalirudin and a GPI would improve outcomes further. For the main part of the trial, the primary end points were the composite of death, myocardial infarction, unplanned revascularization for ischemia, and major bleeding at 30 days. Results were presented for each bivalirudin arm separately compared with the UFH/enoxaparin arm. When bivalirudin alone was compared with heparin/enoxaparin plus a GPI, there was a slight but nonsignificant increase in ischemic events. Bivalirudin suppressed ischemia to the same extent as heparin plus GPI, but with a significantly lower risk of major bleeding.

ISAR-REACT 3

In this trial 4570 patients with stable and unstable angina undergoing PCI were randomized to receive bivalirudin or UFH. The trial examined whether bivalirudin was superior to UFH in patients with stable and unstable angina undergoing PCI after pretreatment with clopidogrel. Primary end points included composite of death, myocardial infarction, ischemia-driven target vessel revascularization at 30 days, or major bleeding during hospitalization. The study demonstrated that in patients undergoing PCI for stable and unstable angina, bivalirudin alone compared to heparin plus GPI resulted in a reduced 30 day rate of major bleeding and net adverse clinical events.

OASIS-5

In this trial 20,078 patients with unstable angina or myocardial infarction without ST-segment elevation were randomized to receive fondaparinux or enoxaparin. Patients were randomly assigned to a study group within 24 hours after the onset of symptoms. Both drugs were used for an average of 5 days. The trial was designed to study the noninferiority of fondaparinux compared with enoxaparin at 9 days. The primary end points included death, myocardial infarction, or refractory ischemia. The primary safety objective was to determine whether fondaparinux was superior to enoxaparin in preventing major bleeding. Patients were followed for a minimum of 90 days and a maximum of 180 days. The secondary end points included death, myocardial infarction, or refractory ischemia, and the individual components of these composite outcomes at 30 days and at 6 months. The trial demonstrated that fondaparinux was similar to enoxaparin in reducing the risk of ischemic events at 9 days, but it substantially reduced major bleeding and improved long-term mortality and morbidity.

There were fewer strokes in the fondaparinux group, and in patients who had a PCI vascular access complications were also reduced: enoxaparin 8.1% vs. fondaparinux 3.3%.

Key Learning Points

• Bleeding complications remain the major problem with antithrombotic therapy.

• The major limitation of UFH is poor clot penetration and a potential risk of heparin-induced thrombocytopenia.

• Low-molecular-weight heparin is a safe and effective alternative to unfractionated heparin for procedural anticoagulation.

• Bivalirudin reduces bleeding compared with traditionally used unfractionated heparin or low-molecular-weight heparin.

• GPIs are necessary in primary PCI when using heparins, but not essential if using bivalirudin.

---

5 | Techniques in Specific Lesions

Left Main Coronary Artery

Essential Angioplasty, First Edition. E. von Schmilowski, R. H. Swanton.
© 2012 John Wiley & Sons, Ltd. Published 2012 by John Wiley & Sons, Ltd.

Introduction

In the early days of balloon angioplasty with bare metal stents, percutaneous intervention of an unprotected left main coronary artery stenosis had poor clinical outcomes with high rates of restenosis and the need for repeat revascularization. In view of the limited data from randomized clinical trials and the lack of standard interventional techniques, both American and European Guidelines recommended surgery as the gold standard for treatment of an unprotected left main stem stenosis. Angioplasty was only recommended for patients not eligible for surgery.

Recent developments in percutaneous coronary intervention (PCI) techniques with new approaches in pharmacological management, along with a decrease in in-stent restenosis (with the introduction of drug-eluting stents), have resulted in better clinical outcomes compared with those early experiences. In consequence, current American College of Cardiology (ACC) guidelines state that unprotected left main stenting is reasonable in patients not eligible for surgery (recommendation Grade IIaB) and may be considered as an alternative to surgery in patients with a low risk of procedural complications and clinical conditions predicting adverse surgical outcomes (recommendation Grade IIbB).

Although existing data from comparative trials support the percutaneous approach with stenting as a safe alternative to surgery in selected patients, widespread use of PCI in left main stem stenosis remains controversial.

Unprotected and Protected Left Main

The terminology of "protected" and "unprotected" refers to the presence or absence of bypass grafts to the left coronary artery. "Unprotected left main disease" refers to a severe (>50%) main stem stenosis with no patent bypass grafts to the left anterior descending (LAD) or the left circumflex artery (LCx). "Protected left main coronary artery" means that there is at least one patent bypass graft to the left coronary circulation.

The following issues should be considered in selecting the best treatment strategy:
• Where is the left main lesion located? Is it an aorto-ostial lesion, a body lesion, or a distal lesion?
• Does the lesion involve the distal left main bifurcation?
• In the case of distal left main lesion:
  – Is the side branch clinically relevant?
  – What access is there to the side branch?
  – Is the side branch lesion severe?
  – What is the side branch size and angle?
• Is the left main long or short? What is the left main diameter?
• Is the left main stenosis an isolated lesion, or are severe lesions also present in other large vessels?
• How many vessels need treatment?

- Is the right coronary artery (RCA) patent, dominant, or chronically occluded?
- What is the left ventricular function?
- Assess the risk profile using the SYNTAX score and the EuroSCORE. Does this help in deciding therapeutic options?
- Is this an emergency or an elective procedure?
- Is the lesion calcified?
- Is debulking needed?
- Is intravascular ultrasound (IVUS)/fractional flow reserve (FFR) mandatory?
- One or two stents? If two stents, which bifurcation technique?
- Bare metal stent or DES? Which DES is optimal?
- Is an intra-aortic balloon pump (IABP) necessary?
- What is the best pharmacotherapy?
- Does the patient need routine angiographic follow-up?
- When should the patient be referred for surgery?

Left Main Anatomy

The left main coronary artery arises from the left aortic sinus of Valsalva and consists of three segments: the ostium, the shaft (the body segment), and the distal segment. The distal segment ends at the LAD/LCx bifurcation. In approximately one-third of all cases a ramus intermedius (intermediate branch) may also be present. The left main is usually short, ranging from 10 to 20 mm, but may reach 40 mm. Congenital anomalies of the left main may also occur (see p. 41).

The location and distribution of the left main plaque as well as vessel anatomy will influence the choice of treatment strategy and these should be considered separately. The most common location of the atheromatous plaque is in the distal segment of the left main, at the bifurcation. An ostial left main lesion and involvement of the body segment are less frequent (Figure 5.1).

Isolated left main disease is very uncommon; most patients also have lesions in at least one other major coronary artery. Isolated left main disease usually has an ostial location.

There are three types of the angle between the aortic lumen and the coronary ostial lumen: right, acute, and obtuse which are normal variations (see Figure 5.2).

Patient Selection

Diagnostic Angiography

The left main should be engaged carefully and gently using a standard Judkins left catheter, avoiding deep cannulation and ensuring the catheter tip is coaxial with the main stem. If the catheter tip points upward to the roof of

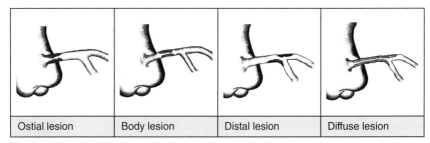

| Ostial lesion | Body lesion | Distal lesion | Diffuse lesion |

Figure 5.1 Left main coronary artery plaque location: ostial, body, distal, and diffuse lesion.

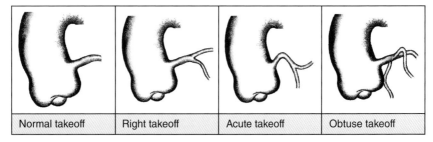

| Normal takeoff | Right takeoff | Acute takeoff | Obtuse takeoff |

Figure 5.2 Variants of left main coronary artery takeoff.

the main stem, there is a risk of main stem dissection. During cannulation of the left coronary ostium, pressure damping may occur. This may be the first sign of an ostial lesion. If this happens, use only limited contrast injection and disengage the catheter immediately (see pp. 238–251).

Start with a projection that displays a glimpse of the left main anatomy on the first injection. The ostium can be visualized best in the left anterior oblique (LAO) cranial view, and the left main body and bifurcation in the right anterior oblique (RAO) or LAO caudal view. Generally, two or three selected views should show the left main adequately enough to decide on further treatment options. If in doubt, use FFR for stenosis significance and IVUS to assess left main size and wall composition. IVUS will also help assess the degree of calcification and involvement of distal branches as well as selection of the correct stent size. Remember that the fewer contrast injections and the shorter the diagnostic procedure, the better. Any risk of ischemia or hypotension may lead to severe complications.

If the left main stenosis coexists with critical occlusion in the RCA, hemodynamic support should be considered. The patient should be admitted to the intensive care unit and reviewed by a cardiac surgeon for possible urgent surgery.

Informed Consent

Where possible, every patient with left main stem stenosis should be discussed in a multidisciplinary team which includes cardiac surgeons.

In every PCI, informed consent is essential. It is necessary to explain clearly that angioplasty for the left main stem stenosis is not a current standard of care. This always takes time, and the procedure should not be performed immediately after diagnostic angiography even if the patient seems to be a good candidate for angioplasty. In view of current guideline recommendations, every patient who is an acceptable candidate for PCI should be fully informed about treatment options, risks, benefits, and potential long-term outcomes. In the case of PCI, the remote possibility of emergency coronary bypass surgery has to be accepted.

It is also important to inform the patient about the need for repeat coronary angiography 6 months after the procedure and that dual antiplatelet therapy will be required for at least 12 months.

In deciding the best revascularization strategy, both patient and lesion characteristics need to be considered. The lesion location (? distal left main) and side branch size and angulation are important. A patient with a heavily calcified left main with a coexisting ostial lesion in the LAD or LCx is more likely to benefit from surgery.

Risk Profile

The lack of established recommendations for left main intervention limits various predictive methods for assessing procedural risk. Although available, they are not used routinely in daily clinical practice.

PCI and surgery have different clinical outcomes depending on the patient risk profile. The role of any risk score based on clinical and angiographic characteristics is a guide to the best treatment.

For many years, procedural and clinical outcomes after left main revascularization were assessed using the EuroSCORE, adopted from surgery for complex left main stem stenosis and multivessel disease. This score was used to assess a risk profile for surgery rather than to select a particular treatment or predict outcomes. Patients with acute coronary syndromes and higher EuroSCORE (>6) seemed at higher risk of death, myocardial infarction, or stent thrombosis than those with EuroSCORE below 6.

Clinical outcomes after left main revascularization are associated not only with the anatomical location of the stenosis within the left main but, more importantly, with the severity and complexity of lesions in other major coronary vessels. Multivessel disease is a determinant of risk particularly in patients undergoing PCI, as the risk of incomplete revascularization is higher than in patients undergoing surgery.

The recently applied SYNTAX score is based on lesion severity and helps guide patient selection for PCI. Results from the SYNTAX trial demonstrated that patients with left main disease and complex lesions (SYNTAX score >33) had a higher rate of death, myocardial infarction, stroke, and

Table 5.1 Overall risk profile assessment in patients with left main coronary artery disease.

	Higher Risk Patient	Lower Risk Patient
Scores	EuroSCORE ≥6	EuroSCORE <6
	SYNTAX score ≥33	SYNTAX score <33
Surgery option	Not suitable for surgery	Suitable for surgery
Clinical factors	Age >75 years	Age <75 years
	Multivessel disease	Isolated left main disease (rare)
	Impaired left ventricular function	Normal left ventricular function
	Impaired renal function	Normal renal function
Angiographic	Large left main diameter >4 mm	Small left main diameter
and	Distal location involving bifurcation	<4 mm
procedural	Chronic total occlusion in the right	Ostial or body location
factors	coronary artery	Right coronary artery dominant
	Left main with heavy calcification	Left main free of calcium
	Two-stent strategy	Provisional stenting

the need for repeat revascularization after PCI in comparison to surgery. However, there were no differences between treatment options in relation to restenosis, death, myocardial infarction, and stroke in patients with low and intermediate SYNTAX scores (<33). Risk profile assessment is shown in Table 5.1.

PCI vs. Bypass Surgery

Randomized trials such as ARTS and ERACI II showed that surgery and angioplasty were equivalent in terms of infarct-free survival, with the risk of myocardial infarction less than 10% and the risk of death less than 1%.

Although PCI and CABG have been shown to be similar in terms of death, myocardial infarction, and stroke at 1 year, higher rates of restenosis and the need for repeat revascularization are greater in PCI patients. Restenosis is part of the overall PCI risk.

Surgery seems to be a better option for patients in whom a suboptimal stenting result is likely, such as patients with complex left main lesions, multivessel disease, or patients who may have difficulties with maintaining long-term dual antiplatelet therapy. It is possible, however, as stent technology develops, that PCI will eventually replace surgery in most patients with left main disease (Table 5.2).

Drug-Eluting Stents

Consistent data from current studies demonstrate that the use of DES in left main stenting results in a significant reduction in angiographic restenosis and repeat revascularization compared with bare metal stenting. Angioplasty outcomes with DES vary due to differences in patient selection and interventional technique as well as lesion location, size of the left main, and general left main complexity. The best results with DES are seen in low-risk patients

Table 5.2 PCI versus surgery in patients with left main coronary artery disease.

PCI Preferable	Surgery Preferable
Normal left main anatomy	Complex left main anatomy, poor distal vessel runoff, severe calcification, tortuosities
Right coronary artery patent	Chronic total occlusion of right coronary artery
Isolated left main	Multivessel disease
Advanced age	Young age
In-stent restenosis of the left main eligible for balloon angioplasty	In-stent restenosis of the left main ineligible for repeat PCI
Emergency procedure, cardiogenic shock	Elective procedure
Compliance with antiplatelet therapy	Antiplatelet therapy contraindicated

with normal left ventricular function and no distal left main bifurcation involvement.

Contemporary Techniques

A few technical considerations:

• Plan your strategy and anticipate the possibility of having to deal with complications such as procedural acute vessel closure.

• Use a 7F or 8F guiding catheter. Use an 8F when dealing with a distal left main lesion.

• Select the two best angiographic projections; assess the TIMI flow and entry angle in both branches when dealing with the bifurcation.

• Assess the size of the LCx and make sure that the RCA is patent.

• Use pre- and postprocedural IVUS in most cases, particularly with a distal left main stenosis.

• Give optimal anticoagulation. During the procedure GPIs may be required. Administer heparin and maintain the ACT between 250 and 300 seconds, or between 200 and 250 seconds if the patient has received a GPI already.

• Direct stenting: In the majority of cases if the lesion is not critical or severely calcified, direct stenting should be performed – often in a distal left main lesion or in an unstable patient to avoid the risk of dissection. In calcified lesions or very tight lesions, predilatation with a small balloon (2.0 mm to 2.5 mm) may be necessary.

• Prepare the lesion if necessary. Rotablation, atherectomy, or cutting balloon should be used in selected patients with calcified or fibrotic lesions.

• Remember that plaques are usually located close to the bifurcation but do not involve the carina itself.

• The majority of left main coronary arteries are larger than 3.5 mm and the stent diameter should never be smaller than 3.5 mm. Do not undersize stents.

It is better to use high balloon pressures and postdilate with a noncompliant balloon to achieve a good result. If in doubt, use IVUS. In ostial lesions, use a stent longer than 10 mm. Flare out the proximal end of an ostial stent with a noncompliant balloon 0.5 mm larger than the shaft balloon.

• DES should be used routinely.
• Always consider provisional stenting. When you need to use two stents, enter the side branch, crossing the main branch stent struts distally.
• When using two stents, always perform a final kissing balloon inflation, inject intracoronary glyceryl trinitrate, and check the angiogram.
• Always follow-up the patient and perform check angiography 6 months after the procedure.

An example of left main stenosis angioplasty is shown in Figure 5.3.

Lesion Location

PCI of left main ostial and body lesions has excellent early and late outcomes (death, myocardial infarction, and repeat revascularization), similar to those of surgery. Distal left main lesions that involve the bifurcation, however, are more challenging technically, and clinical outcomes in this group are inevitably worse. There is a higher risk of procedural complications including acute vessel closure and death, and poorer long-term outcomes with a higher risk of restenosis (particularly within the side branch ostium) and the need for repeat revascularization. For this reason, many patients with a distal left main bifurcation lesion should be considered for bypass surgery.

Provisional Approach or Complex Stenting?

The majority of left main lesions, including some bifurcations, can be treated with provisional stenting. A single stent technique is less demanding and has proven better outcomes, including a lower need for repeat revascularization, than a two-stent approach.

In selected patients, however, two stents may be required. The best two-stent strategy has not been established so it remains at the operator's discretion. The choices for a two-stent technique are shown in Table 5.3. In a two-stent approach, always perform two-step kissing balloon inflation with noncompliant balloons, check the result with IVUS, and use long-term dual antiplatelet therapy.

Ostial Left Main

Ostial lesions are generally difficult. A few considerations should be kept in mind:

• LAO cranial or LAO caudal views are best for ostial left main visualization.
• Good guiding catheter back-up support is needed.
• Stent length for an ostial left main should be longer than 10 mm. A stent shorter than this carries a higher risk of misplacement, migration, or embolization due to its unstable position in the left main coronary artery.

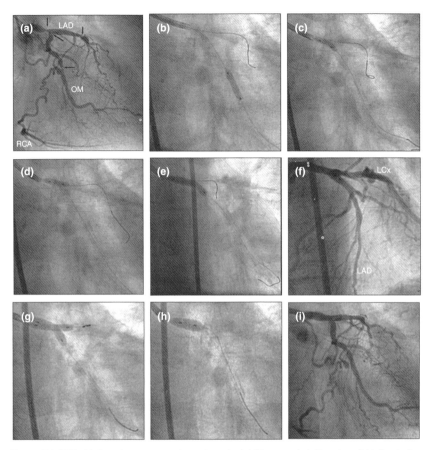

Figure 5.3 PCI of left main coronary artery stenosis. **(a)** Stenoses in left main, mid left anterior descending, ostial left circumflex, and mid obtuse marginal branch arteries (arrows). Retrograde filling of right coronary artery. **(b)** Left anterior descending artery and obtuse marginal branch wired; stent implantation in mid obtuse marginal branch. **(c)** POBA (plain old balloon angioplasty) of ostial left circumflex and left main stenosis. **(d)** POBA of left main and left anterior descending ostium. **(e)** Stent implantation in the left main into proximal left circumflex. **(f)** PA cranial view following stent implantation in the left main stem, the obtuse marginal branch and the left anterior descending artery. **(g)** Final kissing balloon inflation left main stem–left anterior descending–left circumflex. **(h)** Postdilatation in left main stem, wire removed from left anterior descending. **(i)** RAO 30° view, both wires removed. Final result.

• Before stent deployment, disengage the guiding catheter from the ostium and try to achieve an optimal stent position.

• Optimal stent positioning and expansion are essential to prevent acute elastic recoil and late negative remodeling. In case of elastic recoil, sandwich stenting – that is, implanting a second stent inside the existing one – may be effective.

Table 5.3 Choices for two-stent technique in patients with left main coronary artery disease.

Left Main Anatomy	Two-Stent Approach
Short left main	V-stenting
Distal lesion with 60° side branch	Minicrush
	Culotte
Distal lesion with 90° side branch	T-stenting
Significant lesions in the left main and left circumflex and the left circumflex is not suitable for stenting	Left main stenting and left circumflex balloon inflation
Left main disease with left circumflex involvement	Culotte
	V-stenting

• The stent should be placed with approximately 1 mm protruding into the ascending aorta. If it protrudes too far, re-engagement with the guiding catheter may be difficult or impossible and risks deforming the proximal end of the stent.
• The *Szabo technique* (see Figure 5.4) may be of help in achieving optimal stent positioning. In this technique, one wire is advanced into the left main and the second wire (anchor wire) is threaded through the last strut of the stent and placed in the aorta. When the entire stent–anchor wire system is advanced into the ostium, the second wire anchors the stent at the ostium and stops the stent moving forward. When the stent reaches the correct position in the ostium, it can be deployed at low pressure (6–8 atm). The anchor wire is then removed from the aorta and the stent can be deployed fully at high pressure followed by postdilatation with a noncompliant balloon (Figure 5.4).
• Ostial Pro device helps ensure correct stent positioning at the ostium and its complete coverage.
• It is best to perform short high-pressure (16 atm) inflations to limit the duration of ischemia.
• If the result is suboptimal, use IVUS to confirm the stent position and deploy a second overlapping stent.
   To learn more about technical caveats in ostial procedures, see pp. 238–252.

Body of the Left Main
The procedure is usually straightforward, and if the lesion does not involve the bifurcation, a single stent technique is best. In case of bifurcation involvement, provisional stenting is recommended. Short, high-pressure postdilatation with a noncompliant balloon is always necessary.

Distal Left Main Bifurcation
A lesion at the distal left main bifurcation is more difficult technically.
• Often the LCx has to be predilated to prevent plaque shift.
• If the angiogram shows a suboptimal result, provisional stenting of the LCx should be performed.

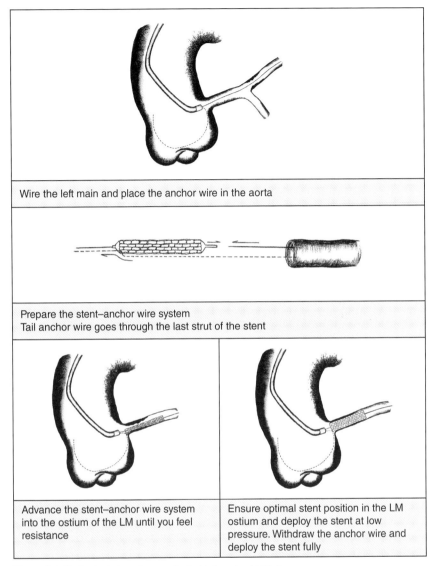

Figure 5.4 Szabo technique in unprotected left main stenting.

• If two stents are required, the optimal strategy is T-stenting or culotte technique (see pp. 204–238).
• The side branch needs to be recrossed distally if possible, before final kissing balloon inflation.
• Final kissing balloon at high pressure with noncompliant balloon is obligatory and must be performed routinely.

• Ideally pre- and postprocedural IVUS should be performed to assess the lesion and vessel size and to check optimal stent expansion and apposition.
• Dedicated bifurcation stents may become an attractive alternative in left main bifurcation stenting; however; there is insufficient data to confirm their superiority over currently used bifurcation techniques.

IVUS Guidance

The application of IVUS in left main stenosis gives invaluable information about the severity of disease, vessel calcification, distribution of atheromatous plaque, and bifurcation involvement. It will also help with stent sizing, optimal stent expansion, and stent apposition to the vessel wall. IVUS findings may also influence further treatment decisions.

Proceed with IVUS as follows:
• Use a 6–8F guiding catheter and avoid deep intubation.
• Give 3000–5000 units of heparin IV and 200 µg GTN before the IVUS transducer is inserted.
• Advance a wire into the left main, either to the LAD or LCx. If the lesion is very tight, first dilate the vessel using a small 2.5 mm balloon to avoid ischemia and then introduce a wire and the IVUS probe.
• Insert the IVUS probe beyond the bifurcation.
• Set up an automatic pull-back at a rate of 0.5 mm/s or, in the case of a long left main, at 1 mm/s.
• If you need to view the left main ostium, disengage the catheter from the left main.

IABP Support

Although there are no specific recommendations as to when IABP should be used, hemodynamic support may be required in complex left main procedures such as distal bifurcation lesions to help maintain coronary and cerebral blood flow. Patients who may benefit from IABP are generally at high risk with impaired left ventricular function, hypotension, or a chronically occluded RCA. In low-risk patients with normal left ventricular function, intra-aortic counterpulsation is usually not required.

Stent Thrombosis and Antiplatelet Treatment

It is important to find a balance between the anti-restenotic effect provided by DES and the potential risk of stent thrombosis. Compliance with dual antiplatelet therapy in all patients treated with DES is essential to avoid stent thrombosis. Data from multiple registries regarding the frequency of definite left main stent thrombosis is consistent and it ranges from 0.5% to 2.7% depending on the type of DES.

Optimal duration of the antiplatelet therapy specific for patients with left main stenosis has not been established and there is no evidence that long-term treatment beyond 12 months reduces death, myocardial infarction, or stent thrombosis in left main lesions. Current guidelines do not support any particular treatment strategy. However, it is suggested that a platelet aggregation check before left main PCI is performed if possible on clopidogrel 75 mg daily. If platelet aggregation is below 50%, the clopidogrel dose should be increased to 150 mg daily (see pp. 174–177).

All patient should receive aspirin and clopidogrel for at least 12 months after the procedure, followed by aspirin 75 mg daily indefinitely.

Follow-Up

Although the use of DES limits the risk of in-stent restenosis, it has not been eliminated completely. There are no recommendations with regard to timing of follow-up angiography. In many centers, all patients undergoing left main stenting routinely have angiographic follow-up at 3–4 months for bare metal stents, and at 4–6 months for DES.

Careful angiographic analysis of the left main is essential to determine the need for any further intervention. In patients with distal left main lesions who have received two stents, restenosis is usually located at the ostium of the LCx, probably because of sharp LCx angulation, gaps between two stents, or stent malapposition. Sometimes the angiographic appearance may suggest restenosis, for example in multiple metal layers (three metal layers after the crush technique), when in fact the ostium is clear if the lesion is assessed in different projections. If in doubt, IVUS may be helpful.

When significant restenosis has been angiographically confirmed, further treatment must be considered. Generally there are three options:
- **Balloon-only angioplasty.** This is preferred for focal restenosis. The drug-eluting balloon may be of value here.
- **Further DES implantation.** This is more suitable for restenosis at the stent margin, but carries a higher risk of recurrent adverse events. A long segment of in-stent restenosis may be managed by sandwich stenting, but, if severe, surgery is advisable.
- **Surgery.** Symptomatic patients with severe restenosis, particularly in the distal left main, will require surgery. Further treatment options must always be discussed with the patient.

TRIALS

MAIN-COMPARE

This was the first long-term study comparing PCI and stenting with bypass surgery. The study evaluated more than 2000 patients with unprotected left main coronary artery who underwent PCI (bare metal stent or DES) or CABG. Results from MAIN-COMPARE data suggested that there is no significant difference in major composite outcomes between stenting and surgery. The risk of death, Q-wave myocardial infarction, or stroke were similar in both groups. However, the rate of target vessel revascularization was significantly lower in the CABG group. The use of IVUS was shown to improve long-term outcomes in the PCI group.

SYNTAX
Data suggest that patients with isolated left main or single vessel disease treated with PCI (paclitaxel DES) had a lower stroke rate and shorter hospitalization time but a higher rate of incomplete revascularization and reintervention compared to the CABG group. There were no significant differences in risk of major adverse cardiac and cerebrovascular events for surgery versus stenting in the groups with low or intermediate SYNTAX scores. However, patients with a SYNTAX score of 33 or higher treated with CABG had significantly lower rates of major adverse cardiac and cerebrovascular events than the comparable PCI group. Although the trial failed to demonstrate noninferiority of PCI to CABG, stenting strategy outcomes at 1 year were equivalent to those seen after bypass surgery.

LE MANS
Results suggest that at 1 year PCI may significantly improve left ventricular function to a greater degree than CABG, with similar rates of major adverse cardiac and cerebrovascular events. This small but important trial showed that, for left main stem stenosis, outcomes following PCI and bypass surgery may be equivalent.

PRE-COMBAT
This is an ongoing multicenter study to compare the safety and efficacy of PCI with sirolimus-eluting stent and CABG for treatment of unprotected left main disease. A primary end point of 1-year major adverse cardiac and cerebrovascular events is expected to evaluate the choice of optimal revascularization.

ISAR-LM
This study randomized high-risk patients (acute coronary syndrome, previous myocardial infarction, previous PCI, multivessel disease, diabetes) with symptomatic left main disease undergoing PCI with DES (Taxus vs. Cypher). One-year follow-up showed no differences in the combined primary end points of death, myocardial infarction, or repeat revascularization in both groups. There were no significant differences in mortality at 2 years and a very low rate of definite stent thrombosis (0.3–0.7%) for both stent groups. Overall major adverse cardiac events at 2 years were similar. Results from ISAR-LM demonstrated that Taxus and Cypher stents provide similar clinical

and angiographic outcomes, and treatment of high-risk patients with left main disease with DES is safe and effective up to 2 years.

EXCEL

In this study 4000 patients with significant left main disease (angiographic stenosis >70% and IVUS minimum luminal cross-sectional area <6 mm^2) and SYNTAX score <33 are randomized to either PCI with Xience Prime stent or to CABG. Clinical follow-up is 30 days, 6 months, and yearly through 5 years. The 3-year primary end point is a composite of death, myocardial infarction or stroke. The 3-year secondary end point is a composite of death, myocardial infarction, stroke or unplanned revascularization. The first patient was enrolled in the third quarter of 2010.

Key Learning Points

- Full informed consent obtained by the operator is essential.
- Lesion preparation and IVUS guidance facilitate the procedure.
- Provisional side branch stenting is recommended in most cases.
- Always use DES and a minimum of 1 year dual antiplatelet therapy.
- Follow-up angiography after 3–9 months is recommended.

Bifurcation Lesions

- Trials, 233
- Dedicated Bifurcation Stents, 235

Introduction

Despite impressive advances in stent technology, the bifurcation lesion can be one of the most complex and demanding in PCI, with a higher risk of complications and a lower rate of procedural success than nonbifurcation lesions. Although DES have been shown to improve long-term results after bifurcation stenting, there is still no consensus on device or technique for all lesions. Bifurcation lesions are common. About 20% of all procedures will involve bifurcations and more than half of them the lesion will involve a side branch.

Basic Bifurcation Anatomy

Branch size obeys Murray's Law for vessel diameters ($PV \times 0.67 = MB + SB$ where PV = proximal vessel, MB = main branch, SB = side branch) (Sherman 1981). The overall mean angle between a main branch and side branch (distal angle or B angle) is $50°$ for non-left-main bifurcations and $95°$ for the left main bifurcation. When the branches form a T shape the distal angle is said to be wide and when they form a Y shape the angle is said to be narrow. The carina is the flow divider that lies between the main branch and side branch and is the region of high flow and high shear stress.

There are a few questions which must be considered:
- Lesion assessment. What is the exact anatomy of the lesion? This should be assessed after intracoronary injection of nitroglycerin.
- Is there severe disease of both branches (true bifurcation lesion)? Is the stenosis dominantly in either main or side branch, or is it just clear of the bifurcation? The Medina classification (see p. 206) is useful in this regard.
- What is the angle of the bifurcation?
- Which is the most important branch?
- What is the clinical importance (size of distribution and vessel diameter) of the side branch?
- How many wires are required?
- What is the severity and length of the side branch lesion, as long severe disease is more likely to need a side-branch stent. Is the ostium of the side branch involved?
- Should the side branch be predilated or not?
- Under what circumstances should the side branch be stented electively?
- If the decision is made to proceed with provisional stenting, when would a second stent be needed?
- Which stent is better – bare metal or DES?
- If the decision is made to proceed with two stents, which technique is the best?
- Is the standard final kissing balloon obligatory? When should two-step kissing balloon postdilatation be used?
- Is IVUS, optical coherence tomography, or FFR assessment necessary?

General Principles with Bifurcation Lesions

• Consider likely antiplatelet therapy compliance and the risk of stent thrombosis. Remember the risk of stent thrombosis with a two-stent bifurcation technique is higher than with a single-stent technique.
• Plan your procedure and be prepared to switch strategy or technique if necessary.
• Optimal radiographic visualization is essential. Assess the bifurcation in at least two views and choose the best working projections that profile the bifurcation.
• Choose a 6F guiding catheter or larger, preferably with extra backup support. You will deal with various devices. An 8F guide is required when two stents need to be deployed simultaneously (crush, simultaneous kissing, V, or Y), but simpler techniques involving only one stent at a time can be managed with a 6F guide.
• Assess the side branch and decide whether to proceed with a strategy of provisional or elective side-branch stenting.
• Generally use two wires – one in the main branch and one in the side branch.
• Prepare the lesion. Predilate or use debulking if necessary.
• Select the best technique for the bifurcation angle. Favor T-stenting in wide-angle bifurcations and culotte stenting if the angle is narrow (<70°).
• When in doubt, keep it simple. Both NORDIC and BBC One trials showed that a provisional stenting strategy was superior to more complex techniques. The fewer layers of metal in the bifurcation, the better.
• You may decide to ignore the side branch if it is small, or the side branch stenosis is mild.
• Use only DES.
• Be aware of the risk of periprocedural infarction caused by side branch occlusion due to carina shift during main branch stenting.
• If in difficulty, concentrate on the integrity of the biggest and most important branch, but aim to keep the side branch open.
• A two-stent procedure must be completed with final kissing balloon postdilatation.
• Using two stents obtains the best angiographic result in both branches but not necessarily the best short-term and long-term clinical outcomes.
• Ensure a minimum of 1 year dual antiplatelet therapy in all patients undergoing bifurcation stenting with DES.

Definition and Classifications

By definition a bifurcation lesion involves a clinically relevant side branch larger than 2.25 mm arising from the main vessel. The plaque may be located either in both branches or in the main vessel only or in the side branch only.

Numerous attempts have been made to classify bifurcation lesions to try to simplify the decision-making process. They are complex, and although valuable in classifying a lesion, do not really help the operator in deciding which technique to use. Their main value is enabling a comparison of techniques and clinical results.

Angulation and Plaque Burden

The bifurcation angle helps determine the best bifurcation strategy, e.g., T-stenting or provisional side branch stenting for wide-angle bifurcations, whereas crush stenting or culotte stenting may be chosen for a narrow-angled bifurcation. Carina/plaque shift is more likely with narrow distal angles, and proper ostial coverage of the side branch during stenting is more difficult or sometimes impossible. The great advantage of T-shape angulation (with the angle between the main vessel and the side branch >70°) is that plaque shift is less frequent and precise stent placement with complete ostial coverage is technically easier. However, wire access to the side branch is sometimes more challenging than in Y-shape angulation, especially if the distal angle is more than 90°. Sometimes the plaque proximal to a side branch with a wide angle can direct the wire away from the side branch, making it impossible to wire the branch. In these situations sometimes predilatation alters the anatomy and allows side branch wire access.

These points are summarized in Table 5.4.

Bifurcation Classification

The *Medina* is the best qualitative classification, simple and easy to remember. It is based on lesion distribution and lesion characteristics. The bifurcation has three parts: main branch proximally, main branch distally, and side branch. Each of these three is graded 0 (normal vessel) or 1 (significant lesion). Classification 1,0,1 would mean stenoses in proximal main branch and side branch, but a normal distal main vessel. This classification, however, has limitations and is not detailed enough to describe the bifurcation lesion itself. The Medina classification is available on the website www. wiley.com/go/essentialangioplasty.com.

Table 5.4 Stent strategy and bifurcation angle.

Distal Bifurcation Angle	Narrow (<70°)	Wide (>70°)
Bifurcation angle shape	Y-shape	T-shape
Side branch wire access	Easier	More difficult
Side branch stent access	Easier	More difficult
Carina/plaque shift into side branch	More likely	Less likely
Complete side branch ostial coverage	Difficult	Easier
T-stenting	Usually suboptimal	Ideal
Culotte or crush stenting	Easier	More difficult

The *MADS* system is based on stenting technique. MADS stands for: *m*ain, *a*cross, *d*istal, *s*ide.

M: Stenting main branch proximally first. Subsequent stents are placed distally in either the side branch or the main branch.

A: Stenting from the main branch across the ostium of the side branch first, followed by T-stenting, reverse crush, or culotte technique if necessary.

D: Distal stents first: either in main and/or side branch, followed by proximal main branch stent if necessary.

S: Side branch stenting first: either at the side branch ostium, or pulled back slightly into the main branch and then crushed with either balloon or stent in the main branch.

The MADS classification is available on the website www.wiley.com/go/essentialangioplasty.com.

Understanding Bifurcation Geometry

Blood Flow, Shear Stress, and Plaque Distribution

Local hemodynamic factors such as turbulent blood flow and shear stress (the force that the fluid flow exerts at the endothelium) influence atherosclerotic plaque distribution and contribute to native disease progression at coronary bifurcations. These result in typical patterns of plaque distribution; e.g., in the distal segment of the main stem plaque distribution is more eccentric, whereas more proximally plaque volume distribution tends to be more concentric.

Changes in the wall shear stress are due to variations in branch angles at the bifurcation. Abnormal shear stress is associated both with progression of atherosclerotic plaque, and also with neointimal hyperplasia. Usually plaque starts in low shear stress areas, only expanding into the high shear stress carina later. High shear (in laminar flow) observed at the carina seems to promote vasodilation, limiting the potential for thrombosis and limiting atheroma development, whereas low shear stress or changes in shear stress direction (in turbulent flow) promote endothelial proliferation, vasoconstriction, atheroma, and platelet aggregation.

Thus, the majority of atherosclerotic plaques are located in areas which are exposed to low shear stress, that is, on the non-flow-dividing walls between the main branch and the side branch, and in most bifurcations the carina itself is usually free of disease. This complex mechanism of plaque distribution at the bifurcation site has an important impact on bifurcation geometry. The carina may develop atheroma late and after atheroma is prominent in other regions of the bifurcation.

Side Branch Angle

Clinical studies vary regarding the impact of side branch angulation on clinical outcomes. These studies are often underpowered for outcome end points. Myocardial damage is more likely if the side branch angle is narrow, because stenting of the main branch may shift the carina into the side branch ostium, causing narrowing or occlusion. Carina shift is less likely with a wide angle (>70). In addition, longitudinal or circumferential shift of plaque after stenting can narrow an unstented branch.

Crossing Through the Side of a Main Branch Stent into the Side Branch

A common problem in treating a bifurcation lesion is side branch access. Difficulties entering the side branch or recrossing the side branch through the main branch stent struts may occur at each step of the procedure, e.g., if the result at the side branch ostium is suboptimal, or before the final kissing balloon inflation. Optimal wire selection and tip shaping as well as a good angiographic demonstration of the ostium are essential. In some cases it is easier to keep the wire in the main branch, passing it beyond the ostium of the side branch, and then pull the wire back until the preformed wide curve drops into the side branch ostium. If there is difficulty recrossing into the side branch after main branch stenting, then localized postdilatation confined to the region of stent overlying the side branch with a larger balloon may enlarge the gaps between struts (see "Proximal Optimization Technique" below).

Proximal and Distal Recrossing

The side branch crossing point contributes to the degree of distortion and the protrusion of struts into the side branch. Crossing into the side branch too proximally leaves the ostium of the side branch with poor scaffolding and with poor ostial coverage. This also causes metal overhang into the main branch, and the result is often not ideal. Distal crossing as close to the carina as possible ensures good ostial side branch coverage and optimizes side branch scaffolding. In addition, it improves the ability to place a side branch stent without gaps in scaffolding (Figure 5.5). Practically however, we often have little control over where the wire crosses and in many cases optimal crossing is not achieved especially if the side branch ostium has become severely narrowed.

Proximal Optimization Technique

If you have difficulty recrossing through the side of a stent into the side branch, you can try the so-called proximal optimization technique (POT) (Figure 5.6), which is not complicated:
• Choose a stent based on the size of the distal main vessel.
• Select a short, oversized noncompliant balloon (ideally, half a size larger).
• Inflate the balloon at the proximal part of the stent, that is, proximal to the carina, to facilitate access through the stent struts to the side branch. This proximal inflation also helps prevent the wire tracking behind the stent (between the stent and the vessel wall).

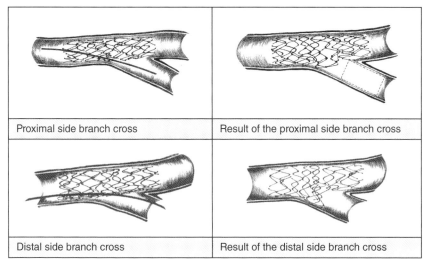

Proximal side branch cross	Result of the proximal side branch cross
Distal side branch cross	Result of the distal side branch cross

Figure 5.5 Technical considerations in bifurcation stenting: Proximal and distal recrossing.

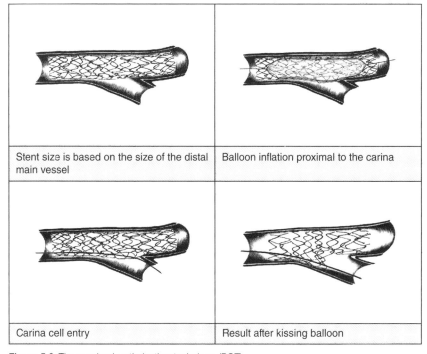

Stent size is based on the size of the distal main vessel	Balloon inflation proximal to the carina
Carina cell entry	Result after kissing balloon

Figure 5.6 The proximal optimization technique (POT).

"Kissing" Balloons

Incomplete stent expansion and stent strut malapposition to the vessel wall may increase the risk of in-stent restenosis, stent thrombosis, and target vessel revascularization. Adequate stent deployment has an important impact on early and long-term clinical outcomes, and final kissing balloon inflation in bifurcation lesions results in better angiographic outcomes and lower rates of major adverse cardiac events. However, one study (NORDIC III) concluded that routine kissing balloon inflation for all single stent deployments was neither beneficial nor detrimental and should be performed at the operator's discretion.

Despite the results from the NORDIC III study, there are many reasons why kissing balloon inflation remains an important part of the procedure.

Although final kissing balloon inflation may not be required in the absence of a tight lesion at the ostium of the side branch after main vessel stenting, in all tight residual side branch lesions (>75% after main branch stenting), or if TIMI flow is reduced, kissing balloon inflation will reduce the physiological significance of these. For this reason, kissing balloon inflation should be performed routinely with any persistent ostial side branch lesion that remains after main vessel stenting or if there is reduction in flow.

Secondly, with a single-stent technique, side branch balloon inflation results in stent distortion. Although the kissing balloon does not eliminate it completely, it helps to correct the distortion, which along with distal recrossing of the side branch ensures better stent scaffolding of the proximal aspect of the side branch ostium. With two-stent techniques, kissing balloons are essential to ensure full expansion at the side branch ostium for optimum scaffolding and drug application (see below).

The procedure itself is straightforward: always use a noncompliant balloon, and choose a balloon size that is the same size as the vessel (usually a slightly smaller diameter balloon for the side branch). First place a balloon in the side branch so that it protrudes into the side branch and extends into the main branch but not proximal to the stent. Advance another balloon (shorter than the main branch stent) to the main branch so it lies within the main branch but not extending beyond the confines of the stent. Inflate the balloons simultaneously (Figure 5.7).

The balloons should be deflated simultaneously or distortion may occur.

Note that the conventional final kissing balloon technique may not ensure full expansion of a side branch ostium. This can be improved by using the two-step kissing balloon inflation described below.

Two-Step Kissing

Compared with standard kissing postdilatation, two-step kissing balloon postdilatation improves stent expansion at the side branch and reduces the restenosis rate and repeat revascularization.

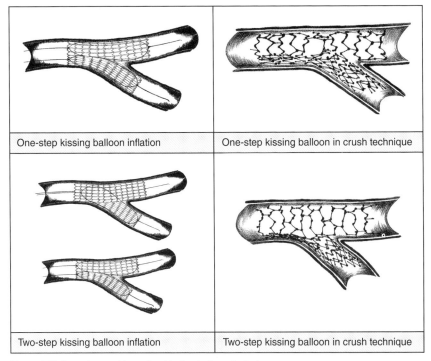

One-step kissing balloon inflation	One-step kissing balloon in crush technique
Two-step kissing balloon inflation	Two-step kissing balloon in crush technique

Figure 5.7 One-step and two-step kissing balloon technique.

Use noncompliant balloons sized for the distal vessel. For the first step, select a balloon that is a quarter size smaller than the distal side branch vessel and advance it to the side branch so that its proximal end lies in the main branch. Advance the main branch noncompliant balloon to the main branch. The balloons should lie entirely within the stents to avoid vessel damage outside the stents. Inflate the side branch balloon to high pressure (>20 atm, perhaps 24 or 26 atm) and deflate. Inflate the main branch balloon to moderate pressure and deflate.

The second step is simultaneous balloon inflation at low pressure to correct any distortion caused by sequential balloon inflation (Figure 5.7). The balloons should be deflated simultaneously to prevent reintroduction of stent distortion. This approach has been shown to improve results in all side branch angles.

Technical Considerations

Adequate visualization of the bifurcation lesion is essential for assessment of both vessels and choice of treatment strategy. The angiographic projection should minimize foreshortening and vessel overlap and display the side branch ostium to enable easy wire access and adequate stent positioning. Optimal bifurcation projections are described in detail on pp. 25–40.

Lesion Assessment and Preparation

A few important practical tips should be considered when dealing with bifurcation lesions:

• Assess the morphology of the bifurcation lesion based on the classifications given above.
• Assess the size of both branches, side branch angulation, plaque location, and the length and severity of the lesions.
• Be aware that side branches are usually larger than they appear on angiography.
• Use of IVUS is very helpful. It allows detailed lesion assessment and an accurate choice of stent size and stent apposition. Good stent expansion is very important.
• If IVUS is not available, ensure high pressure postdilatation.

Predilatation of bifurcation lesions is very important and should be performed for a variety reasons.

Carina Shift or Plaque Shift

Although in the majority of patients the carina is not involved with atheromatous plaque, data from CT angiography has demonstrated that a small amount of carinal atheroma may be present in up to one-third of bifurcation lesions, particularly if the total plaque burden is high. A stenosis which appears to be only in the main branch and crosses a side branch without involving its origin may turn into a bifurcation problem with the first balloon inflation.

The major cause of side branch narrowing after main branch treatment is "carina shift," meaning displacement of the carina across the side branch ostium. In addition, shifting of atheroma proximally or distally into the side branch ostium potentially complicates the procedure. Side branch narrowing is more likely if there is side branch ostial disease or the side branch angle is shallow.

Predilatation of the Main Branch

Predilatation of the main branch has several potential advantages and should always be considered if the upstream vessel is tortuous or the stenosis is tight or calcified. First, predilatation allows better vessel and lesion assessment, which gives valuable information about optimal stent length and diameter as well as stent position. Secondly, an adequately prepared vessel will make stent insertion easier. Finally, predilatation has been shown to reduce ischemic incidents during stent implantation.

Predilatation of the Side Branch
The side branch should be predilated if a two-stent technique is planned, but is not recommended for provisional side branch techniques because the inevitable damage and small dissection in the side branch may prevent wire recrossing into the side branch. Some experts disagree with this approach and do predilate.

Predilatation of the side branch must be performed carefully as it carries a risk of dissection, which will complicate the entire procedure and influence outcome. If dissection does occur, rewire the side branch through the struts of the main vessel stent and perform stent implantation.

Debulking
Rarely, debulking with rotational atherectomy may be needed to prepare the vessel, especially if it is heavily calcified. The great advantage of debulking is that the atherosclerotic plaque is removed before stent deployment. This has proved to reduce the risk of carina or plaque shift into the side branch ostium. It also facilitates stent apposition with a lower inflation pressure and ensures adequate stent expansion. Debulking is usually a complex procedure with the potential of an increased rate of procedural complications such as vessel perforation or myocardial infarction. Temporary RV pacing is required for rotablation (rotational atherectomy). Debulking techniques require good operator skills and careful device selection.

Two Wires
The most common mistake during bifurcation PCI is to use a single wire. In the majority of bifurcation procedures both the main branch and the side branch should be wired routinely.

Side branch wiring is very important for following reasons:
• To protect the side branch from occluding due to carina or plaque shift.
• To modify or to reduce the angle between the main branch and the side branch, which facilitates side branch recrossing.
• To identify the side branch ostium if the side branch is occluded.

A wire placed in the side branch helps keep the side branch open during main branch dilatation. If the side branch is occluded, the second wire will serve as a marker and will help identification of the side branch ostium. There is evidence that a wire in the side branch helps preserve its patency and improves clinical outcomes, reducing periprocedural myocardial infarction and the need for repeat intervention. Furthermore, insertion of the second wire influences the bifurcation geometry by reducing the angle between the main branch and the side branch, which facilitates side branch rewiring.

Side Branch Problems
The frequency of side branch occlusion during a bifurcation procedure remains high. Several mechanisms responsible for side branch occlusion have been observed:

• **Carinal/plaque shift.** As mentioned above, in some cases the side branch may be compromised due to carina or plaque shift, either during predilatation or during stent positioning.

• **Side branch dissection.** The risk of side branch dissection is always higher when dealing with small vessels (diameter <2.5 mm). The side branch may also be dissected during balloon inflation or stent deployment in the main branch. Wide side branch angulation also increases the risk of side branch dissection. Side branch dissection may prevent rewiring.

• **Side branch spasm**, particularly at the ostium, may also occur due to adjacent main branch balloon inflation or stent deployment or vigorous wire manipulation. The side branch may be difficult to enter with a wire, and good angiographic visualization, selection of a hydrophilic wire, and precise shaping of the wire tip help to facilitate side branch access. A word of caution about hydrophilic wires: try to avoid deploying a main branch stent with a hydrophilic wire in the side branch, as these wires are more likely to be damaged or broken than conventional wires when as a standard part of a provisional strategy one is trapped (jailed) outside the main branch stent.

• **Jailing of the side branch ostium** by stent struts.

• **Side branch occlusion.** There are some angiographic predictors of possible side branch occlusion which should be considered:
  – Narrow bifurcation angle that is less than 50°
  – Ostial side branch stenosis
  – Length of side branch stenosis
  – Small side branch diameter (<2.5 mm)

The risk of side branch occlusion can be decreased by appropriate stent size selection (stent diameter should be based on the distal reference diameter). The diameter of the main branch stent can be then increased proximal to the carina by kissing balloon postdilatation.

Which Vessel Should Be Wired First?
From a practical point of view it is sensible to advance the first wire into the less accessible and more challenging branch. Whereas wiring the main branch is usually straightforward, side branch access may become more difficult. If you fail to enter the side branch, reshape the tip of the wire, change the wire type, or use techniques described above.

When two wires are used, it is important to be able to identify which wire is which outside the patient and on the catheter table. Some operators keep the wires in the same position on the table as on the monitor to facilitate identification. Others make a small bend on the proximal end of one of the wires. Most operators will separate the wires on the table with a drape. An

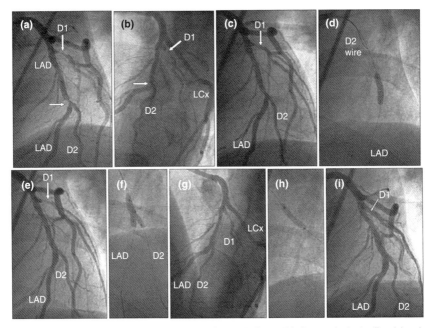

Figure 5.8 Bifurcation left anterior descending/second diagonal lesion angioplasty. Provisional T-stenting (additional stenting of D1 lesion). JL3.5 8F guide. **(a)** PA cranial view. Tight stenosis in proximal first diagonal (D1), stenosis in mid left anterior descending artery (LAD) at bifurcation with second diagonal (D2). **(b)** LAO cranial view to show both lesions (arrows). **(c)** PA cranial view. LAD and diagonal wired. Result of balloon dilatation (3.0 × 15 mm balloon) of both vessels. **(d)** PA cranial view. Diagonal wire withdrawn. LAD stent deployed (3.5 × 15 mm). **(e)** PA cranial view. Result of LAD stenting. Good LAD result. Fair result at D2 origin without additional D2 stenting. **(f)** PA cranial view. D2 rewired through LAD stent. Kissing balloons in LAD and D2 (3.5 × 13 mm balloons). **(g)** LAO cranial view. Final result in LAD and D2. (LAD stent and D2 POBA). **(h)** PA cranial view. Stenting of D1 stenosis with 3.0 × 12 mm stent. **(i)** Final result.

alternative is to attach different colored torquers to the wires to avoid confusion and possible inadvertent withdrawal of the wrong wire. Whichever technique is chosen, the wires must not be mixed up!

Wire exchange can be made easier by tip shaping to facilitate access to the side branch through the main branch stent struts (see pp. 96–97).

An example of bifurcation lesion angioplasty (provisional side branch stenting) is shown in Figure 5.8.

Bifurcation Techniques

Treatment of bifurcation lesions can be divided into three categories: "keep it open" (side branch open), provisional side branch stenting, and two-stent strategies. Provisional stenting remains the most recommended initial treatment option.

One Stent or Two Stents?

This decision should be based on side branch characteristics. The following issues need to be considered:

• Is it a true bifurcation?
• How large is the side branch?
• Is the side branch clinically relevant and supplying a significant area of myocardium? Is the side branch contributing much?
• Is the side branch severely diseased?
• Does the lesion extend beyond the ostium?

Side Branch Assessment

In most cases side branch lesions are relatively short (<3.5 mm in length), located close to the bifurcation, and do not involve the carina. In general, treatment may be needed if the side branch is larger than 2.5 mm and becomes occluded. If the side branch diameter is very small (<2.0 mm) a "keep it open" strategy is the only option (Figure 5.9).

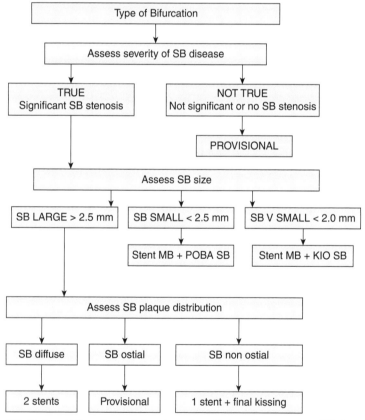

Figure 5.9 Choice of bifurcation technique based on side branch assessment. KIO, keep it open; MB, main branch; POBA, plain old balloon angioplasty; SB, side branch.

"Keep It Open"

Sometimes it is necessary to keep the side branch open without rewiring, predilatation, stenting, or postdilatation. This strategy is required when the side branch is not suitable for stenting (smaller than 2.0 mm) or is clinically unimportant, or when the side branch has ostial or diffuse disease.

To deal with this type of bifurcation, proceed as follows:

- Use a 6F guide.
- Wire both branches. Keep a wire in the side branch to maintain side branch patency.
- Predilate only the main branch.
- Stent the main branch, leaving wire in the side branch so that it is outside the main branch stent (trapped).
- Do not rewire the side branch as it may result in dissection.
- Do not postdilate the side branch as this may cause side branch occlusion due to elastic recoil or plaque shift.
- Postdilate only the main branch, with a wire left in the side branch.
- Remove side branch wire.
- Check result and consider provisional strategy if necessary.

Provisional Side Branch Stenting

Provisional stenting remains the gold standard technique for most bifurcation cases, and the majority of bifurcations lesions can be treated successfully with one stent. Essentially, the main branch is stented first and the side branch is stented afterwards only if necessary after kissing balloon dilatation.

When Is It Necessary?

The principle is to stent the side branch only if a severe stenosis and reduced flow is present in the side branch after main branch stenting. Generally, side branch stenting is appropriate if:

- the vessel diameter is reasonably large (2.5 mm or larger), or
- TIMI flow grade is 0 or 1 in the side branch after main branch stenting, or
- there is a greater than 70% stenosis in the side branch.

Assessing the side branch ostium by fractional flow reserve (FFR) is recommended but not widely used in practice.

In the single-stent strategy, correct stent sizing is important for a good result. The stent placed in the main vessel should be sized according to the distal, not proximal main vessel diameter (see p. 111).

Provisional Stenting Step by Step

- Use a 6F guiding catheter.
- Wire both branches.
- Predilate the main branch only. The side branch should not be predilated, because potential side branch dissection may prevent wire entry into the side branch.

- Stent the main branch across the side branch ostium, leaving a wire in the side branch.
- Check on angiography.
- If the result in the main branch and the side branch is optimal, gently remove the jailed wire from the side branch and finish the procedure.
- If the result is not satisfactory, leave the jailed wire in the side branch and recross the side branch (the most difficult part) with the main branch wire. Then withdraw the jailed wire into the main branch and recross the main branch stent with this wire (ie wire swapping).
- Dilate the side branch, then follow with kissing balloon postdilatation to improve side branch stenosis and flow, correct main branch stent distortion, and scaffold the side branch ostium.
- Withdraw the balloons leaving both wires in place.
- Check angiography.
- Assuming an excellent main branch result and TIMI grade 3 flow in side branch, do nothing more (see Figure 5.8).
- If the final result is unsatisfactory a second stent may be required.

Assess TIMI flow, side branch size, percentage of residual stenosis, and FFR if possible, and check if the side branch has been dissected. A second stent in the side branch is needed if:

- The side branch still shows slow flow (TIMI < 3).
- The side branch diameter is 2.5 mm or larger.
- The residual stenosis is great than 70% (carinal/plaque shift).
- FFR is below 0.75.
- The side branch is severely dissected.

This strategy, although relatively simple, has some limitations. Sometimes side branch wiring is very difficult or impossible, which leaves the vessel untreated. Even if side branch wiring is successful, advancing a balloon or stent to the side branch may fail and the side branch has to be left unstented.

Two-Stent Strategies

Although major adverse cardiac events have been reduced by advances in bifurcation techniques and the introduction of drug-eluting stents (DES), a two-stent approach is a complex procedure and carries a higher risk of adverse events compared with simple stenting. New studies (BBC ONE) have shown that, although there is no difference in mortality and target lesion revascularization between one- and two-stent strategies, a two-stent approach results in a higher rate of periprocedural myocardial infarction. Therefore, achieving an optimal final result is critical to a good long-term result.

There are a few situations in which an elective two-stent technique can be considered:

- The side branch is reasonably large (>2.5 mm) with ostial disease extending more than 5 mm from the carina.

• The side branch is clinically important, supplying a significant area of myocardium.
• The side branch has a flow-limiting dissection.
  In addition:
• The choice of technique depends on the angulation of the side branch.
• T-stenting is best when the distal angle is wide.
• After side branch stenting, the side branch should be postdilated with a noncompliant balloon at high pressure.
• A final kissing balloon inflation, usually at low pressure, is mandatory.

General Considerations
There are a few general rules which apply to all two-stent techniques:
• Most techniques can be carried out through a 6F guide but an 8F guide is needed for V stenting, SKS (simultaneous kissing stent), and most crush stenting.
• Consider administration of a glycoprotein IIb/IIIa inhibitor (GPI) for very complex stenting or suboptimal results.
• Recrossing into the side branch is very important and should performed carefully and precisely. Use a standard Pilot 50, BMW or stiffer Asahi wire.
• Before recrossing into the side branch with a wire, dilate the main vessel stent with balloon at moderate pressure.
• Postdilate both branches sequentially at high pressure using a noncompliant balloon (main branch first, then the side branch). Some advise against high pressure postdilatation because it may rarely be very difficult or impossible to remove the side branch wire and there is a risk of wire fracture.
• Always perform final one- or two-step kissing balloon inflation for optimum stent expansion, especially side branch ostial expansion. Afterwards use a short noncompliant balloon and inflate the proximal stent for correction of oval-shaped proximal stent distortion caused by kissing balloon inflation.
  A few two-stent techniques are available, but none offers obvious advantages (Table 5.5).
• T-stenting and T-stenting with protrusion (TAP)
• Crush and minicrush
• Culotte stenting
• V-stenting
• Simultaneous kissing stent technique (SKS)
• Y-stenting, also called the Helquist procedure
  If provisional stenting is required, the optimal strategy is to use the T-stenting technique. When a decision has been made to treat the bifurcation with two stents, the next best techniques are culotte, minicrush, or V-stenting.

Table 5.5 Bifurcation techniques: advantages and disadvantages.

Technique	Advantages	Disadvantages
V-stenting	Both branches protected Rewiring not needed	Stenosis of the proximal vessel Poor side branch ostium coverage
Crush	Side branch ostium fully covered Both branches patent immediately	Rewiring side branch Three strut layers
Reverse crush	Suitable for any anatomy Complete ostium coverage	Recrossing needed Three strut layers at carina
Culotte	Very good side branch ostium coverage	Time consuming Rewiring both branches Two strut layers at carina
Simultaneous kissing stents	Technically simple Both branches protected Rewiring not required Proximal lesion covered	Suitable only for large vessel with small angle Stent implantation proximally or distally to kissing stents
T-stenting with protrusion	Very good side branch ostium coverage Technically easy Rewiring not needed	Struts protruding in to main branch

T-Stenting (see Figure 5.10)

This strategy is ideal for bifurcation lesions if the disease in the main branch is proximal to the bifurcation and the side branch angle at the origin is wide, for instance 90°. The first stent is positioned at the side branch ostium without protruding into the main branch, followed by a second stent deployed in the main branch. Both branches should be dilated and a balloon may be left in the main branch, which helps locate it later on. The stent in the side branch should be deployed with its proximal end at the side branch ostium. Try to avoid stent protrusion into the main branch. The wire and balloon are removed from the side branch and a second stent is advanced into the main branch. At the end the side branch is rewired, before the final kissing balloon inflation.

Advantages and Disadvantages Classic T-stenting needs two stents. It is best if the side branch origin is at 90° and the main branch lesion extends proximal to the bifurcation. If the side branch angle is narrow this is not the technique of choice. There is the risk that there will be incomplete stent coverage of the angle between the main and side branches at the ostium. This small gap in scaffolding and drug application may be the site of restenosis. This can be limited by correct rewiring of the side branch. When recrossing from the main branch into the side branch, the wire should cross distally near the flow divider so that, after postdilatation, struts protrude optimally from the main branch into the side branch, minimizing the gap in scaffolding between the

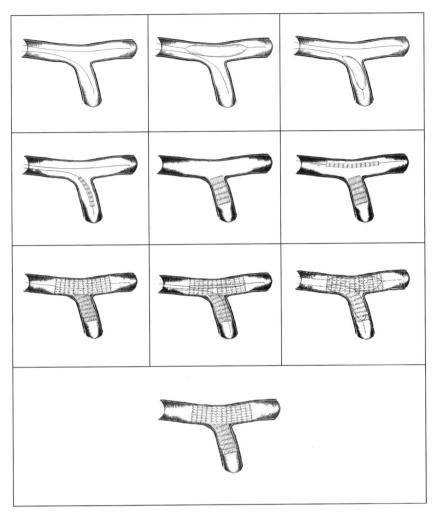

Figure 5.10 T-stenting technique.

main branch and side branch stents in narrow distal angled bifurcations (see above). The alternative is to use the, TAP technique but with this technique there is protrusion of side branch stent struts into the main branch.

T-Stenting Step by Step (Figure 5.10)
- Use a 6F guiding catheter.
- Advance a wire into the main branch and another to the side branch.
- Predilate both branches.
- Two stents are used. The side branch stent is advanced first, avoiding protrusion into the main branch.

• Some operators inflate the main branch balloon at low pressure to facilitate positioning of the side branch stent, but this may require a guide larger than 6F.
• The side branch stent is deployed and the wire and the balloon are removed from the side branch.
• The main branch stent is advanced next and deployed across the side branch (T-formation). After deployment, the deflated balloon and the wire are still in the main branch.
• The main branch balloon may need to be removed, because sometimes its crossing profile is too wide to allow kissing postdilatation through a 6F guide.
• The side branch is rewired through a single layer of the main branch stent struts and a balloon is advanced into the side branch for the final kissing balloon inflation.
• Final kissing balloon inflation.

T-Stenting and Protrusion
T-Stenting and protrusion (TAP) is a modified version of the T-stenting technique and is an elective side branch strategy. It is most suitable for a bifurcation lesion with a narrow distal angle of 60° or less. The great advantage of this approach is full scaffolding and drug application to the side branch ostium. The final kissing balloon modifies the angulation of the side branch stent struts protruding into the main branch if the side branch balloon is deflated first. A potential disadvantage is that side branch stent struts protrude into the main branch.

TAP Step by Step (Figure 5.11)
• Use a 6F guiding catheter.
• Wire and predilate both branches.
• The main branch stent is advanced first.
• Recross into the side branch through the single layer of the main branch stent struts. This is the most difficult part of the technique.
• Predilate through the side of the main branch stent, then advance the second stent into the side branch.
• Withdraw the side branch stent, allowing it to protrude slightly (1–2 mm) into the main branch. Side branch stent protrusion into the main branch prevents gaps and ensures full coverage of the ostium by placing the proximal stent edge at the proximal border of the ostium.
• Deploy the side branch stent, then carry out kissing postdilatation.

Crush Techniques
In majority of centers, crush technique has been replaced by culotte, minicrush stenting, or T-stenting. There are a few modifications of the classic crush technique, such as minicrush, step crush, and internal crush. All of these

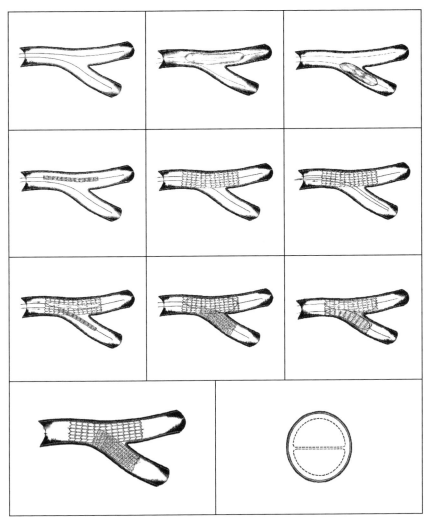

Figure 5.11 T-Stenting and protrusion (TAP) technique.

techniques require final side branch rewiring and high-pressure side branch dilatation as part of two-step kissing balloon postdilatation.

Classic Crush and Minicrush An 8F guide is needed. In the classic crush technique, two stents are positioned together. The side branch stent is deployed first ,and deployment of the main branch stent crushes the side branch stent. Kissing postdilatation follows.

Advantages and Disadvantages: Crush deployment is easy, quick, and ensures side branch patency. However, kissing balloon postdilatation, which is essential for the best clinical outcomes, is difficult and in trials is not achieved in significant proportion of patients. The difficulty lies with rewiring the side branch, which is the major disadvantage of the technique. There is the potential for gaps in scaffolding and drug application close to the side branch ostium. Late results do indicate a small percentage of late side branch occlusions, and early comparative studies suggest the culotte technique may be superior in cases where two stents are required (NORDIC study). Inevitably in the crush technique there are three layers of struts in the crushed portion, with increased vessel damage and increased antiproliferative drug dose with DES to that region of vessel wall.

Classic Crush Step by Step (Figure 5.12)
• Use a 7F or 8F guiding catheter; 8F is best from the femoral artery. You may just manage with a 7F guide, but it is not possible with a standard 6F guide.
• Wire both branches and predilate both branches.
• The side branch stent positioned first across the side branch ostium must be long enough to cover the side branch lesion.
• The main branch stent is positioned next, with its proximal marker more proximal than the proximal marker on the side branch stent, i.e., covering it.
• The side branch stent is pulled back very slightly so that approximately 3 mm are in the main branch. Do not deploy this stent yet!
• Check in two views that the stents are correctly positioned.
• Deploy the side branch stent first. Check angiogram for side branch patency.
• Remove side branch balloon and wire if there is a good stent lumen and no distal side branch dissection on angiography.
• Deploy the main branch stent at high pressure (>20 atm). This crushes the protruding 3 mm of the side branch stent. Check the angiogram.
• Rewire the side branch stent through the side of the main branch stent. This is the most difficult maneuver because there are two layers of struts across the side branch ostium and it may be impossible.
  Two-step kissing postdilatation is now performed:
• First advance a noncompliant balloon into the side branch stent (after pre-dilatation to separate struts) and postdilate across the ostium at high pressure (>20 atm).
• A second noncompliant balloon is then advanced down the main branch to postdilate the main branch stent at high pressure. Then simultaneous kissing balloon inflation is performed at low pressure.

Minicrush (Modified T-Stenting) This technique limits the extent of multiple layering of crushed struts compared with the classic crush. The most favorable clinical outcomes have been shown with a narrow side branch angle of <50°. However, the minicrush technique can be successfully used in both T-shaped and Y-shaped bifurcations. Always perform final two-step kissing balloon postdilatation.

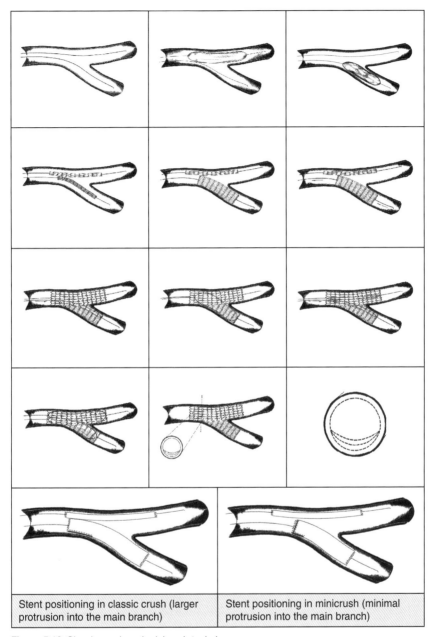

Stent positioning in classic crush (larger protrusion into the main branch) | Stent positioning in minicrush (minimal protrusion into the main branch)

Figure 5.12 Classic crush and minicrush techniques.

Step Crush This is similar in principle to the classic crush but is a staged procedure which allows the use of a 6F guide from either the femoral or the radial route: essentially one stent at a time. The side branch is stented first, but is crushed with a main branch balloon only. If at this stage there is balloon predilatation into the side branch, struts are partially cleared from the side branch ostium, which makes crossing easier after main branch stent deployment. The main branch stent is then deployed, followed by kissing postdilatation.

Step Crush Step by Step (Figure 5.13)
• Use a 6F guide.
• Wire and predilate both branches.
• Position the stent in the side branch (as in classic crush above, or as in minicrush), protruding the stent slightly into the main branch.
• Position a noncompliant balloon in the main branch and keep it there if the guide will accommodate a balloon and a stent at the same time. Otherwise, do not try to place a balloon in the main branch.
• Deploy the side branch stent first and check angiography. If the side branch appears satisfactory, remove the side branch wire and balloon.
• Inflate the main branch balloon, crushing the protruding 3 mm of the side branch stent that lie in the main branch.
• Remove the wire and the balloon from the main branch. Check angiogram.
• Wire the side branch stent through the single layer of crushed struts across the ostium and carry out balloon dilatation into the side branch, opening up the struts.
• Position the stent in the main branch across the side branch ostium, fully covering the protruding side branch stent.
• Deploy the main branch stent and remove the deploying balloon.
• Then proceed as in the final stages of the classic crush technique, rewiring the side branch with a one-step or two-step kissing balloon procedure as follows:
• Rewire the side branch stent through the side of the main branch stent.
• Perform two-step kissing inflation: first advance a balloon into the side branch stent and postdilate it at high pressure (20 atm), then perform classic kissing postdilatation.

Advantages and Disadvantages This is a crush technique that can be performed through a 6F guide, avoiding the need to upsize to a larger guide catheter. It has more stages than the standard crush procedure. It allows the radial operator the use of a crush technique.

Internal Crush (Reverse Crush) This is a provisional two-stent technique, a modification of TAP (described above), that involves main branch and ostial side branch stenting. It is usually used in cases where there is a suboptimal

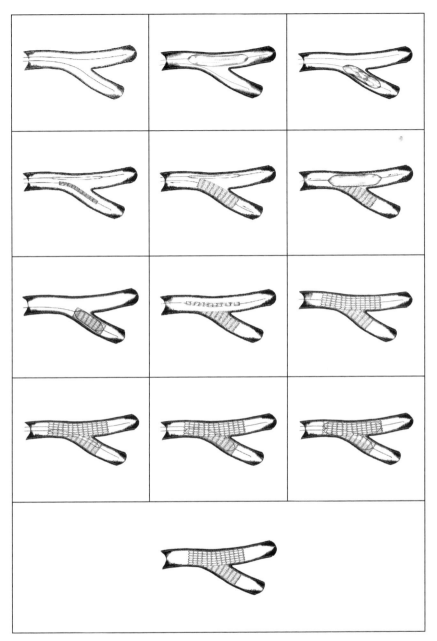

Figure 5.13 Step crush technique.

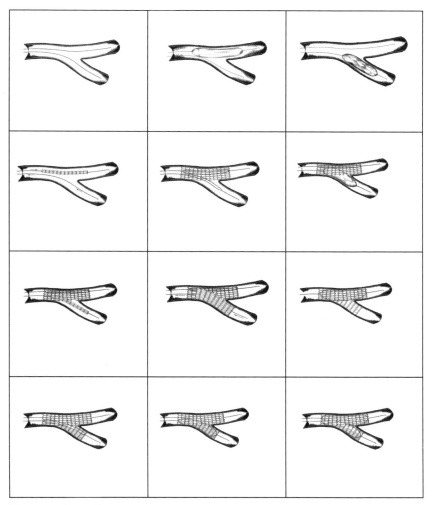

Figure 5.14 Internal/reverse crush technique.

final result with a need for a second stent, rather than as an elective procedure.

Advantages and disadvantages are as in the step crush technique.

Internal or Reverse Crush Step by Step (Figure 5.14) This is potentially a provisional side branch stenting strategy.
- Use a 6F guide.
- Advance wires into both branches and predilate both branches.
- Advance a stent into the main branch but do not deploy it yet. Remove the side branch wire.

- Deploy the main branch stent across the side branch ostium, and remove the main branch balloon.
- Rewire the side branch through the main branch stent struts and advance a balloon into the side branch. This may bedifficult.
- When the side branch has been successfully recrossed, inflate the balloon in the side branch, then withdraw the balloon. Advance a stent into the side branch.
- Position the side branch stent with minimal protrusion, pulling it back about 2–3 mm into the main branch.
- Deploy the side branch stent. Check angiogram.
- If the result is satisfactory, remove the side branch wire.
- Now advance and inflate a main branch balloon at 20 atm, crushing the short protruding segment of the side branch stent (>20 atm).
- Then proceed as in the final stages of classic crush: rewiring the side branch with a two-step kissing balloon procedure. It is easier to cross into the side branch now because the struts have been partially cleared from the main branch earlier in the procedure.

Culotte Technique
The culotte technique is most suitable for a bifurcation lesion with main branch disease which extends proximal to the bifurcation and a side branch with an approximately 60° angle or less at the origin. The culotte is a technique which gives good coverage of the side branch ostium and widely patent branches, at the expense of a double layer of metallic struts in the proximal main branch. Although it involves two stents, they are delivered separately and it is possible to use a 6F guide. This technique is more demanding on the nerves as for a short while one vessel (usually the main branch) remains unstented but jailed by stent struts. If it is not possible to cross through the side of the first stent to the jailed vessel, there is a risk of vessel occlusion. With wide distal bifurcation angles the T technique is preferred. In comparison with the crush technique, the culotte technique has a lower combined rate of restenosis, death, myocardial infarction, target vessel revascularization, and stent thrombosis (NORDIC culotte vs. crush trial).

Advantages and Disadvantages This technique ensures a metal coverage of the bifurcation, but with a double layer of stent in the proximal main branch. Two rewiring maneuvers are needed to complete the procedure and this may just not prove possible. Secondly, it is preferable to choose a stent with an open cell design to allow full expansion of the gap through which a second stent must pass. Most contemporary stents have potential cell sizes (potential areas between struts) that are sufficiently large for culotte deployment without constriction.

Culotte Technique Step by Step (Figure 5.15)
- Use a 6F guide.
- Wire and predilate both branches.

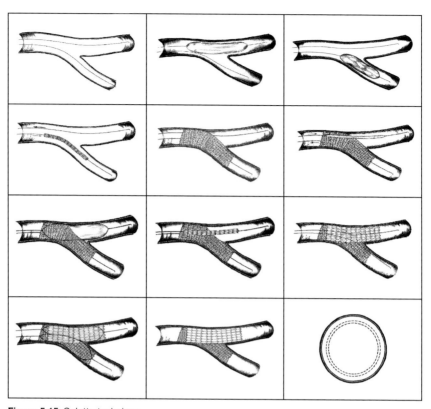

Figure 5.15 Culotte technique.

- Position and deploy a stent into the branch with the sharpest angulation (usually the side branch) while retaining the wire in the other branch.
- Check angiogram. If satisfactory, remove side branch wire and redirect it into the main branch through the side of the deployed side branch stent. Remove the trapped wire. Then advance a noncompliant balloon through the side of the side branch stent into the main branch.
- Position the main branch balloon through the side of the side branch stent and dilate this new opening in the side of the stent with a noncompliant balloon. Remove this balloon over the wire.
- Now advance a second stent through the side of the side branch stent into the distal main branch.
- Deploy this second stent in the main branch.
- Rewire the side branch through the side of the main branch stent struts.
- Advance a balloon into the side branch and perform final kissing balloon postdilatation.

Simultaneous Kissing Stents Technique
Essentially an 8F guide is needed to deploy two stents simultaneously: either in a Y manner (shotgun, or Helqvist technique) or in a V formation. The V stent technique (see below) is preferable, with minimal or no protrusion of the stents into the main proximal branch, thus avoiding the central division of a main lumen by two layers of stent struts (a metal neocarina). The technique for the two procedures is very similar, just differing in the length of stents protruding into the proximal main branch. V-stenting needs a large disease-free proximal vessel and Medina 0,1,1 disease distribution.

Advantages and Disadvantages SKS is a relatively simple technique with the advantage that balloon inflation of the stents is in itself a kissing balloon procedure. The disadvantage of Y-stenting is the neocarina of two layers of struts in the main branch, which especially in smaller-caliber vessels may lead to stent thrombosis.

SKS Step by Step (Figure 5.16)
- Use an 8F guide via the femoral artery.
- Wire both branches and predilate both branches.

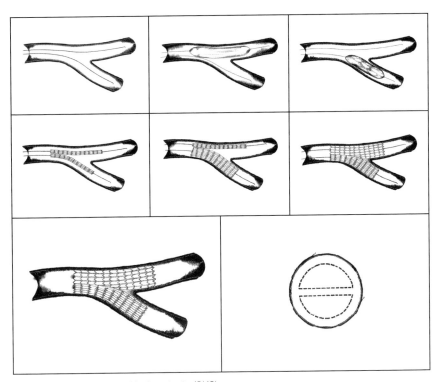

Figure 5.16 Simultaneous kissing stents (SKS).

- Assess the stent size from the side branch size, not the main branch size.
- Position a stent in each branch. The stents do not have to be the same length or diameter, but in both the V and the Y stent procedure the proximal stent markers must be absolutely adjacent to each other (check in two views if in doubt).
- Inflate the side branch stent first, then the main branch.
- Pull the balloons back several millimeters so that they do not protrude distally beyond the stents. Inflate each balloon sequentially, then together to postdilate.
- Remove both balloons and recheck angiography.

V Stenting

This technique is useful for only a very small number of bifurcation lesions. It is most suitable for Medina 0,1,1 bifurcations with an ample-sized main branch. It is thus suitable for dilatation of a very short left main or of a left main stem bifurcation where the main disease is in the ostium of the LAD and LCx, but the main stem itself is disease-free. V-stenting is a relatively simple technique with the advantage that balloon inflation of the stents is in itself a kissing balloon procedure. The disadvantages are the need for a large guiding catheter (8F) and the possibility of two adjacent layers of stent metal dividing the main branch if the Y formation is used (see advantages and disadvantages of SKS above), which may be prone to thrombosis. The technique is similar to SKS, just differing in the length of stent protruding proximally into the main branch.

V-Stenting Step by Step (Figure 5.17) Use V-stenting when dealing with the left main with large branches and proceed as follows:
- Use an 8F guide via the femoral artery.
- Wire both branches and predilate both branches.
- Assess stent sizes from the side branch sizes, not the main branch size.
- Advance a stent to the main branch and one to the side branch. The first stent should be advanced slightly more distally to facilitate the insertion of the second stent.
- Pull both stents back to the bifurcation, creating a V-shape, and make sure that the proximal markers are absolutely adjacent, then deploy the stents at low pressure. Sequential inflations with the deploying balloons can postdilate the stents. Final simultaneous inflation is needed to correct distortion.
- The limitation of V-stenting is the problem of possible upstream dissection in the main branch.
- Stenting of upstream main branch dissection usually results in the procedure turning into a crush procedure, when the final result is usually suboptimal.

Y-Stenting or Helqvist Procedure

This involves stenting the main branch up to the bifurcation, then deploying stents in the branches using the V-stenting technique described above. It can

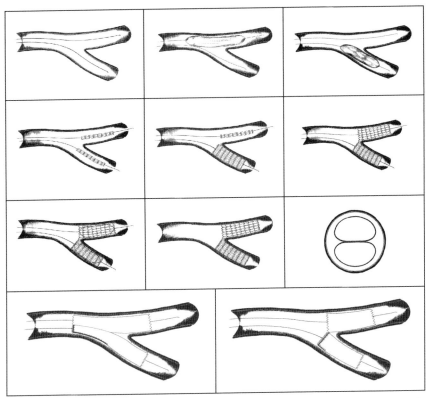

Figure 5.17 V-Stenting. Lowermost images show stent positioning in SKS technique (left) and in V-stenting (right). Place proximal markers at the same position together.

be used in Medina 1,1,1 bifurcation disease and in addition prevents the potential problem of main branch dissection with V-stenting in Medina 0.1.1 disease treatment.

Trials
Although both simple and complex stenting techniques provide optimal stent apposition when correctly performed, studies suggest that a simple stenting strategy is better than a complex one.

NORDIC I
This study, along with the BBC ONE trial (see below), has had a major influence on how bifurcation lesions are treated. Both support a simple strategy of a single stent in the main branch with side branch stenting only if necessary. In the Nordic I trial, 413 patients with straightforward bifurcation lesions were randomized to a single stent to the main branch or a double-stent strategy. The simple single-stenting strategy was associated with reduced

procedure and fluoroscopy times and lower rates of procedure-related biomarker elevation.

BBC ONE

In this study 500 patients were randomized to either a simple strategy (provisional T-stenting) or a complex strategy (crush or culotte techniques) using paclitaxel-eluting stents. At 9 months clinical follow-up there was a significantly higher rate of death, myocardial infarction, and revascularization in the group randomized to the complex strategy. These results supported a simple strategy of main branch stenting with provisional side branch stenting for straightforward bifurcation lesions.

NORDIC Complex Bifurcation Stenting Study

In this study 424 patients were randomized for bifurcation treatment by either a crush or culotte technique using sirolimus-eluting stents. At 6-month clinical follow-up there was no significant difference between the two groups with regard to death, postprocedural myocardial infarction, or revascularization. Both the crush and culotte arms had excellent clinical and angiographic results, but the incidence of in-stent restenosis was significantly higher in the group randomized to the crush technique.

CACTUS

In this study 350 patients were randomized to either provisional T-stenting or the crush technique. A limitation of this trial is the high rate, 31%, of patients randomized to provisional T-stenting, receiving a side branch stent so that the control arm was not treated as simply as in the NORDIC or BBC ONE trials. There was no significant difference in primary clinical outcomes in terms of death, myocardial infarction, and revascularization between the two groups.

NORDIC III

In this study 477 patients with bifurcation lesions were randomized to provisional T-stenting with or without final kissing balloon inflation. The primary end points at 6 months were death, myocardial infarction, target lesion revascularization, and stent thrombosis. A strategy of routine kissing balloon inflation did not improve early clinical outcomes in low-risk patients compared with a strategy of no kissing balloon inflation. However, there were no disadvantages to final kissing balloon inflation.

SEA-SIDE

In this study 150 consecutive patients with bifurcation lesions underwent sirolimus-eluting versus everolimus-eluting stent implantation using provisional TAP stenting. The purpose was to compare outcomes with sirolimus- and everolimus-eluting stents and to evaluate whether a residual side branch stenosis was associated with postinterventional inducible ischemia in patients with complete revascularization. Early outcomes demonstrated that more than 50% stenosis in a side branch was strongly associated with postprocedural inducible ischemia. Secondly, final kissing balloon inflation was associated with absence of residual inducible ischemia.

Key Learning Points

- Medina is the simplest and the best qualitative classification for lesion distribution.
- Side branch predilatation is recommended in complex, calcified lesions.
- Always use two wires. Always use drug-eluting stents. Always perform final kissing balloon dilatation.
- Provisional stenting remains the gold standard in the majority of bifurcation lesions.

Dedicated Bifurcation Stents

The limitations of the conventional stent techniques in bifurcations described above and the demands on the operator indicate a need for dedicated bifurcation stents. These are in their infancy, but in time adequate devices will be developed and their use will increase and supersede current techniques. A tailored and simple technique should improve outcomes not only in complex procedures such as a distal left main or acute myocardial infarction with a bifurcation lesion, but also in a simple LAD-diagonal bifurcations with a narrow angle.

Currently available conventional drug-eluting (DES) techniques have many disadvantages, such as multiple metal layers leading to potential excessive vessel damage and drug dose. In addition, the side branch is not truly protected, and it may not be possible to cross from the main branch through the side of a stent to treat the side branch. Some strategies using conventional DES are complex to perform and may not be attempted by the low-volume operator. Conventional DES techniques are likely to result in disturbed flow. Dedicated stents should facilitate and simplify the procedure and subsequently improve outcomes.

Besides protecting the branches, the design of the optimal bifurcation stent should consider both the geometry and the various anatomical variations of the bifurcation, particularly the complexity of the transition zone between the main branch and the side branch. Currently the frequent need to cross through the side of the main branch stent struts to access the side branch in the classic two-stent approach is the most difficult part of the procedure. This may not longer be needed as with many dedicated designs the side branch is prewired. There is also a chance that the ostium of the side branch will be better supported by fully expanded struts. Consequently, stent positioning and deployment may be improved, which will help avoid all the problems associated with stent malapposition or overexpansion. It is also important in bifurcation stenting to ensure optimal side branch ostial scaffolding. Finally, the dedicated bifurcation stent will limit the number of metal layers and, hopefully, as a result, late thrombosis of the side branch.

Many of the bifurcation stents available or in trials are not drug eluting. Two exceptions are the Devax biolimus stent and Nile Croco paclitaxel-eluting stent. The design is either a bifurcation Y stent, side branch stent only, or main branch stent with side branch access. Stents are delivered either over one wire or over two wires. Stent delivery over two wires is more difficult, and although they provide good protection of the side branch, there is a risk of wire wrap (twisting) and wire bias that prevents the side branch component of a dedicated device from rotating, aligning, or delivering.

Categories of Dedicated Bifurcation Stents

Main Branch First Approach The most commonly used device is the Devax Axxess carina-sparing stent. The stent consists of a self-expandable drug-eluting stent with a bioabsorbable polymer and provides good opening of the side branch ostium by pushing plaque away from the flow divider (carina), which is usually spared from atheroma. An 8F guide is needed. The Axxess stent has excellent long-term clinical and angiographic results in nonrandomized trials. The great advantage of this device over provisional side branch stenting is that it provides safe and certain side branch access for additional stenting if necessary.

Main Branch and Provisional Side Branch Stenting Approach These types of stents ensure optimal access to the side branch and are most suitable for provisional side branch stenting. The device is delivered over two wires and consists of two independent catheters: the main branch with balloon and stent and the side branch with balloon only. A few devices are available:

- *Nile Croco* either polymer-free paclitaxel-eluting or bare metal stent. It allows kissing balloon inflation to limit proximal overexpansion. The stent consists of two independent balloons with a lumen for a rapid exchange for two wires. 6F-compatible.
- *Abbott* everolimus-eluting side-branch access stent (*Pathfinder*) partially supports the side branch ostium. It limits wrap by delivering the stent to the lesion over a single wire, then when it is close to the bifurcation, the second wire is advanced from a protected side port into the side branch. Its limitations are that it does not truly protect the side branch as it delivers the stent to the lesion over a single wire. Its second problem is that it must passively rotate to align with the side branch and this may be limited by wire bias, the oval cross-sectional nature of the device, crossing profile, and by plaque.
- *Taxus Petal* paclitaxel-eluting stent has unique "petal" elements that protrude into the side branch ostium, providing mechanical support and applying drug. The delivery system has a cylindrical main branch component and a droplet-shaped balloon that deploys the petal elements into the side branch ostium. It is 7F-guide compatible. It protects the side branch because it delivers the stent over two wires, but the delivery over two wires can be difficult.

The device must rotate passively to deliver and align with the side branch ostium. The FIM Taxus Petal trial showed that the device was effective if delivered, but delivery was difficult and frequently unsuccessful because of wire wrap, wire bias, and crossing profile. A torquable shaft in development overcomes these problems as the operator can actively rotate the device, overcoming wire wrap and wire bias, align the device, and deliver it appropriately to the bifurcation. It has a potential role in left main disease as it functions well in wide distal angled bifurcations. It could be coated with everolimus and could be made 6F compatible.

• *BRANCH* trial dedicated device. This bare metal stent has a "trouser" design constructed by linking three component stents derived from the Driver design. It is 7F compatible. It delivers over two wires so has the same unacceptable delivery issues as the Petal, although like the Petal it protects the side branch.

• *Y-Med Side-Kick* consists of a fixed wire for the main branch and a movable wire for the side branch. 5F compatible.

• *TriReme* delivery system consists of a main and a side branch wire and a crown that extends into the side branch, providing some ostial support. It has a torquable shaft and is easy to use. Side branch support length is limited, but it does conform to the funnel shape of the side branch ostium.

Elective Side Branch First Approach These systems have been designed to treat a side branch and do not allow provisional side branch stenting. The self-expanding ostium side branch device *Capella Sideguard* is a coronary side branch stent compatible with a 6F guide which is optimal for wide bifurcation angles (>45°).

Another example is the *Tryton* side branch stent. This is a cobalt chromium stent (2.5 mm side branch), balloon expandable, 6F guiding catheter compatible, that in essence facilitates a culotte approach, with the *Tryton* extending from the main branch into the side branch. *Tryton* consists of three zones which match bifurcation anatomy: distal side branch, transition zone at the carina, and the main branch zone, called the collar. The main branch zone has a minimal amount of metal and allows the delivery of a conventional stent of operator choice into the main branch. It is relatively easy to use and is 6F guide compatible. It is delivered over a single wire, so does not suffer from issues of wire wrap and wire bias and does not need to rotate to align. It is not drug eluting; whether this is a problem is not established. Its limitation is that it precludes a provisional side branch stenting strategy.

Dedicated Bifurcation Stent Trials
DIVERGE In this study 302 patients with bifurcation lesions were treated with the Axxess stent followed by additional sirolimus-eluting stent to the side branch(es) as required. At 9 months clinical follow-up major adverse cardiac event rate was an encouragingly low 7.7%, stent thrombosis rate was low, and the angiographic restenosis rate was only 6.4%. The percentage of

neointimal volume obstruction for the Axxess-covered area was 4.3% as measured by IVUS.

PETAL In this first-in-man study, 28 patients with bifurcation lesions were treated with the Taxus Petal paclitaxel-eluting dedicated bifurcation stent. At 30 days one patient presented with acute myocardial infarction. At 1 year target vessel revascularization was 11.1%, target lesion revascularization was 7.4%, and there were no deaths, Q-wave myocardial infarctions, or stent thromboses. This study demonstrated relatively low stent deliverability (73.5%) but with satisfactory clinical and angiographic outcomes in situations where stent delivery was achieved successfully.

BRANCH Study In this first-in-man study, 45 patients with bifurcation lesions were treated with the Medtronic Bifurcation Stent (MBS) followed by postprocedural IVUS assessment. Major adverse cardiac events at 30 days included two non-Q myocardial infarctions (4.4%) but no death, thrombosis, or target lesion revascularization by IVUS. The MBS provides adequate stent coverage and expansion at the carina and side branch ostium. The limitations of this device were the same as for the Petal stent, namely delivery difficulty due to wire wrap and wire bias and the limited ability of the device to rotate to align with the side branch.

Key Learning Points

• Dedicated bifurcation stents should facilitate and simplify the procedure and subsequently improve outcomes.
• Dedicated bifurcation stents will limit the number of metal layers and hopefully, as a result, late thrombosis of the side branch.
• Many of the current bifurcation stents are not drug eluting.

Ostial Lesions

Introduction

Although ostial lesions represent less than 10% of all PCI lesions, they remain a challenge for the interventional cardiologist. The ostial lesion is difficult technically, frequently with a suboptimal result. In addition, the restenosis rate is high. This is due to various factors including a large plaque burden and a tough often calcified lesion. Stent positioning is challenging, so that some part of the lesion may not be scaffolded, and even if optimal stent expansion is achieved, recoil is more frequent than in nonostial lesions. Neointimal hyperplasia adds to the potential for restenosis. A further problem is the high rate of complications such as dissection, rupture, acute closure, or the need for repeat revascularization, compared with PCI to nonostial lesions.

Profiling the ostium at angiography is often difficult and may affect diagnosis, treatment strategy, stent positioning, and outcomes. Difficulties in achieving a stable guide catheter position and maintaining position during the procedure are frequent. Moreover, balloon inflation in the ostium of the left main carries a risk of dissection extending into the aorta. In addition, there is a risk of left main coronary artery dissection during dilatation of the ostium of the LAD or the LCx. Ostial lesions are not suitable for direct stenting because of the importance of optimum preparation before stenting. Drug-eluting stents are preferable because of lower rates of restenosis and repeat intervention. Balloon angioplasty alone is not recommended because elastic recoil is a frequent problem in coronary ostia.

Many questions arise when a true ostial lesion is encountered:
- What is a geographic miss and how can I avoid it?
- In case of coexisting ostial and distal lesions, which lesion should be treated first?
- How do I achieve a stable guide catheter seating position?
- What should I do when the guide catheter repeatedly slips out?

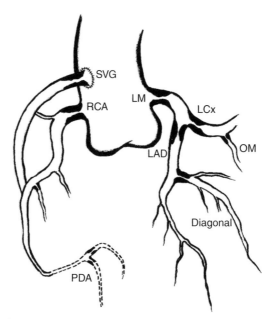

Figure 5.18 Classification of ostial lesions. Aorto-ostial lesions: saphenous vein graft (SVG), right coronary artery (RCA), left main coronary artery (LM). Non-aorto-ostial lesions: left anterior descending artery (LAD), left circumflex artery (LCx). Branch ostial lesions: left circumflex/oblique marginal (OM), left anterior descending/diagonal (LAD), right coronary artery/posterior descending artery (PDA).

- Should I use a buddy wire or other backup technique?
- How can I achieve optimal stent placement?
- Which technique should I use to achieve the best stent position?

Definition

By definition an ostial lesion is a narrowing that arises within 3 mm of the origin of the vessel and often involves a bifurcation. These are classified according to the type of vessel involved (Figure 5.18):

- *Aorto-ostial disease* involves native vessels such as ostial left main and ostial RCA or the ostium of bypass grafts arising directly from the aorta.
- *Non-aorto-ostial disease* refers to an ostial location of coronary arteries not arising directly from the aorta, such as LAD, LCx, or intermediate.
- *Branch ostial location* refers to all the ostial lesions that involve branches of the major coronary arteries, such as diagonals from the LAD, marginals from the LCx, and PDA from the RCA.

Recognizing a True Aorto-ostial Lesion

There are several clues in the recognition of a true aorto-ostial lesion:

- Difficulty in coronary intubation
- Heavy calcification in the proximal vessel visible without contrast injection

- Pressure damping as soon as the catheter enters the coronary artery
- No reflux of contrast into the aorta even with a vigorous coronary injection (see Figure 5.20)
- Clearly visible ostial narrowing on angiography (see Figure 5.36)
- Spasm excluded with intracoronary glyceryl trinitrate (GTN) injection (see below)

Catheter Selection and Aorto-ostial Engagement

The best guiding catheter for aorto-ostial lesions should not be aggressive; a standard Judkins guide is used successfully by many operators. Judkins shaped guides are often easier than other shapes to engage and disengage at will. If the Judkins guide does not provide adequate support in RCA intervention, a modified Amplatz left or right may be helpful. It is important to proceed carefully, avoiding deep intubation, wedging within the lesion, and vigorous manipulation. This may cause trauma, ischemia, dissection, or vessel closure.

Side holes in a guide can be very useful with aorto-ostial lesions, because the contrast exiting the holes can outline the aorta adjacent to the ostium and enhance identification of the true position of the ostium. The operator can easily drill side holes near the distal end of the guide by holding the sharp tip of a scalpel against the guide and rotating the blade.

Different shaped guide catheters are required when dealing with bypass grafts. While good guide support is a priority, the ability to engage and disengage is also important. Commonly used catheters are left or right bypass graft shapes and the Judkins right shape.

Sufficient backup support by the guiding catheter is important. Sometimes cannulation with standard 6F catheters is difficult or impossible, and even attempts with different catheters may fail. Even if a catheter is engaged successfully it may inadvertently disengage. Therefore, passive backup techniques are essential in ostial lesion procedures. One of the available options is a Proxis catheter, which has been designed for proximal embolic protection of a saphenous vein graft. Many operators prefer the coaxial double catheter technique, also called mother–child backup. This technique provides good catheter backup support and is helpful not only in aorto-ostial lesions, but also in cases of severe tortuosities proximal to a treated lesion, or in patients with a dilated aorta or takeoff anomalies. This technique requires two guiding catheters, the outer (the mother catheter) and the inner (the child). All backup techniques are described on pp. 85–92.

Predilatation and Debulking

Ostial lesions are usually tough, calcified, and fibrotic and may be prone to dissection. These calcified plaques may limit full stent expansion or there may be elastic recoil. Hence, good lesion preparation is a priority. Predilatation should be performed routinely, either with a standard noncompliant balloon or, in the case of a severely calcified lesion, with a cutting balloon. Sometimes it is necessary to use a standard balloon to facilitate cutting balloon passage. It has been shown that predilatation with a cutting balloon significantly reduces target vessel revascularization in ostial LAD lesions (FLEXI-CUT study, 2006).

It is important to withdraw the guiding catheter fractionally into the aorta before stent deployment so that the stent is not partially deployed in the guide. There are several techniques to disengage the guide. Guide rotation – for instance counterclockwise for the right Judkins shaped guide – will usually disengage the guide from the right coronary artery. Another technique to back the guide off from the ostium while retaining device position across the ostial lesion is to push forward on a distally placed guide wire.

If balloon predilatation is inadequate, and especially if a noncompliant balloon or cutting balloon is not adequately expanded, then rotational atherectomy is recommended before stenting. Prior debulking of the plaque reduces the potential risk of carina or plaque shift and is more likely to result in optimal stent expansion. Debulking, however, also carries some risk of complications. While most ostial lesions require stenting, debulking alone may be enough in small vessel lesions.

Ostial Lesion or Coronary Spasm?

In some cases coronary spasm can be misinterpreted as ostial disease, particularly in the RCA. To differentiate this, assess the lesion in at least two projections, avoiding overlapping and foreshortening. Ostial coronary spasm often occurs following deep guiding catheter cannulation, but may be triggered even by even gentle engagement with a catheter tip. Coronary spasm will usually respond to intracoronary nitroglycerin injections of 200 μg. Two or three of these injections should be administered directly to the ostium to rule out spasm.

Ostial Lesion and Distal Lesion

Sometimes ostial and distal disease coexist in one artery. In these cases, treat the distal lesion first and then deal with the ostium. There are two reasons for doing so. Firstly, when a stent is placed in the ostium, loss of the guiding catheter position is likely and re-engagement may be very difficult or impossible. Secondly, after stent implantation in the ostium, all further devices need to be advanced through this stent to reach the distal lesion. This may cause stent trauma and influence long-term outcome.

Stent Positioning

The main concern during ostial lesion PCI is achieving exact and precise stent placement. The main difficulty is poor visualization of the ostial lesion and problems maintaining a stable catheter position with normal cardiac motion. The lesion should be fully covered. It is important to make sure that the

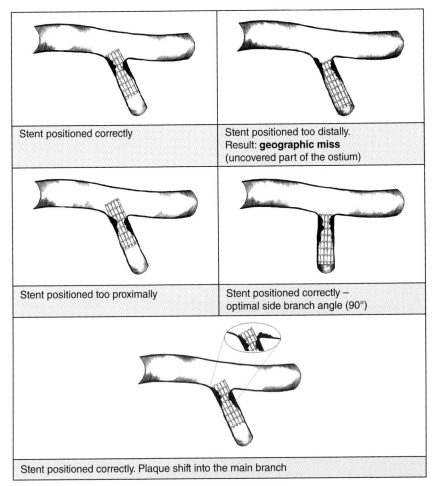

Stent positioned correctly	Stent positioned too distally. Result: **geographic miss** (uncovered part of the ostium)
Stent positioned too proximally	Stent positioned correctly – optimal side branch angle (90°)

Stent positioned correctly. Plaque shift into the main branch

Figure 5.19 Stent positioning in ostial lesions.

proximal part of the stent covers the ostium. If the stent is placed too proximally, excessive stent protrusion into the aortic lumen makes re-engagement of the guiding catheter or subsequent restudy at a later date difficult and carries the risk of stent damage. On the other hand, if the stent is placed too distally, part of the ostial lesion is uncovered by stent, which carries the risk of restenosis (see below, "Geographic Miss").

Note that the bifurcation angle matters, and the narrower the side branch angle, the more difficult it is to achieve an optimal stent position. With a T-shaped bifurcation, the stent can be placed in the ostium with minimal risk of protrusion, whereas in a Y-shaped bifurcation this can be impossible (Figure 5.19; see also pp. 204–233).

Geographic Miss

"Geographic miss" means leaving a part of the ostial lesion uncovered by a stent. This results in failure to treat the lesion, and may result in a higher rate of complications such as acute closure or early in-stent restenosis. The part of the lesion that has not been fully covered by the stent often requires a second stent.

Geographic miss usually occurs with incorrect stent positioning, and precise stent placement can be difficult. To avoid this you need to select an angiographic projection which displays the proximal position of the stent marker. Then gently disengage the catheter from the ostium. If stenting the right coronary artery, remember to achieve disengagement by anticlockwise rotation or by pushing the wire forward. Some operators inflate the stent at very low pressure (2–4 atm) to stabilize the stent and limit movement during the cardiac cycle. This also allows repositioning before final deployment, which facilitates stent positioning before implantation.

Dissection and Carina Shift

One of the most common pitfalls during stent implantation of the ostial lesion is carina shift. Stent positioning, initial balloon inflation, or stent implantation will always carry the potential risk of carina shift into the main branch, causing narrowing (Figure 5.18). In addition, there is evidence that stenting itself leads to redistribution of the plaque. Therefore, adequate lesion preparation with predilatation with a standard balloon alone, or with a standard balloon and cutting balloon, followed by debulking may prevent plaque displacement and facilitate stent positioning and full expansion. A buddy wire may also help protect the vessel. After successful stent implantation, postdilatation with a noncompliant balloon at high pressure should be performed routinely in every ostial lesion. The proximal end of the ostial stent in aorto-ostial lesions should be flared using this balloon or one 0.5 mm larger than the main vessel. In this way the stent may adapt to the funnel shape of the aortic ostium.

General Technical Considerations

Both disengagement and re-engagement of the guiding catheter are important parts of the procedure and should be performed safely and efficiently. Accidental loss of guiding catheter position is frequent, and dealing with re-engagement requires time and experience, although once a guide wire has been advanced to the distal vessel this is usually not a challenge.

Catheter Disengagement

During aorto-ostial intervention, the guiding catheter has to be disengaged from the coronary ostium to allow full stent expansion (Figure 5.20). This difficult maneuver may result in inadvertent dislodgment of the wire and stent from the coronary artery. There are several steps which can be followed. First, assess the lesion in at least two orthogonal projections avoiding overlapping and foreshortening. Then try disengaging the catheter. Once the proximal stent marker reaches the tip of the catheter, gently pull back the catheter along with the stent and wire and inject some contrast to establish the correct stent position. If you fail and the whole system slips out of the ostium, engage the catheter again and use a buddy wire for more stable backup.

Significant guide catheter disengagement will limit visualization because of poor contrast opacification. A very short disengagement length can allow contrast to outline the aorta adjacent to the ostium and demonstrate precisely its position and its relationship to the stent before deployment. The correct stent position should be ensured and confirmed in at least two angiographic projections. Some operators make holes in the tip of the guide catheter to improve visualization of the ostium.

Difficulties with Catheter Re-Engagement

The best way to re-engage the catheter is to leave the balloon (which has just delivered a stent into the ostial lesion) in place and re-engage a catheter coaxially over the balloon. This should be performed slowly, but some clockwise rotation may help in the right coronary ostium. When this succeeds, withdraw the balloon. If this technique fails, use a buddy wire to stabilize the whole system and try to advance the catheter again.

Difficulties with Stent Expansion

In some cases stent expansion may be inadequate because of heavily calcified plaque remaining in the vessel. If the vessel has not been predilated using a cutting balloon or rotablator and difficulties with stent deployment occur, the best option is to postdilate the stent at high pressure with a noncompliant balloon. IVUS may be useful to assess the lesion before stent deployment and to check stent apposition after intervention.

Summary of General Principles in Ostial Lesions

A few general principles are summarized below:
- Engage a catheter in the ostial lesion, avoiding excessive manipulation.
- Ensure a stable catheter seating position,
- Select a wire. In most cases a routinely used workhorse wire is adequate. Hydrophilic wires are suitable for tortuous lesions but offer less support. Sometimes a second buddy wire is needed to provide extra support, stability, or to serve as a marker during stent positioning.
- If there is a coexisting distal lesion, remember to treat this first.
- Advance the wire slowly into the vessel, then advance a standard compliant balloon and predilate the lesion. Assess the lesion again and decide if debulking is required. Consider pros and cons and take into account possible carina shift during stent positioning, particularly if the lesion is heavily calcified.

- If the guiding catheter is not stable, use the mother–child technique or a buddy wire.
- When the lesion has been prepared, choose the optimal projections for stent positioning.
- Place a stent in the vessel. IVUS guidance may be helpful in selecting the best stent.
- Always disengage the catheter from the ostium during stent deployment in the aorto-ostial lesion. This will cause temporary instability and poorer visualization, but will greatly improve stent expansion and apposition.
- After stent implantation, re-engage the ostium and postdilate the stent, flaring out the proximal end in aorto-ostial stents.

Study the stent before introduction into the body to determine the relationship of the end of the stent to the balloon marker. With some designs the stent overlies the marker and in others there is a gap of even several millimeters between stent and marker. This information is important for accurate stent placement.

An example of a right coronary artery ostial lesion angioplasty is shown in Figure 5.20 and of a left coronary artery in Figure 5.36 (p. 287).

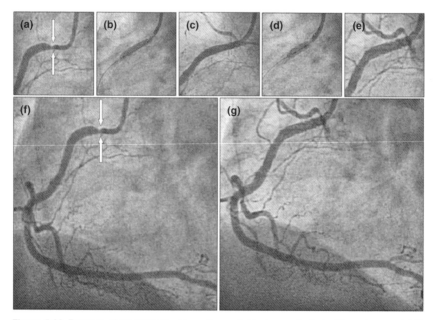

Figure 5.20 Example of the right coronary artery ostial lesion angioplasty. Upper images: LAO view. JR4 8F guide catheter. **(a)** Ostial stenosis (arrows) after 200 μg GTN injection. No contrast reflux into aorta. **(b)** POBA (plain old balloon angioplasty) 3 × 15 mm balloon. Note guide catheter withdrawn slightly into aorta. **(c)** Result of stenting of ostial lesion with 3.5 × 16 mm stent. Note contrast reflux into aorta. **(d)** Postdilatation of ostium with short 4 × 8 mm noncompliant balloon. **(e)** Final result. Lower images: Right coronary artery ostial lesion **(f)** before PCI and **(g)** after stent implantation.

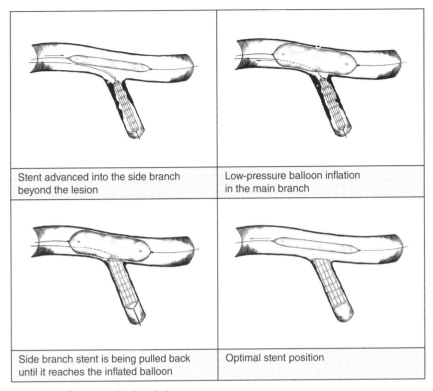

Stent advanced into the side branch beyond the lesion	Low-pressure balloon inflation in the main branch
Side branch stent is being pulled back until it reaches the inflated balloon	Optimal stent position

Figure 5.21 Stent draw-back technique.

Special Techniques

Stent Draw-Back Technique

This technique applies to non-aorto-ostial lesions such as left anterior descending, left circumflex coronary artery, or intermediate artery, ideally with a relatively wide angle. A second balloon placed opposite the ostium of the treated vessel helps to avoid plaque shift into the main vessel and proximal stent extension. The balloon should be inflated at low pressure to prevent potential vessel trauma and risk of future restenosis.

Stent Draw-Back Step by Step (Figure 5.21)
- Use a 7F catheter.
- Predilate the lesion and use debulking if necessary.
- Advance a stent into the side branch beyond the lesion.
- Use a compliant balloon and place it in the main branch across the side branch ostium. The balloon must be long enough to fully cover the side branch ostium.

• Inflate the main branch balloon at low pressure (4–6 atm). This allows manipulation of the stent and optimal positioning covering the ostium without protrusion.
• Keep pulling back the stent from the side branch until the inflated balloon is reached with a good stent position.
• Now expand the stent in the side branch.
• Deflate both balloons and postdilate the side branch with a noncompliant balloon at high pressure (16 atm).

Ostial LAD Stenting

The ostial LAD lesion is one of the most difficult to treat. Device delivery and balloon or stent deployment may cause trauma to the left main. The major concern during ostial LAD intervention is optimal stent positioning and full ostial coverage. It is important to assess the lesion in two orthogonal projections, avoiding foreshortening and overlapping. The RAO caudal view usually offers the best visualization. Although every effort should be made to treat the LAD ostium exclusively, sometimes protrusion of the stent into the left main is inevitable. Likewise, the left circumflex artery can be compromised during the procedure. This requires balloon inflation into the LCx, followed by stenting if necessary and subsequent kissing balloon postdilatation. Wire protection of a dominant circumflex in ostial LAD cases before stent deployment is advisable.

Szabo Technique

This technique is best described using the LAD–LCx bifurcation as an example with the lesion in the LAD ostium. Stenting the ostial LAD lesion is usually difficult and there is still no standard technique applicable to this lesion. If the angle between LAD and LCx is narrow, obtaining an optimal stent position is very difficult and the risk of carina shift is high. The potential advantage of the Szabo technique is that it offers optimal stent positioning without proximal protrusion or compromising the side branch, and provides full ostial coverage. A second wire which serves as an anchor fixes the stent in the ostium of the target vessel to facilitate positioning.

This technique has also important limitations. The side branch wire, when removed, pulls the struts proximally across the ostium of the nonstented artery and widens the cells proximally in the stent, reducing scaffolding and drug application where these are most needed. The preinterventional check is very important as, if the lesion extends proximal to the bifurcation, the Szabo technique is not suitable.

There are a few important technical considerations:
• The wire should be inserted through the last stent strut gently to avoid balloon damage. This complication will result in stent underexpansion or failure of expansion.
• The passage of the stent–anchor wire system should be slow as any upward protrusion of the stent strut will cause resistance, preventing proper

positioning. Some operators prefer to place a stent in the ostial lesion before the stent–anchor wire system is advanced, in order to check stent deliverability.
• The anchor wire should be withdrawn slowly and carefully. The wire may dislodge the stent from the balloon.

Szabo Technique Step by Step (Figure 5.22)
• Use a 7F catheter and establish a stable, well-seated arterial engagement. A large guiding catheter is needed to ensure stable backup and to reduce resistance during insertion of the stent system.

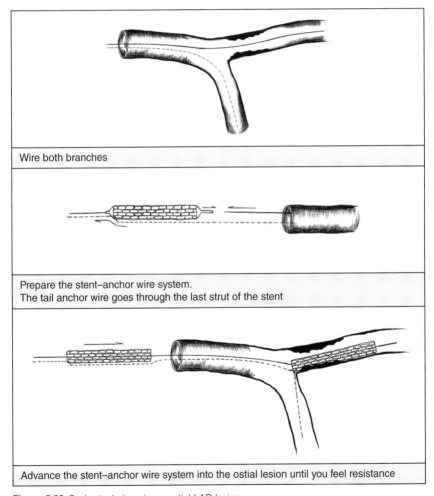

Wire both branches

Prepare the stent–anchor wire system.
The tail anchor wire goes through the last strut of the stent

Advance the stent–anchor wire system into the ostial lesion until you feel resistance

Figure 5.22 Szabo technique in an ostial LAD lesion.

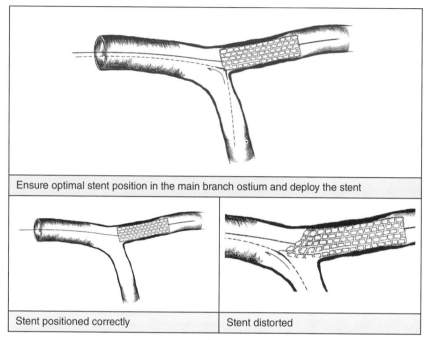

Ensure optimal stent position in the main branch ostium and deploy the stent	
Stent positioned correctly	Stent distorted

Figure 5.22 *(Continued)*.

• Advance a wire into the main branch and one to the side branch if dealing with bifurcation, and into the aorta when you are treating an aorto-ostial lesion. The wire in the side branch is called the anchor wire.

• Choose a stent, inflate it slightly up to 1 atm, and carefully thread the stiff end of the anchor side branch wire through the last strut of the main branch stent. Proceed carefully to avoid stent balloon damage.

• Now advance the stent–anchor wire system into the ostial main branch lesion. Keep going until resistance is felt, then stop. This means that the side branch anchor wire prevents further forward movement and the stent has reached the proper position.

• Check the stent position in the angiogram. Ensure a correct stent position and deploy the stent at low pressure (6–8 atm).

• Remove the anchor wire from the side branch and deploy the stent fully at high pressure.

• Postdilate the vessel with a noncompliant balloon at high pressure.

Ostial Pro Stent System

The Ostial Pro is a nitinol device that allows precise stent placement at the aorto-ostial lesion. Once the wire crosses the ostial lesion and the stent is correctly positioned, self-expanding legs are advanced distally to the tip of the catheter. These expanded legs prevent entry of the catheter into the treated vessel and stabilize the tip of the guide proximal to the aorto-ostial plane.

Complications

Ostial Dissection
Most aorto-ostial dissections result from catheter-induced injury to the ostium due to forceful manipulation of the guiding catheter. Contrast injection causes further extension. IVUS is a useful tool for evaluation of the entry point and extent of the dissection and should be performed if available. In case of difficulties with engagement, change the guide catheter or choose one of the support techniques. e.g., mother–child technique, rather than keep manipulating. Remember that in the right coronary artery dissection is more likely to occur during disengagement than during insertion. This is particularly the case with Amplatz guides in the RCA. To minimize the risk, always disengage a catheter from the ostium by slight anticlockwise rotation or by pushing the guide wire forward. Stent deployment usually seals off the dissection entry point. In aorto-ostial dissection cases where dye is seen to collect and track up the aortic wall, rapid stent deployment in the ostium is necessary to seal this.

Side Branch Closure
Heavily calcified lesions located either in the side branch ostium or extending from the side branch into the main vessel increase the risk of side branch closure and risk side branch loss. A significant side branch should be always protected with a second wire (see p. 213). In case of occlusion, first inject 100–200 µg of GTN to exclude coronary spasm. Recheck the angiogram. Simultaneous balloon inflation in both branches is often helpful to maintain vessel patency.

Vessel Dissection
Vessel dissection usually occurs on the edge of the stent, particularly if the plaque is significant and severely calcified. If high inflation pressure is needed, try to select a stent diameter which is 0.5 mm smaller than the vessel diameter and then use an adequately sized balloon to postdilate the lesion.

Restenosis
This is a difficult situation as treatment strategies are limited. In each case IVUS should be performed to assess ostial stent coverage and the possible causes of restenosis, e.g., stent underexpansion. In restenotic lesions, stent implantation is one option, but balloon angioplasty at high pressure or use of a cutting balloon is preferable. If the patient is symptomatic with severe lesions in other major coronary arteries, surgery may be necessary.

Key Learning Points

• One of the first signs of the presence of the ostial lesion is pressure damping.

• When dealing with an aorto-ostial lesion, disengage the catheter before stent deployment.

• Lesion preparation is important, with predilatation followed by debulking to help prevent carina shift and to ensure the lesion is fully expandable.

• Check the stent before introduction to learn about the relationship of the stent to the balloon marker. With some stent designs the stent overlies the marker, and whereas with others there may be a gap of several millimeters.

• Where there is a coexisting distal lesion, treat the distal lesion first and then the ostial lesion.

• Ostial lesion PCI carries a high risk of restenosis.

Chronic Total Occlusion

Introduction

A chronic total occlusion (CTO) remains one of the most difficult of all angioplasty targets and the reason many patients are still referred for bypass surgery. Although in many centers the success rate is lower than for standard angioplasty of coronary stenoses, data from Japan show average procedural success rates of 95%. Successful recanalization is dependent on appropriate patient selection, detailed analysis of the coronary angiogram, and choice of an optimal strategy. The procedure requires patience and time.

There is enough evidence now that reopening of a CTO is of long-term benefit, with symptom relief, electrical stability, and improvements in left ventricular ejection fraction and regional wall motion. There is increased tolerance to possible future coronary events and long-term reduction in rates of myocardial infarction and cardiac death. There is also improvement in event-free survival. Recurrence and reocclusion rates are higher than with other coronary lesions.

It is important to become familiar with CTO procedures right from the beginning. A simple CTO requires minimal technical skills and basic knowledge, and every interventionist should be capable of performing this. However, a complex chronic occlusion, particularly with the retrograde approach, requires considerable experience and a skilled operator.

A few basic principles should be considered:
- Is the CTO lesion complex? What are the lesion age and characteristics?
- Based on angiographic, patient, and procedure-related factors, is there any realistic chance of procedural success?
- What is the success/failure balance and what is the risk of the procedure?
- Do I have enough time for the procedure?
- Which is the best working projection?
- Which guiding catheter will give the best backup support?
- Should I always use an over-the-wire balloon or microcatheter?
- Do I need simultaneous contralateral injection?
- Which wire should I select at the beginning of the procedure?
- Do I need to shape the wire?
- Which wire should I use if the first wire fails to cross the lesion or enters the false lumen?
- What do I do if the wire goes subintimally?
- Which stent do I have to use after successful recanalization: bare metal or drug eluting?
- Which antithrombotic agents should I use?
- What do I do if crossing the lesion is unsuccessful?
- When should I stop the procedure?

Definition

This definition has been agreed by the EuroCTO Club. A chronic total occlusion can be recognized in a vessel with TIMI 0 flow with angiographic or clinical evidence or a likelihood that the occlusion has existed for 3

Table 5.6 Definition of chronic total occlusion (CTO) and evidence and indications for PCI.

CTO Definition	Evidence and Indications for PCI
Definite	Angiographic evidence of total occlusion ≥3 months
Probable	Symptomatic angina or ischemia in the CTO region
	Absence of other lesions which might be responsible for symptoms
Possible	Angiographic CTO, but no recent deterioration in symptoms

months or longer. The duration of the occlusion is often difficult to determine.

A chronically occluded lesion is considered suitable for PCI if angiographic and clinical evidence is present as shown in Table 5.6, and a successful final result is possible based on angiographic predictors. In multivessel disease it is important to assess the potential chances for successful complete revascularization.

Patient Selection

Patients who are potential candidates for a CTO procedure should be selected carefully. Medical history and clinical examination are essential (renal insufficiency? diabetes? peripheral vascular disease?). Additional tests, e.g., ECG, echocardiography, Doppler ultrasonography, stress echocardiography, positron emission tomography, (PET) or MRI may be required.

• Symptomatic patients with a large ischemic area, heart failure, or arrhythmia should be considered in the first instance as patients in this group benefit from the procedure the most.

• Asymptomatic patients with small vessels or occlusions which will be technically very difficult to cross (e.g., very long or tortuous, heavily calcified, without a visible distal end) are not suitable for a CTO procedure.

Prediction of Success and Failure

The success/failure balance should always be assessed individually based on various angiographic factors summarized in Table 5.7 and shown in Figure 5.23. Some parameters increase the chances of a successful procedure, whereas others may lead to failure.

Inability to Cross the Lesion

Procedural failure is usually caused by difficulties with wiring, or inability to cross the lesion or to reach the distal end of the vessel. The diagnostic angiogram should be reviewed in detail to assess the occluded segment and find the location of the distal re-entry. Attention should be paid to the characteristics of the proximal and distal caps, presence of tortuosities and calcification in the treated segment, relation to a side branch or side branches, length of the lesion, and presence of distal collaterals. Long

Table 5.7 Factors associated with probability of procedural success in PCI of chronic total occlusion.

More Likely to Succeed	Less Likely to Succeed
Vessel diameter ≥3.0mm	Vessel diameter ≤3.0mm
Tapering of proximal stump	Blunt ended/squared off stump
Convex distal stump/cap	Tapering of distal cap
Short occlusion ≤20mm	Long occlusion ≥20mm
Straight vessel	Tortuous vessel
No side branch at proximal cap	Side branch at proximal cap
No calcification seen	Heavy calcification
Good distal vessel opacification	Poor distal vessel opacification
No multiple occlusion	Multiple occlusion
No distal vessel disease	Severe distal vessel disease
No ostial location	Ostial location
Minimal tortuosity proximal to occlusion	Severe tortuosity proximal to occlusion
Normal renal function	Renal insufficiency
First attempt	Previous attempts
Occlusion 3–6 months	Occlusion >2 years

lesions, particularly with poor distal visualization, are very difficult to cross.

CTO With and Without Blunt Stump

There is evidence that a tapered proximal stump indicates the presence of antegrade microchannels, which increase the chances of successful crossing.

Although microchannels are present in almost half of chronically occluded lesions, it is easy to miss them with bridging collaterals. If the presence of antegrade microchannels is confirmed, penetration of the proximal cap is often easy and the wire should cross them successfully. If there is a blunt stump, however, penetration of the proximal cap is more complicated and usually, if the side branch is large enough, requires IVUS guidance. The most vulnerable point is the lesion entry, as the wire can easily enter a false lumen.

Which Guiding Catheter?

In PCI of a CTO lesion, femoral access is usually used to facilitate introduction of a larger-lumen guiding catheter and wider device application. The choice is always individual and based on operator experience and personal preferences. Some operators prefer a radial approach with the lower access site complication rate and earlier ambulation after the procedure. Whichever access is chosen, good guiding catheter stability and support are essential.

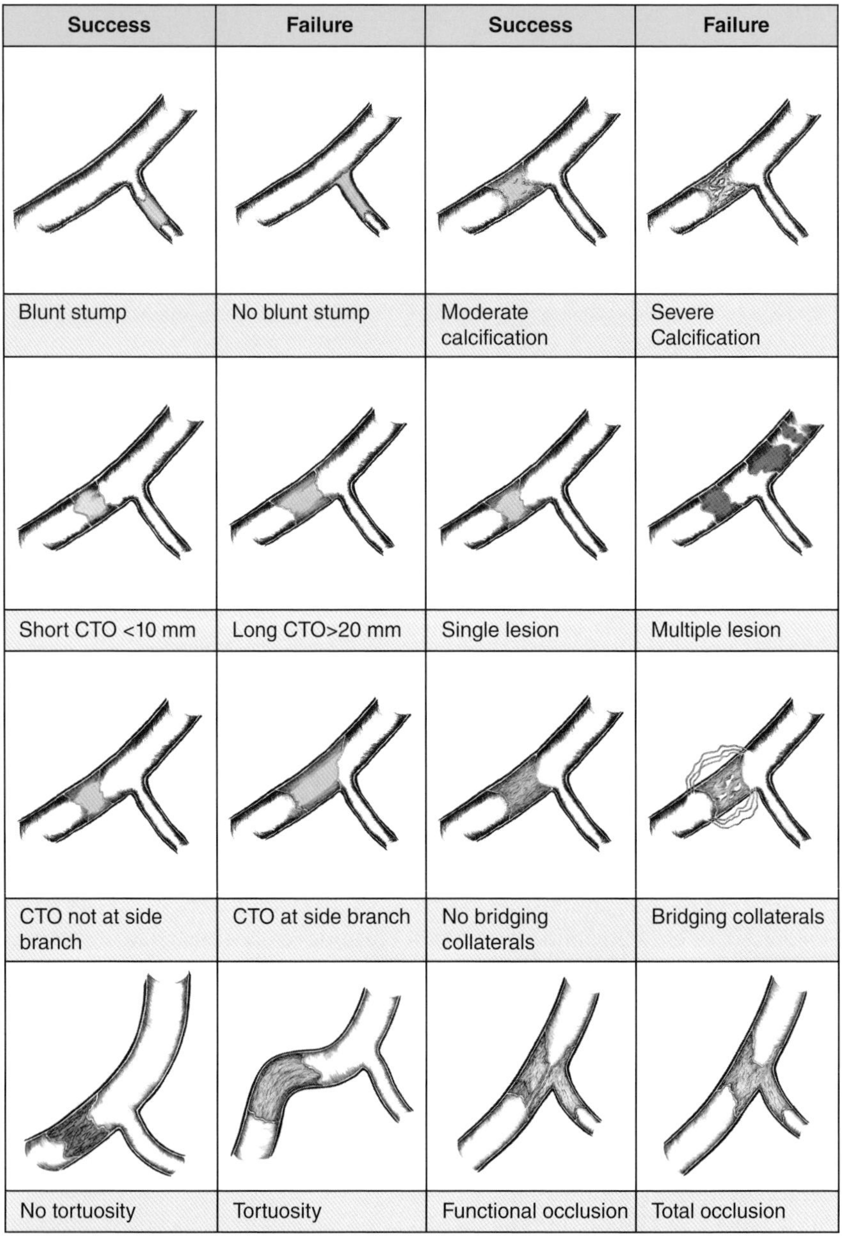

Success	Failure	Success	Failure
Blunt stump	No blunt stump	Moderate calcification	Severe Calcification
Short CTO <10 mm	Long CTO>20 mm	Single lesion	Multiple lesion
CTO not at side branch	CTO at side branch	No bridging collaterals	Bridging collaterals
No tortuosity	Tortuosity	Functional occlusion	Total occlusion

Figure 5.23 Predictors for procedural success or failure based on angiographic lesion morphology.

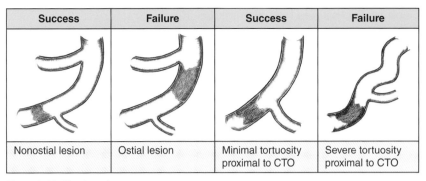

Success	Failure	Success	Failure
Nonostial lesion	Ostial lesion	Minimal tortuosity proximal to CTO	Severe tortuosity proximal to CTO

Figure 5.23 (*Continued*).

Table 5.8 Choice of guide catheter for CTO PCI.

Coronary Artery	Guiding Catheter
Right coronary	JR4, AL1
Left anterior descending	EBU
Left circumflex	AL2

AL, Amplatz left; EBU, extra backup; JR, Judkins right.

A properly selected catheter will provide maximum support and stability and optimal backup power. The commonly used guide size is 7–8F (7F for the majority of procedures, 8F for complex procedures). These guides provide strong backup and optimal passive support, and allow wider application of devices such as IVUS or covered stent in case of perforation. If IVUS is planned, an 8F guiding catheter is needed.

Deeply engaged smaller catheters, e.g., 5F or 6F, provide great active support and many operators use them for easy procedures. However these are not suitable for complex PCIs, e.g., parallel wire technique with two over-the-wire catheters and two wires.

For contralateral injection, using a retrograde approach, a 4–5F catheter should be advanced via the contralateral femoral artery.

The choice of the type of catheter is also very important. The most commonly used catheter for the RCA is the Judkins right. The deep intubation or anchor techniques described below provide good support. The Amplatz left can also be used successfully, and this is the best option for the RCA with a shepherd's crook takeoff. For an occlusion in the LCA, the standard Judkins guide is not recommended as its backup support is not sufficient. The best choice is EBU or XB, which provides great extra backup. For the circumflex artery, Amplatz left 2 or 3 is a good choice (Table 5.8).

Support Techniques (see also pp. 85–90)

Anchor balloon techniques and side branch techniques provide not only strong support for the guiding catheter but also an effective way to cross the distal part of the CTO lesion (the anchor balloon technique is commonly used in non-CTO cases). The following strategies can help optimize the procedure:

• **Anchor balloon in the target vessel for strong guide backup.** Anchoring a balloon proximal to the occlusion, either in the target vessel or in the side branch, helps achieve adequate catheter stabilization and wire support. This is a simple technique. Advance a wire into the target vessel proximal to the CTO lesion, then advance a small 1.5 mm balloon and deploy the balloon at low pressure. Keep the balloon in the vessel and proceed further.

• **Anchor balloon in the side branch for strong guide backup** *(Figure 5.24)*. Advance a wire into the side branch (nontarget vessel) proximal to the CTO lesion, then insert a small 1.5 mm balloon and deploy the balloon at low pressure. Alternatively, a over-the-wire balloon inflated proximal to the CTO lesion provides strong backup support for wire manipulation.

• **The trapping technique.** Balloon inflation inside the guiding catheter will help fix and maintain the wire position.

• **Target vessel balloon technique to cross the distal part of the CTO.** Advance a wire into the target vessel proximal to the lesion, advance a 2.5–3.0 mm balloon and deploy it at low pressure (4–6 atm). Keep the deployed balloon in the vessel and continue to penetrate the distal part of the CTO lesion.

• **Side branch balloon technique to cross the distal part of the CTO** *(Figure 5.25)*. In this technique the balloon serves not as an anchor, but to make a crack in the distal part of the CTO lesion. Advance a wire into the side branch,

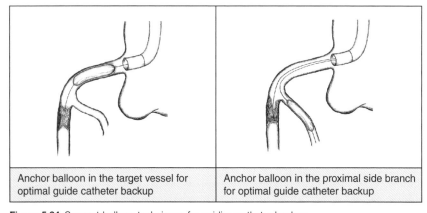

| Anchor balloon in the target vessel for optimal guide catheter backup | Anchor balloon in the proximal side branch for optimal guide catheter backup |

Figure 5.24 Support balloon techniques for guiding catheter backup

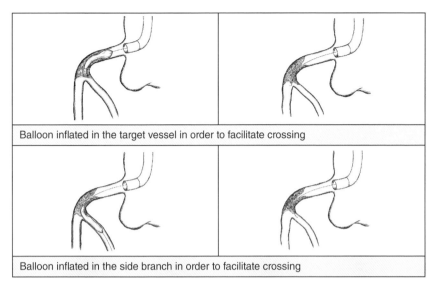

Balloon inflated in the target vessel in order to facilitate crossing

Balloon inflated in the side branch in order to facilitate crossing

Figure 5.25 Support balloon techniques to facilitate crossing of the CTO lesion.

crossing the CTO lesion along the vessel wall. Advance a small 1.5 mm balloon and place the balloon in the entry of the side branch. Deploy the balloon at low pressure. Withdraw the balloon and try to enter the CTO lesion through the crack made by the balloon.

Which Guide Wire and Balloon?

Good wire selection simplifies the procedure and increases the chance of successful crossing.

Traditional CTO-dedicated wires have a tapered tip with strong penetration capability and good torquability (Confianza, Shinobi, Cross IT), whereas softer wires provide good trackability and are suitable for tortuous vessels (Fiedler, Asahi). There are two types of CTO-dedicated wires: the more aggressive hydrophilic wires and the more controllable hydrophobic wires. Hybrids are also available but are rarely used.

• *Hydrophilic wires* are wires coated with polymer, which provides excellent torquability but at the cost of minimal tactile feel. There is always a potential risk of dissection, particularly if the wire enters the false lumen and the balloon is inflated subintimally. Hydrophilic wires are preferable for tracking the subintimal channels with the support of a second parallel wire which will access the true lumen. The most commonly used are Whisper, Pilot, Choice PT, and Shinobi.

• *Hydrophobic wires* are noncoated wires which provide better tactile feel and therefore are more controllable, with lower risk of complications. Commonly

Table 5.9 Choice of wire depending on type of the occlusion.

Type of Occlusion	Choice of Wire
Recent CTO	HT Intermediate, PT wire, Pilot 50, Cross-IT 100, Miracle
CTO >12 months	HT Standard, Cross-IT 200, Confianza, Shinobi
Tortuous CTO	Fielder, Whisper, Pilot 50, Shinobi
Calcified CTO	Fielder XT, Cross-IT 400, Miracle 12 g, Confianza Pro
In-stent CTO	HT Standard, Pilot 200, Cross-IT 200, Shinobi
SVG CTO	Pilot 200, Cross-IT 200
Crossing microchannels	Whisper, Pilot 50, PT wire, Cross-IT 100, Confianza, Shinobi
Retrograde approach	Fielder XT, FC, Confianza Pro , Miracle 3 g

used hydrophobic wires include the Asahi Miracle, Confianza, and Cross-IT.

It is sensible to start the procedure with a moderately soft wire, e.g., a floppy wire to enter the segment proximal to the occlusion and probe its proximal part. This wire, however, is not capable of crossing a true CTO, and long, forceful manipulation may only result in subintimal tracking and complications. After the initial probing, as the procedure progresses, it is necessary to switch to a more aggressive, stiffer wire with greater penetrating ability. The last choice is always a stiff, tapered wire. This graded approach is relatively safe and carries a low risk of vessel injury.

Stiffer, more aggressive CTO-dedicated wires are likely to achieve passage through a tough CTO cap, and some operators prefer this approach. Whichever approach you choose, remember to use an over-the-wire catheter for better wire support, to prevent wire kinking and prolapsing, and to facilitate multiple wire exchanges during the procedure. The choice of wire depending on the type of the occlusion is shown in Table 5.9.

Balloon Selection

In terms of balloon selection, the smaller the size of the balloon, the better. The smallest, Nan (0.85 mm) has no marker, but Falcon (1.00 mm) or Apex Push (1.50 mm) have markers and have good visibility.

Tornus Catheter

This catheter has been designed to break down very hard tissue, particularly when delivery of an antegrade support device into the CTO is difficult. Tornus is a metallic 2.6F catheter with extra backup support with the wire. It provides a special anchor effect and allows penetration of tight, calcified and long lesions which a balloon is unable to cross. This also has great pushability. It is made from eight steel wires stranded over each other.

In order to advance the catheter, you need to rotate it counterclockwise up to the maximum, and as you feel it move, stop rotating and advance a wire.

Then keep advancing the catheter again until you reach the distal lumen. Remember that Tornus should always be used with stiffer wires such as Asahi or Miracle. A floppy wire is not an option. Although many operators use the Tornus catheter specifically for CTO lesions, it can also be useful for some other very severe but not chronically occluded lesions, and is very effective in lesions which have previously proved uncrossable. It also facilitates exchanging wires and advancing balloons.

IVUS-Guided Procedure

IVUS is of great value in CTO procedures to help identify the wire position and guide the wire to re-enter the true lumen from the subintimal track. IVUS can also be helpful in assessing the lesion characteristics and to identify the proximal cap. An IVUS guided procedure however, carries a potential risk of dissection or perforation and should be performed by experienced operators.

Example of a chronic total occlusion angioplasty is shown on Figure 5.26.

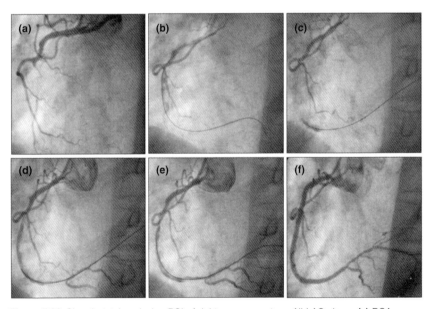

Figure 5.26 Chronic total occlusion PCI of right coronary artery. All LAO views. **(a)** RCA injection shows tapered stump of CTO just distal to origin of RV branch. **(b)** Miracle wire through occlusion positioned in posterior descending artery. Slight contrast filling to margin and small marginal branch fills. **(c)** Miracle wire now in LV branch distally, therefore likely to be in true lumen. **(d)** Right coronary artery injection; hazy vessel to margin. Posterior descending artery just visualized. **(e)** Following further long balloon dilatations from occlusion to beyond crus. Flow improved. Dissection proximal to crus. **(f)** Final result following deployment of four Xience stents. From distal to proximal: 2.75 × 23, 3.0 × 28, 3.0 × 28, and 3.5 × 18 mm, and postdilatation with Quantum Maverick balloons.

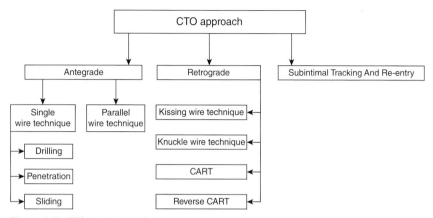

Figure 5.27 CTO techniques. CART, controlled antegrade and retrograde subintimal tracking.

CTO Techniques

Over the last 10 years CTO techniques have changed and developed hugely. With increased operator experience and advances in CTO-dedicated devices, many chronic occlusions left untreated in the past are now considered treatable. Contralateral injection is used routinely if filling from distal collaterals is present.

There are two wire-based approaches for CTO revascularization: antegrade and retrograde (Figure 5.27). Subintimal tracking and re-entry is an alternative, but is rarely used because of the high risk of complications. The majority of CTO lesions can be treated with the antegrade approach. However, in selected cases, or after an unsuccessful first antegrade attempt, a retrograde technique is required. Various additional simple techniques such as an anchor balloon and side branch balloon approach can support either an antegrade or a retrograde strategy.

These technical points and tips may be helpful in dealing with CTO lesions:

• Dealing with CTO lesions usually requires a longer time than a standard procedure, and a good rule is not to start the procedure as the last case of the day.

• Always perform CTO with a partner.

• Plan your strategy, be patient and willing to change it if necessary.

• Every technique should be taken as a preparation towards the next step.

• Preprocedural assessment is very important. Consider the risk of the procedure, access to the CTO (easy/difficult), possibility of retrograde access, presence of channels, etc.

• Use orthogonal projections and assess the lesion carefully in at least two views.

• Give heparin and maintain ACT above 300 seconds. Check ACT every hour.
• Perform a collateral injection if distal filling is present from the opposite artery.
• An over-the-wire balloon catheter should be used routinely.
• CTO-dedicated devices should facilitate the procedure
• Always start with a floppy wire, and switch to an increasingly stiff wire if progress is inadequate.
• A tough CTO usually requires stiff wire that is stiffer than Miracle 3.0 g.
• Shape the wire precisely; the tip curve for drilling and penetration should be at 45–60°.
• Block the false lumen by inserting a second wire using the parallel wire technique.
• If a balloon will not cross the lesion, use a second wire for support. If this does not help. switch the guide for greater support: e.g., Judkins right 4 to Amplatz left 1 if dealing with the RCA.
• Always check the angiogram before balloon inflation. You have to be absolutely sure that the wire is placed in the true lumen before balloon inflation.
• Preserve the side branch when dealing with a CTO bifurcation lesion. Avoid suboptimal stenting and pay attention to the point of crossing into the side branch. Use IVUS if necessary.
• If the wire keeps entering the side branch, switch to a stiff straight wire, use support catheter or IVUS guidance.
• Stop the procedure for the following reasons:
  – Contrast dose is higher than 600 ml.
  – Cumulative radiation dose is higher than 5 Gy.
  – Total procedure time is longer than 90 minutes.
• If complications occur: first, manage these and stabilize the patient. Another attempt can be considered in a few weeks' time.
• The procedure can be considered a technical success if TIMI 3 flow has been restored and residual stenosis is less than 50%.

Contralateral Injection

Bilateral injection by simultaneous injections in the right and left coronary system helps improve distal visualization and assess the distal side of the CTO lesion. Although visibility of collaterals may become poorer during the procedure, due to wire manipulation, even very poor collaterals are helpful in marking the distal vessel and in detecting potential dissection or perforation. Advancing a balloon into a perforated vessel will result in severe bleeding and can lead to tamponade. Sometimes it is difficult to find distal collaterals, and identification of a specific collateral channel (e.g., a connection between RCA and LAD through the conus branch) may solve the problem.

Table 5.10 Single wire techniques.

Approach	Wire Manipulation	Wire Selection	Type of Lesion
Controlled drilling	Probe back and forward and gently rotate	Softer wires, stepwise increase: Floppy Pilot 50-200 Miracle 3 g–6 g–12 g Asahi 3 g–6 g Cross-IT 100–300	Easy CTO: lesion with discreet entry point, straight forward
Penetrating	Probe forward with minimal rotation	Stiffer wires stepwise increase: Miracle 6 g–12 g Confianza 9 g tapered tip Confianza Pro 9 g,12 g Cross-IT 400,	Complex CTO: fibrotic, calcified lesion in a relatively straight segment
Sliding	Probe gently with minimal rotation	Pilot 50–200 Whisper, the floppiest wire Shinobi, the stiffest wire, best torquability Fielder family	Lesion with microchannels or anticipated microchannels

Antegrade Approach

The choice of strategy with the antegrade approach is determined by the type of lesion and vessel anatomy. The technique initially selected often requires modification or revision during the procedure. There are two available strategies: single wire technique and parallel wire technique.

The single wire approach is the initial attempt to cross the occlusion, manipulating one wire with various techniques. The parallel wire technique is an effective way to deal with situations when the wire enters a subintimal track (i.e., a false lumen). Support catheters such as a microcatheter or over-the-wire balloon catheter greatly facilitate the procedure.

Single Wire Technique

This approach requires precise wire manipulation (controlled drilling, penetrating, and sliding) and use of various wires (Table 5.10). It is always good to start with a floppy wire and switch progressively to a wire with greater strength and stiffness, e.g., Miracle 3 g – 6 g – 12 g. Sometimes a small 1.5 mm balloon deployed in the proximal side branch can facilitate the procedure. CTO-dedicated wires are stiffer and more aggressive than conventional PCI wires, and rapid advancement or rotation must be avoided.

Controlled Drilling This is a useful technique to help deal with simple CTO lesions with a discrete entry point. Drilling probes the lesion more precisely than penetration by backward and forward wire movement with slight rotation. Start drilling the lesion with a moderately floppy wire and increase wire stiffness during the procedure if necessary. Miracle Bros family wires are a good choice.

Penetrating This should be performed if the entry point is blunt and the lesion is tough and resistant. The technique provides directional control of the wire tip and is based on direct firm probing forward with minimal rotation of the tip. The wire should be stiff and tapered to penetrate heavily calcified lesions, e.g., Confianza.

Sliding Sliding is based on simultaneous minimal rotation and minimal probing and is useful particularly in crossing microchannels or subtotal occlusions. Sliding requires a polymer-coated wire with a longer and less angulated tip, e.g., for microchannel tracking Fielder FC/XT is a good option.

Parallel Wire Technique

This is a penetration technique used to deal with the problem of a wire entering a false lumen (subintimal track). Progress during crossing the lesion should be checked frequently in multiple angiographic projections to monitor this subintimal track. The first wire enters the false lumen and the second parallel wire detects and probes the true lumen – finally crossing the lesion. The distal cap can be penetrated at its central point based on the position of the first wire. In some cases the second parallel wire may also enter the false lumen, which often happens on the opposite wall of the vessel. The optimal solution in such situations is to withdraw the first wire from the false lumen and try to find the true lumen, leaving the parallel wire in the false lumen. This is the seesaw technique (see below).

Parallel Wire Technique Step by Step (Figure 5.28)

• Use a Miracle or Confianza Pro wire; shape the tip, trying to match the vessel angle with the bend in the wire.
• Draw the wiring line before advancing the wire and follow the pathway.
• Advance the first wire into the vessel and, using the penetration technique, go subintimally, creating a false lumen. When entering it, manipulate the wire for a while to enlarge the false lumen.
• Keep the first wire in the false lumen. There are several reasons for this. First, the wire will serve as a marker and will help advancement of a second wire. Second, it will occlude the path into the false lumen. Finally, it will enhance the passage of the second wire into the true lumen.

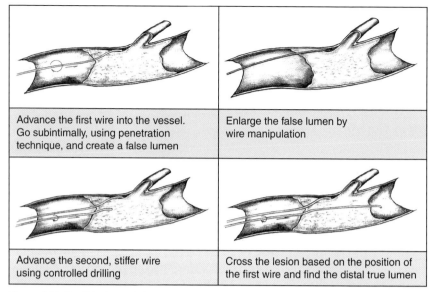

Advance the first wire into the vessel. Go subintimally, using penetration technique, and create a false lumen	Enlarge the false lumen by wire manipulation
Advance the second, stiffer wire using controlled drilling	Cross the lesion based on the position of the first wire and find the distal true lumen

Figure 5.28 Parallel wire technique.

• Advance the second, stiffer wire parallel to the first wire using the controlled drilling maneuver (see above).
• Cross the lesion, using the position of the first wire as a marker, and find the distal true lumen.
• Check the angiogram.
• If the result is not satisfactory, e.g., if the second wire enters another subintimal track, withdraw the first wire and try to enter the true lumen. This is the *see-saw technique* (Figure 5.29).
• Do not advance a balloon until you are absolutely sure of the position of the wire. Check the wire position in at least two orthogonal views and assess distal filling from collaterals.
• If you are sure that the wire has reached and is in the true lumen, switch to a softer wire and advance a small 1.25 mm balloon. A wire in true lumen should be able to enter side branches easily (see Figure 5.26). Perform the first dilatation and check the result with angiography.
• If the result is satisfactory, switch to a larger balloon and perform a second dilatation. Give 100 µg GTN and check with angiography again.
• If the result is satisfactory, deploy a DES.
• If the stump is not present and the occlusion is very long (longer than 20 mm), this technique may fail. IVUS guided re-entry may be helpful.

Retrograde Approach

This is an alternative technique suitable for selected patients with complex CTO in whom an antegrade attempt has failed. Often the distal cap of the

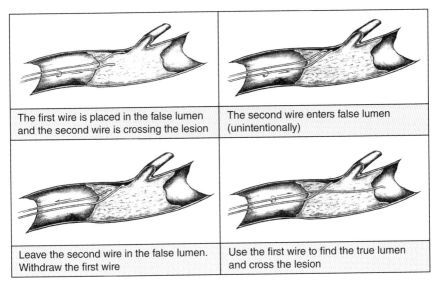

The first wire is placed in the false lumen and the second wire is crossing the lesion	The second wire enters false lumen (unintentionally)
Leave the second wire in the false lumen. Withdraw the first wire	Use the first wire to find the true lumen and cross the lesion

Figure 5.29 See-saw technique.

occlusion is softer than the proximal cap, and although the procedure is technically more demanding, the chances of procedural success are relatively high. The retrograde approach should be selected only for the RCA or the LAD coronary artery as it requires appropriate selection of collateral channels.

In about half the patients with a CTO lesion the retrograde approach is not feasible. The most common reason is poor visualization of the distal collaterals. If the channels are visualized and crossed successfully, the distal vessel beyond the CTO can be entered and the chronically occluded lesion can be crossed retrogradely. An antegrade wire is used to cross a lesion, whereas a retrograde wire serves as a marker and creates a channel for the wire approaching antegradely.

Equipment Selection
- **Guiding catheter.** Usually a 7F, short (80–85 cm) catheter is required to ensure deep seating and strong backup. The best choice is EBU for the LAD coronary artery and JR for the RCA.
- **Microcatheter.** This is a supportive device that helps overcome tortuosities in the collaterals and is needed for superselective injection to visualize channels. The great advantage is clear visibility of the tip and good tracking ability.
- **Wire selection and crossing the channel.** A polymer-coated, steerable slippery wire such as Fielder FC/XT is most suitable. It provides good support and prevents kinking of septal collaterals, allowing safe septal dilatation. The wire tip should be shaped before advancing. The first step is to cross

collaterals with a wire targeting the distal vessel. After crossing collaterals, a stiffer wire such as the Confianza Pro may be needed to penetrate the distal cap.

- **Balloon.** Once the retrograde wire is positioned in the distal vessel and is definitely in the true lumen, a microcatheter or a small over-the-wire balloon (diameter 1.25–2.0 mm) can be advanced for septal dilatation. This should be done slowly and carefully and the balloon must be inflated at very low pressure (2–3 atm).

Collateral Channel Selection

- **Collateral injection.** A retrograde procedure should start with a collateral injection. Once the microcatheter is placed in the septal branch, slowly inject 100 μg GTN with contrast. This should be performed carefully to avoid the risk of dissection.
- **Collateral connections.** Collateral vessels may be connected either with the distal segment of the same vessel or with other collaterals, for example septal, epicardial, or atrial channels or grafts. Commonly used septal branches include LAD-posterior descending, LAD–posterolateral and LAD–left circumflex
- **Collaterals assessment.** Assessment from multiple projections is important as channels are often bendy and have various patterns. The continuous connection grade scale (Table 5.11) is helpful to describe collateral visibility and characteristics.
- **Crossing collaterals.** Successful crossing is dependent on good selection of CTO-dedicated devices. The guiding catheter should be short (shorter than 85 cm) with strong support, whereas the microcatheter for collateral visualization should be rather long (>145 cm). Septal branches suitable for a retrograde approach must be easily visible (CC1/2) and not very bendy. If septal branches are difficult to visualize, a Fielder wire may be very helpful. Shape the tip and advance the wire carefully, avoiding extensive pushing.

Table 5.11 Continuous connection grade scale for assessment of septal collaterals.

CC0	Connection not visible
CC1	Connection visible
	Thread-like size
	Mild tortuosity
	Mild corkscrew morphology
CC2	Connection clearly visible
	Mild tortuosity
	Mild corkscrew morphology

Adapted from R. G. S. Werner.

Kissing Wire Technique

In this bilateral technique one wire is advanced into the target vessel crossing the CTO lesion antegradely through the microchannels, while the second wire goes retrogradely. The retrograde wire serves as a marker for the antegrade approach. Both wires should move inside the channels. This technique is rather demanding and is rarely used.

Controlled Antegrade and Retrograde Subintimal Tracking (CART) Technique

This is subintimal tracking performed simultaneously from both sides of the occluded lesion (antegradely and retrogradely). The antegrade wire goes from the proximal true lumen into the CTO lesion, reaching the false lumen. The retrograde wire is advanced from the distal true lumen into the CTO lesion through the best collateral channel and then also tracks subintimally (Figure 5.30). It is possible to recognize the moment when the wire enters the subintimal track by decreased resistance felt on the tip of the wire.

Once the wire reaches the subintimal path, inflate a small balloon at low pressure on the retrograde wire to make a crack in the chronic lesion, deflate it, and leave the deflated balloon in place. This will help keep the subintimal track open and will provide a stable platform.

At this point the antegrade wire and the retrograde balloon, both placed subintimally at the CTO site, can be connected (Figure 5.30). The antegrade

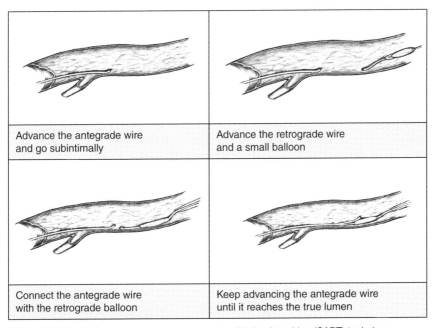

| Advance the antegrade wire and go subintimally | Advance the retrograde wire and a small balloon |
| Connect the antegrade wire with the retrograde balloon | Keep advancing the antegrade wire until it reaches the true lumen |

Figure 5.30 Controlled antegrade and retrograde subintimal tracking (CART) technique.

wire should be advanced a little further along the deflated retrograde balloon in order to reach the distal true lumen. At the end, perform septal injection to assess septal collaterals.

CART Technique Step by Step
• Advance the first wire antegradely and go subintimally.
• Advance the second wire, e.g., Miracle 3g, go retrogradely, and create subintimal dissection.
• Advance a small balloon retrogradely and inflate the balloon at low pressure (2–3 atm).
• Deflate the balloon and leave the deflated balloon in place to keep the subintimal track open.
• Keep advancing the first antegrade wire, targeting the deflated retrograde balloon.
• Connect the antegrade wire with the retrograde balloon, both subintimally, and keep advancing the antegrade wire until it reaches the distal true lumen. This should happen automatically.
• Check the result on multiple projections to ensure optimal alignment and confirm that the wire is placed in the true lumen. This is very important.
• Inflate balloon and deploy DES.

Reverse CART Technique
In the reverse CART technique the antegrade wire goes subintimally as above. However, the subintimal crack is made by an antegrade balloon positioned at the proximal part of the CTO lesion. This approach is safer than CART and it helps avoid collateral complications as the anchoring balloon is advanced antegradely. Reverse CART is often helpful when the CART technique fails, e.g., the retrograde balloon will not enter the distal true lumen due to severe calcifications or tortuosities.
Proceed as follows:
• Assess the septal collaterals and find the best track to cross them.
• Advance the first wire retrogradely and find a subintimal track.
• Insert the second wire and a small balloon antegradely, go subintimally, and inflate the antegrade balloon at low pressure.
• Deflate the balloon and leave it in place.
• Keep advancing the retrograde wire, targeting the deflated antegrade balloon.
• Connect the retrograde wire and the antegrade balloon, both subintimally, and keep advancing the retrograde wire until it reaches the proximal true lumen. This should happen automatically.
• Ensure optimal alignment and proceed further as in the CART technique.

Knuckle Wire Technique
This technique is similar to the STAR technique (see below) but using a retrograde wire (Figure 5.31). The retrograde wire is advanced first into the distal

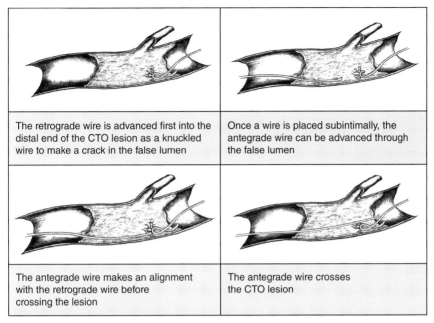

The retrograde wire is advanced first into the distal end of the CTO lesion as a knuckled wire to make a crack in the false lumen	Once a wire is placed subintimally, the antegrade wire can be advanced through the false lumen
The antegrade wire makes an alignment with the retrograde wire before crossing the lesion	The antegrade wire crosses the CTO lesion

Figure 5.31 Knuckle wire technique.

end of the CTO lesion as a knuckled wire in order to make a crack in the false lumen (Figure 5.31). Once the wire is placed subintimally, the antegrade wire goes through the false lumen, forms a loop, and makes an alignment with the retrograde wire.

The best way to create the knuckle, or loop, is to keep advancing the wire subintimally until resistance is felt. Then a slight push and rotation should result in a knuckle. A soft hydrophilic wire, e.g., Whisper or Pilot, seems to be optimal.

Subintimal Tracking and Re-entry (STAR) Technique

This approach is rarely used and should only be considered if traditional techniques have been unsuccessful or if surgery is not an option. This technique carries a higher risk of perforation compared to other CTO techniques. There is also a risk of occlusion of side branches located proximal to the distal re-entry and is therefore more suitable for the RCA.

It is sensible to use a stiff hydrophilic wire, e.g., Miracle 3 g or 6 g, through the 1.5 mm over-the-wire balloon catheter, creating a subintimal dissection, and then switch to a hydrophilic wire, e.g., Pilot. The tip of the wire should be shaped to minimize risk of vessel injury. Then the wire re-enters the true lumen of the vessel distal to the occlusion by multiple balloon inflations.

Failure to Cross the Lesion

If the lesion is uncrossable and the procedure is not successful, the patient may need to be referred for surgery. This is most beneficial for symptomatic patients with ST changes or demonstrable ischemia in the CTO area or in multivessel disease if angioplasty cannot achieve complete revascularization.

Complications of CTO Angioplasty

In general the risk of complications during CTO angioplasty is low. However, the following problems may occur:

• **Perforation, dissection.** Mechanical vessel damage is the most common problem in CTO angioplasty. This is often caused by aggressive manipulation while crossing the lesion with a stiff wire. Specific treatment is usually not necessary as a small hematoma absorbs spontaneously.

• **Hemorrhage.** Intraluminal tracking does not cause severe hemorrhage, and dilatation of the true lumen followed by stent implantation will solve the problem. If the wire enters a false lumen, however, the balloon must not be inflated and the best solution is to dilate a balloon proximally and to stop the bleeding by reversing heparin with protamine sulfate. Severe bleeding is rare, but may occur, e.g., due to channel rupture. This should be treated with proximal balloon inflation or suction with a penetration catheter.

CTO procedures require routine administration of heparin. Other agents such as abciximab, other GPIs, or bivalirudin can be given only after successful crossing when the distal flow is fully restored, as there are no antidotes which immediately reverse the anticoagulation effect of these agents.

• **Subepicardial hematoma** usually requires coil embolization.

• **Myocardial infarction** is rare, but may occur, e.g., due to occlusion of collateral channels which compromises collateral flow.

• **Other complications** such as coronary rupture, fistula to the right or left ventricle, or cardiac tamponade may also occur, and in these situations emergency surgery is required. Immediate ligation of the perforated vessel is needed, followed by grafting where appropriate.

Trials

OAT

In this trial 2166 patients with total occlusions of infarct-related arteries were randomized to either routine PCI plus stenting and medical therapy or medical therapy alone, 3 to 28 days after their myocardial infarction. Patients with significant left main or three-vessel disease, angina at rest, hemodynamic or electrical instability, NYHA class 3 or 4 heart failure, or shock were excluded from the trial. At follow-up, the estimated 4-year cumulative primary event rate – a composite of death, reinfarction, or heart failure – did not differ between the PCI group and the medical group. Although, individually, rates of death and rates of heart failure were also no different between the two groups, the rate of nonfatal reinfarction tended to be higher among PCI-treated patients. In secondary end point analyses, the difference in nonfatal reinfarction rates between the two groups reached statistical significance. Do not attempt to reopen an occluded coronary artery late after a myocardial infarction in an asymptomatic patient.

TOSCA-2

A total of 381 patients enrolled in the OAT study were included in the TOSCA-2 ancillary study, in which coronary and left ventricular angiography was performed 1 year after randomization.

The study demonstrated that 83% of PCI-treated patients had patent infarct-related arteries at one year, compared with 25% in the medical therapy group. Left ventricular ejection fraction improved in both groups, but with no significant differences between the two groups. Change in left ventricular end-diastolic volume index was lower in the PCI group, suggesting that PCI had a favorable effect in terms of reducing ventricular enlargement.

PRISON II

In this study 200 patients with coronary arteries that were totally occluded for at least 2 weeks with evidence of ischemia were randomized to undergo PCI with either DES (sirolimus-eluting stent) or bare metal stent. The primary end point was in-segment angiographic binary restenosis at 6 months, and the secondary end points at 3 years included clinical restenosis, major adverse cardiac events, and target vessel failure. This study demonstrated that a sirolimus-eluting stent for total coronary occlusion was associated with reduced rates of restenosis and major adverse cardiac events at 3 years compared with a bare metal stent.

Key Learning Points

- A CTO procedure requires more time than a standard PCI and should not be left as the last case of the day.
- Plan the procedure; assess success/failure factors; be patient and willing to change strategy if necessary.
- Choice of strategy should depend on the availability of retrograde access.
- Every step and every technique should be an integral part of the strategy and a preparation towards the next step.
- Perform collateral injections from the opposite artery if distal filling is present.
- Do not attempt a CTO procedure in an asymptomatic patient late after a myocardial infarction.

Grafts and Conduits

Saphenous Vein Graft Angioplasty

Introduction

The coronary vein graft is a very different structure from the native coronary artery and carries its own problems. Almost 10% of PCIs are in saphenous vein grafts (SVGs), and angioplasty if possible is preferable to repeat bypass surgery. SVG patency is time limited; about 50% will be occluded and may need repeat revascularization 10 years after surgery. This is mostly due to atherosclerotic plaques, thrombus formation, or deposition of lipids. Atheroma in a vein graft tends to be bulky and friable, and instrumentation easily causes distal embolization of atheromatous fragments and microthrombi. The vein graft wall itself may be friable and more prone to rupture. The restenotic lesion itself (more common than in native vessels) is more lipid-rich than the restenotic lesion in native vessels and is softer than plaques from native coronary vessels. In addition, vein grafts may have a large luminal diameter, sometimes associated with a sharp step-down in diameter at the distal anastomosis, which can make balloon sizing for the distal anastomosis stenosis difficult.

Lipid-lowering therapy and antiplatelet therapy are required in all patients who have had bypass surgery with a vein graft. Repeat bypass surgery is often difficult and carries a higher risk of complications, perioperative myocardial infarction, and mortality than the initial operation. The success of redo surgery at relieving angina is less – particularly in elderly patients with comorbidities. Angioplasty is also more demanding, with increased rates of no-reflow, acute myocardial infarction, distal embolization, and restenosis with poorer early outcomes than with native-vessel PCI. In selected cases, new CTO techniques used in a native vessel may help improve myocardial perfusion and symptoms enough to avoid the need for SVG angioplasty.

Principles in Vein Graft Angioplasty

In view of the these problems, there are a few caveats in vein graft PCI:
• Proceed carefully in old degenerative vein grafts and avoid vein graft rupture.
• Plaque manipulation may cause embolization.
• Good flow is much more important than a perfect cosmetic result.
• Be prepared for no-reflow during balloon angioplasty and stenting (more likely in vein grafts than native vessels).
• Distal runoff is important: additional dilatation of distal disease in the native vessel may be necessary to ensure this (see Figure 5.34).
• Choose a suitable guide catheter and ensure good support, particularly in tortuous vein grafts (multipurpose, Amplatz left).
• A 6F guide is large enough for a protection device, which should be used.
• Avoid predilatation if possible, with its risk of distal embolization of plaque fragments. Attempt direct stenting.
• Use thrombectomy devices to remove fresh thrombus.
• Use DES only in smaller grafts (3.0 mm or less), but bare metal stents should be used in larger grafts.
• There is no evidence to support the use of covered stents. These are only indicated for graft rupture.
• Avoid oversizing (see Figure 5.32).
• Avoid high-pressure inflation if possible.
• Consider new CTO techniques to open an occluded native vessel.
• Ensure prolonged dual antiplatelet therapy after DES implantation.

When to Proceed

Any case where a graft PCI is being considered should be discussed with a cardiac surgeon. A surgical option should be excluded as these cases are rarely suitable for emergency PCI. The decision usually rests on the quality of the native vessels and on information from either stress echocardiography or myocardial perfusion imaging. Is there reversible ischemia in the relevant territory, or is the area essentially just scar tissue?

If there is multivessel disease with several grafts already occluded, and reasonable distal target vessels, then redo CABG should be considered as the first-choice strategy. Patients with disease of a single graft or comorbidities precluding surgery should be managed with PCI as the first option, with continued medical treatment considered as the alternative. It must always be remembered that angioplasty is treating symptoms and has not been shown to affect prognosis in these cases.

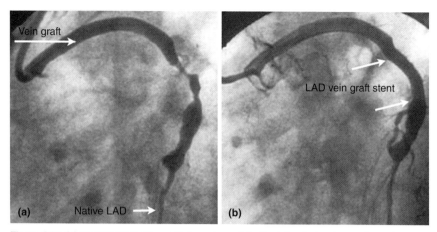

Figure 5.32 **(a)** Degenerative change in the vein graft to the left anterior descending artery (LAD). **(b)** LAD vein graft after stent implantation The stent has been deliberately slightly undersized (see text).

Guide Catheter Support

Guide support is very important for successful balloon and stent delivery. In a tortuous vein graft, particularly with a steep angle, stent delivery can be very difficult, and it is important to select the optimal guide and ensure stable seating. Amplatz, left coronary bypass (LCB), Judkins right, or even a LIMA guide for a graft with a vertical takeoff can be used successfully for left vein grafts and multipurpose catheters for the right vein graft. In a high takeoff from the aorta, a multipurpose catheter or Judkins right would be an initial choice.

Drug-Eluting or Bare Metal Stent?

This remains a controversial area, with little evidence favoring DES in SVG PCI to guide us. In most randomized trials assessing DES, SVG lesions were excluded.

There are two major concerns about DES in this subset of lesions; long-term safety and long-term efficacy. First, the mechanism of in-stent restenosis is different in SVG than in native arteries. Secondly, there is potential delay in endothelial healing after DES, which may lead to a higher risk of acute, subacute, and late thrombosis.

Although DES provide lower early risk of restenosis and show better results than bare metal stents (BMS) in reducing target vessel revascularization at 9 months, there is a "catch up phenomenon" and in 2 years time the benefit is usually lost or at least diminished. The RRISC trial randomized 75 patients with vein graft disease to either a drug (sirolimus)-eluting stent or BMS, using embolic protection in most patients. The primary end point was 6 month late stent loss, which was significantly lower in the DES group.

Target vessel revascularization was similarly significantly better in the DES group.

Although this data appears to favor DES in vein graft disease, there are three caveats with this study:

1. Large vein grafts (>4.0 mm) were excluded (approximately 20% of the registry).

2. Three-year follow-up of this group raised concerns of the long-term safety of DES in vein graft disease. There were 11 deaths (7 cardiac) in the DES group at a median follow-up of 32 months, and none in the BMS group. Definite stent thrombosis was found in 5% of the DES group vs. 0% in the BMS group.

3. The initial benefit of reduced target vessel revascularization in the 6 month analysis was not maintained in the secondary long-term follow-up analysis.

On this evidence, bare metal stenting is recommended for vein graft disease. There may be a case for the use of DES in small vessels, but data from more randomized studies with larger numbers are needed. In new studies, DES show similar long-term results to BMS in respect of death/myocardial infarction and target vessel revascularization.

The main concern with SVG PCI is that almost 40% of SVG fail again in 12–18 months after BMS implantation. This is mostly due to restenosis or thrombus at the treatment site, or simply disease progression in another segment in the vein graft. Results from ARRIVE Registry (2009) showed that 2-year vein graft vessel revascularization using the Taxus DES was higher than in native vessels, but lower than with BMS, with a failure rate of almost 40% by 18 months. DES do not prevent a high 1-year mortality rate in SVG stenting and do not prevent progression of disease in other vein graft segments.

Some interventionists use DES routinely in de novo lesions, others prefer BMS. If graft restenosis occurs in a BMS stent, DES are preferable as additional or sandwich stents.

Generally, direct stenting is recommended in SVG procedures to avoid the risk of distal embolization. However, in some cases, such as tortuous or heavily calcified lesions, predilatation is required. It is important not to over-size the balloon to prevent potential dissection or vessel rupture. When the stent is expanded successfully, high-pressure postdilatation with a noncompliant balloon is necessary in these cases.

Distal Protection

Embolization remains the primary cause of vascular obstruction and poor outcomes in vein graft PCI, with increased infarct size and higher risk of death. Vein graft PCI is one of the few confirmed indications for distal protection. Embolization may occur spontaneously due to plaque rupture or as a result of mechanical injury which leads to thrombus fragmentation. Embolic protection reduces the risk of no-reflow and the embolization rate by up to

50%, and also the 30-day rate of major adverse cardiac events (SAFER, FIRE trial). Nevertheless, devices themselves carry a risk of vessel injury and embolism,e.g., during primary crossing. Three types of devices which have been successfully tried are discussed below, but none has proved superior to the others.

Proximal Occlusion and Flow Reversal
Inflation of a balloon proximal to the graft stenosis prevents any flow of blood down the graft (Figure 5.33). When the stenosis has been dilated and stented, aspiration of this stagnant pool of blood and embolic material can be performed through the same catheter. The PROXIMAL randomized trial of the Proxis Embolic Protection System showed that this device was noninferior to distal protection devices, with a 30-day rate of major adverse cardiac events of 9.2% for the Proxis device and 10% for the distal protection devices. Advantages and disadvantages of proximal balloon protection are listed in Table 5.12.

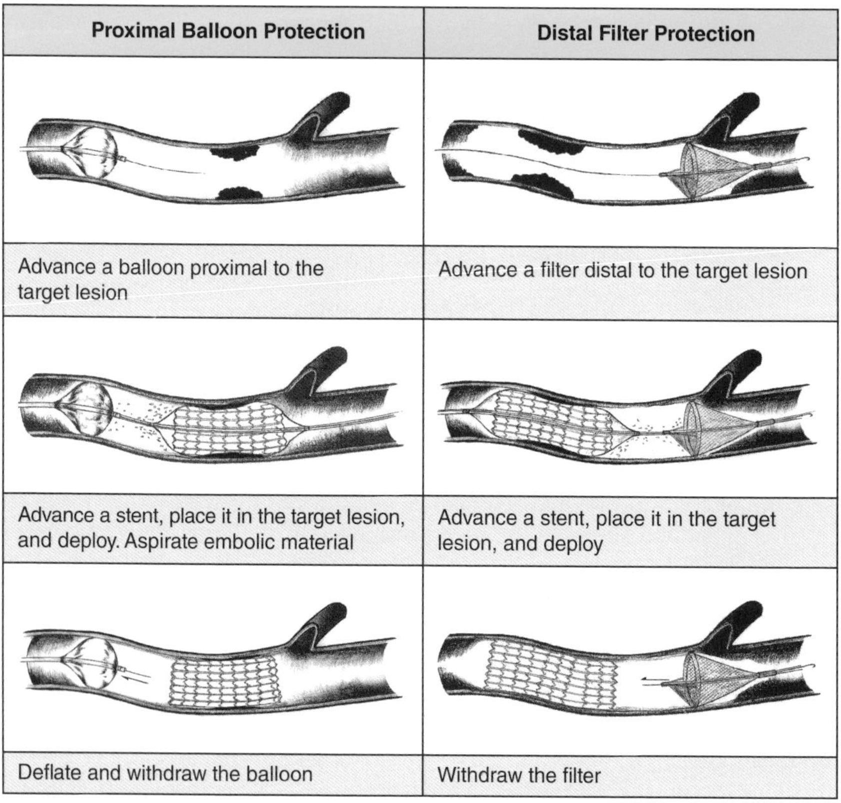

Proximal Balloon Protection	Distal Filter Protection
Advance a balloon proximal to the target lesion	Advance a filter distal to the target lesion
Advance a stent, place it in the target lesion, and deploy. Aspirate embolic material	Advance a stent, place it in the target lesion, and deploy
Deflate and withdraw the balloon	Withdraw the filter

Figure 5.33 Proximal balloon protection and distal filter protection.

Table 5.12 Advantages and disadvantages of proximal balloon protection.

Advantages	Disadvantages
Good myocardium protection during procedure	Myocardial ischemia during procedure
Contrast suspension	Antegrade flow not preserved
Aspiration of large thrombus fragments	Not suitable for ostial lesions
Landing zone not required	

Table 5.13 Advantages and disadvantages of distal balloon protection.

Advantages	Disadvantages
Easy to cross a lesion	Vessel damage caused by balloon
Able to aspirate large fragments	Poor torquability
Stable trap of thrombus remnants	Antegrade flow not preserved
Compatible with devices	Poor contrast imaging during procedure
	Risk of intolerance
	Landing zone required

Distal Occlusive Devices and Filters

Distal Protection Balloon (Distal Occlusion) A small, low-pressure balloon is first inflated in the distal (normal) part of the vein graft, once again blocking all antegrade flow. The graft angioplasty is then performed, and finally the contents of the graft are aspirated before the distal balloon is deflated. The SAFER trial compared this device with BMS alone. There was a highly significant reduction in 30-day major adverse cardiac events in the distal protection arm compared with BMS. The main benefit was the reduction in periprocedural myocardial infarction. Advantages and disadvantages of distal balloon protection are listed in Table 5.13.

Distal Filter Protection (Distal Filters) This device is similar to the distal protection balloon, and the filter is similarly positioned distally in the graft beyond the stenosis and catches embolic material in its porous net (Figure 5.33). The filter does not completely occlude the graft during deployment, unlike the other two devices above. A major limitation of distal filter devices is the need for a landing zone with a good sized distal vessel. The device is quite bulky and it may be difficult to advance it across the lesion, particularly in a tortuous vein graft. The 30-day rate of major adverse cardiac events showed the filter was noninferior to the distal protection balloon in the FIRE trial. Advantages and disadvantages of distal filter protection are listed in Table 5.14.

There is no doubt that graft PCI should include an embolic protection device, but on present evidence there appears to be nothing to choose between

Table 5.14 Advantages and disadvantages of distal filter protection.

Advantages	Disadvantages
Antegrade flow preserved	Unreliable trap of thrombus remnants
Good contrast imaging during procedure	Risk of clogging
Easy to use	Risk of catheter embolization before filter is used
	Landing zone required

these three devices. Interventionists need to learn how to use one of these devices in spite of their expense. Their use in graft PCI needs to increase as only about one-quarter of graft PCI procedures actually include one.

Covered Stents and Abciximab

Two strategies have failed: covered stents and abciximab.

Covered Stents

Theoretically a stent covered in polytetrafluoroethylene (PTFE) should be the answer to friable bulky atheroma by trapping it in the graft wall and preventing distal embolization. Unfortunately, four randomized trials have each failed to show any benefit of covered stents over BMS in vein grafts, and meta-analysis of these trials has shown a trend to an increase in restenosis with covered stents. Their use has been abandoned except in the rare occurrence of coronary perforation.

Abciximab

In theory, a GPI should be of value in reducing platelet emboli and new thrombus formation in vein graft angioplasty. Unfortunately, meta-analysis of five randomized trials using abciximab in bypass grafts has not shown a clinical benefit in using this drug. It cannot be recommended on a routine basis but is still used in cases with a high thrombus burden.

An example of a saphenous vein graft angioplasty is shown in Figure 5.34.

Complications of SVG Procedures

The major problem with saphenous vein graft angioplasty is the high rate of in-stent restenosis and periprocedural adverse cardiovascular events. Despite all the rules that apply to SVG intervention, such as crossing the lesion without predilatation, immediate use of distal protection devices, and use of DES, the rate of complications is still high. This is mostly due to the degenerative change in vein grafts and bulky thrombotic or atherothrombotic lesions. Sometimes the entire lesion including thrombus may fragment, shift, and embolize distally.

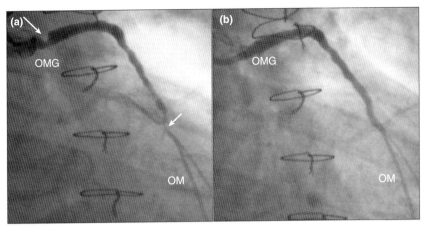

Figure 5.34 **(a)** Severe stenosis (long arrow) at the origin of the obtuse marginal graft (OMG) and degenerative disease (short arrow) in the distal graft with anastomosis stenosis. **(b)** Final result after stenting: 2.5 × 16 mm and 3.0 × 16 mm Taxus stent in distal obtuse marginal graft and 5 × 13 mm Ultra bare metal stent proximally.

Distal Embolization

Distal embolization results in periprocedural myocardial infarction and increased long-term mortality. The main causes of embolization are spontaneous plaque rupture, and mechanical plaque fragmentation. The risk should be assessed on the basis of vessel morphology. Thrombus is often present.

A few caveats may help avoid distal embolization:
• Initial aspiration is very important and should be performed before selection of a distal protection device.
• Protection by a balloon occlusion and aspiration system has been shown to facilitate the SVG procedure. Incomplete retrieval of emboli may result in embolization with secondary spasm and platelet aggregation. This leads to no-reflow.
• The stent should be long enough to cover the entire lesion, and occasionally a covered stent may be needed.
• Finally, a GPI should also be considered if it is felt there is a thrombus burden.

No-Reflow

This usually occurs in old degenerate vein grafts or thrombotic lesions as a result of distal embolization and platelet aggregation which may lead to myocardial infarction, arrhythmias, and death. No-reflow is less common in arterial grafts than in vein graft PCI. Distal filter devices have been shown to reduce no-reflow in vein grafts and should be routinely used if technically feasible. The use of intravenous GPIs which are of benefit in native coronary intervention (particularly primary PCI) have failed to improve outcomes in vein graft PCI. No-reflow is usually reversible after aggressive treatment with adenosine, calcium channel blockers, and/or nitroprusside (see pp. 294–296). However, it may be resistant to treatment, resulting in severe myocardial damage. In some cases, particularly if the lesion is large and thrombotic, pretreatment with intracoronary verapamil 200–300 µg may reduce the risk.

Vessel Rupture

Although very rare, this is a life-threatening complication that may occur during complex and more aggressive intervention such as using a cutting balloon to deal with in-stent restenosis, selection of too large a balloon or stent, or high-pressure dilatation. Sometimes, however, even predilatation may cause dissection or rupture. Graft rupture may lead to mediastinal hemorrhage, tamponade, and cardiac arrest. Immediate deployment of a covered stent may be life-saving. Emergency surgery with ligation of the graft is usually required.

In-Stent Restenosis

Vein graft angioplasty is associated with a higher risk of in-stent restenosis compared with native coronary arteries. Although DES decrease the risk of restenosis in the native coronary, data from vein graft stenting are still limited.

Trials

ARRIVE SVG

In this study 457 patients had PCI of a SVG with one Taxus Express stent. The aim of this study was to examine the incidence of clinical events after implantation of the Taxus Express paclitaxel-eluting stent in SVG lesions. This study showed that SVG patients have significantly more baseline comorbidities/complex disease than simple-use patients undergoing native coronary intervention or other expanded-use patients. They had higher 2-year rates of mortality, myocardial infarction, and definite/probable stent thrombosis than the simple-use group. They also had higher 2-year adverse event rates, including significantly higher mortality than other expanded-use patients. Treatment with a paclitaxel-eluting stent seems to offer a reasonable therapeutic option in this group of patients.

SOS

This is a prospective, randomized, multicenter trial comparing the Taxus DES with Express BMS in SVG intervention. The purpose was to compare the 12-month angiographic outcomes and 24 clinical outcomes between DES and BMS in this subset of lesions. Use of DES resulted in significant reduction in 12-month angiographic restenosis, target lesion revascularization, and target vessel failure, and showed trends for lower target vessel revascularization and myocardial infarction. No difference was observed in mortality and stent thrombosis.

CAVEAT II

In this study 305 patients were randomized to directional coronary atherectomy (DCA) or percutaneous transluminal coronary angioplasty (PTCA) for lesions with more than 60% diameter stenosis in vein grafts larger than 3 mm in diameter. The purpose of this study was to identify the predictors and sequelae of distal embolization in SVG intervention. The study demonstrated that SVG DCA was associated with greater angiographic success and less need for repeat intervention than was PTCA, but at the cost of more acute complications – notably, distal embolization. In SVG intervention, distal embolization was more common after DCA than after PTCA and in lesions containing thrombus. In-hospital adverse events were more frequent after distal embolization. At 12-month follow-up, adverse event rates were also higher in patients with distal embolization.

Key Learning Points

- Every vein graft case should be discussed with a cardiac surgeon.
- Predilatation carries a risk of distal embolization.
- Direct stent if possible.
- Avoid stent oversizing.
- Use DES for small vein grafts, and BMS for large vein grafts
- Proceed carefully in old degenerative vein grafts to avoid vein graft rupture.
- Always use an embolic protection device.
- Ensure prolonged dual antiplatelet therapy after DES implantation.

Left Internal Mammary Artery Graft Angioplasty

Introduction

The majority of patients undergoing bypass surgery receive a LIMA (left internal mammary artery) graft to the LAD and vein grafts to the remaining arteries. LIMA is preferred as a graft mostly because of its better patency rates (approximately 90% at 10 years), but also because of lower rates of myocardial infarction and mortality compared to saphenous vein grafting. Stenoses in the LIMA itself are rare. The most common site for a LIMA graft stenosis is at the distal anastomosis, usually into the LAD.

Common Problems

LIMA angioplasty can be a particularly challenging problem for several reasons:
- A femoral approach is preferable, but the left radial will have to be used if there is severe iliofemoral disease.

- The origin of the LIMA from the left subclavian artery is a delicate area and easily traumatized by a guide catheter.
- Access to the LIMA origin may be difficult if the left subclavian artery is tortuous or stenosed. It can be predicted before the procedure by taking the blood pressure on both arms. A bruit beneath the left clavicle or a difference of more than 20 mmHg between the systolic pressure in the two arms may indicate a subclavian stenosis.
- There may be a step down in vessel size, with a large LIMA anastomosed to a smaller LAD.
- The LIMA itself is often tortuous.
- LIMA spasm may be a problem.
- LIMA angiography is painful for the patient and adequate analgesia will be needed.

In view of these problems, any case involving a LIMA graft stenosis should be discussed with a cardiac surgeon in case there is a clear case for regrafting. If a PCI seems the best option, then consider:

- Can I use the left radial approach?
- Which guiding catheter should be selected and how can the graft be engaged?
- Which is the best angiographic projection for the LIMA and the subclavian artery?
- Is there a significant lesion in the distal anastomosis?
- Is the native LAD still patent, and, if so, is there a chance of dilating this LAD stenosis through the native vessel and leaving the LIMA graft alone?
- Is the LIMA tortuous?
- Should the lesion be predilated before stenting?

Coronary Angiography Projection

Visualize the graft end to end, especially the distal anastomosis. The PA cranial or LAO cranial projections give good views of the whole graft and LAO 90° gives the best view of the anastomosis. An ostial stenosis is rare. If one is suspected, select the LAO 60° or RAO 45° view. Subclavian artery angiography is also important if a subclavian artery stenosis is suspected.

Guiding Catheter

- Femoral access is preferable.
- The left radial approach is necessary when femoral access is impossible, when the left subclavian artery is tortuous, or when there is an acute angle between the subclavian artery and the LIMA.
- From the left radial approach use a 90 cm, 6F internal mammary artery (IMA) guiding catheter.
- From the femoral artery use a 6F Judkins right (JR4) or 6F LIMA guide initially. If the pressure drops on intubation, switch to a side hole guide (JR4 SH).

• Do not feel it is necessary to intubate the LIMA origin deeply. Although this may result in better angiographic pictures, spasm and injury to the LIMA ostium may occur.
• Deep intubation with the LIMA guide will not be needed for backup as the stenosis is usually too far distal to make backup with the guide catheter relevant.
• Cannulation can be facilitated by giving GTN before the procedure. Proceed gently.
• LIMA cannulation is challenging if there are tortuosities of the subclavian artery. In this situation it is best to use a Judkins right guiding catheter and enter the LIMA in the 60° LAO view.

Guide Wire
• A wire with good steerability is a first choice. Use a polymer tip (PT)-coated wire or high-torque floppy wire.
• The tortuosity of the LIMA will be more easily negotiated with a PT wire.
• The use of an over-the-wire catheter with a flexible shaft will help negotiate tortuosities.

Predilatation, Crossing, and Stenting
• Balloon selection should be based on vessel length and tortuosity. A longer-shaft balloon (150 cm) or short (90 cm) guide may be needed.
• Always predilate the distal anastomosis stenosis. A high-pressure noncompliant balloon may be needed as these stenoses can be remarkably tough.
• Further dilatations may be needed in the distal LAD to ensure adequate runoff.
• Crossing the tortuous vessel with a standard wire will straighten the vessel, which may result in spasm, flow reduction and consequently poor visibility. Some operators place a Transit exchange catheter distally and then remove the wire. The Transit catheter is very flexible and prevents straightening or spasm, allowing better angiographic assessment.
• Use DES.
• Size the stent from the size of the LAD not the LIMA, aiming to get half the stent in each vessel.
• Postdilate with a high-pressure noncompliant balloon, if necessary flaring out the proximal half of the stent in the bigger LIMA.

Tortuosities and the Distal Anastomosis
A severely tortuous LIMA is one of the major predictors of procedural failure. When this occurs, it is important to select a longer catheter to reach and visualize the distal segment of the artery. The anastomosis with the LAD is the commonest site for obstructed flow and a vulnerable site to deal with. Tortuosities may also cause subtotal vessel occlusion and wire access through the lesion may be difficult or impossible. In this situation surgery will need

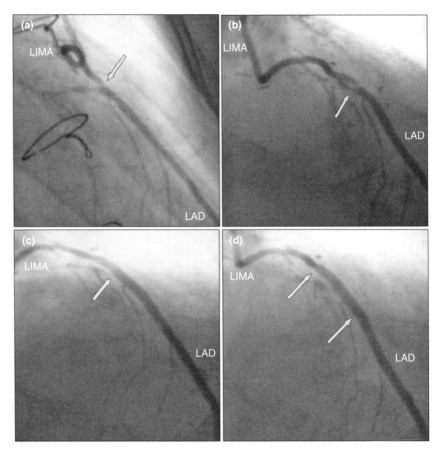

Figure 5.35 Example of left internal mammary artery (LIMA) graft angioplasty. **(a, b)** LIMA distal anastomosis stenosis to the left anterior descending artery. **(c)** Stented with a 2.75 × 16 mm Taxus stent through LIMA. **(d)** Final result.

to be considered. Tortuosities also increase the risk of spasm, dissection, or abrupt closure during wire manipulation. A hydrophilic wire should be selected to facilitate the passage and reduce the risk of complications.

An example of LIMA graft angioplasty is shown in Figure 5.35.

Complications
Procedural success in LIMA graft PCI is more than 80% and complications are rare. However, distal embolization, dissection, abrupt closure, or myocardial infarction may occur, and in some cases emergency surgery is the only option.

• **Spasm.** The LIMA graft is very prone to spasm. Catheter engagement and wire manipulation should be gentle and careful, particularly if the graft is tortuous. If this happens, inject intracoronary GTN or verapamil and check with angiography.

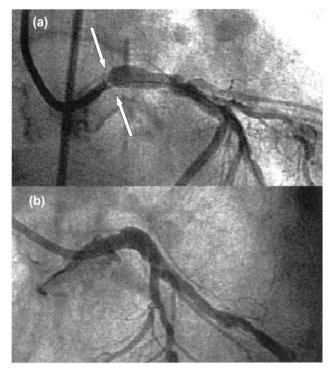

Figure 5.36 Ostial left main stem stenosis in an 84-year-old woman. **(a)** RAO view pre-stenting. JL3.5 guide with a PT extrasupport wire. Minimal dye reflux into aorta. **(b)** LAO cranial view post-stenting with a 4.0 × 13 mm bare metal stent, post-dilated with a 5.0 × 8 mm noncompliant balloon. Some dye reflux now visible.

- **Perforation.** This is a very rare but potentially fatal complication which will lead to major bleeding and tamponade. The most common reason is high-pressure stent deployment.
- **Restenosis.** Compared to SVG, restenosis rates of the internal mammary artery are lower but vary widely. This is probably due to different character-istics of their smooth muscle cells and the high production of endothelial vasodilators.

Key Learning Points

- Always discuss a LIMA graft case with a cardiac surgeon.
- Femoral or left radial access.
- The LIMA graft is often tortuous.
- Access to the LIMA origin may be difficult due to left subclavian artery tortuosities.
- The distal anastomosis with the LAD is the commonest site for a stenosis.
- Always predilate the distal anastomosis stenosis.
- Size the DES from the LAD distal to the lesion.
- Always postdilate the stent.
- Spasm, perforation, and restenosis are the most common complications.

6   Complications

With increasing operator experience, advances in interventional techniques and technology, complication rates are falling, but there are still many potential problems to trap the unwary. Effective prevention, quick recognition, and correct management are essential.

Contrast Reactions

- Introduction, 288
- Management, 289

Introduction

Reactions to contrast agent can be either cardiotoxic or anaphylactoid. The risk increases in patients with an atopic disorder or previous contrast reaction. Always check this possibility when obtaining consent.

Essential Angioplasty, First Edition. E. von Schmilowski, R. H. Swanton.
© 2012 John Wiley & Sons, Ltd. Published 2012 by John Wiley & Sons, Ltd.

• *Cardiotoxic reactions* are related to contrast properties such as osmolality and may present as hypotension and bradycardia.

• *Anaphylactoid reactions* (due to histamine release) differ in mechanism, but not in manifestation from anaphylactic reactions, which are immune-complex-mediated. Newer contrast agents have resulted in fewer reactions, and major contrast reactions are rare.

Minor reactions include urticaria, itch, and erythema.

Moderate reactions include angioedema, laryngeal edema and bronchospasm, and hypotension.

Severe reactions include shock with respiratory and cardiac arrest.

Management

• *Mild reactions* such as urticaria usually do not need treatment, and if the patient is hemodynamically stable, angiography can be continued. With moderate urticaria, diphenhydramine 25–50 mg PO/IM/IV, or chlorpheniramine (chlorphenamine) 10 mg PO/IV should be given.

• *More severe reactions* such as bronchospasm, laryngeal edema, or severe hypotension necessitate the following treatment:

– Oxygen (6–10 l/min).

– Establish femoral vein access quickly if not already available.

– Epinephrine 1 ml of 1 : 10.000 in 10 ml IV slowly every minute (equivalent to 0.1 mg), up to 1 mg if needed.

– Antihistamine (e.g., diphenhydramine 50 mg IV)

– Corticosteroids (e.g., hydrocortisone 200–400 mg IV)

– Volume if hypotensive: 1 l normal saline run in quickly followed by a further 1 l if necessary.

– Atropine 0.6–2.4 mg IV for bradycardia.

– Right ventricular pacing wire may be needed.

– Call for an anesthetist.

Patients with previous contrast reactions are at higher risk of subsequent reactions. In these patients, pretreatment with oral steroids and diphenhydramine 25–50 mg or chlorphenamine 8 mg three times daily starting 24 hours before the procedure is recommended. Alternatively, these drugs can be given intravenously just before the procedure.

Femoral Access Site Problems

The following access site complications may occur:
- Overt bleeding.
- Hematoma, including retroperitoneal bleeding.
- Femoral artery pseudoaneurysm.
- Arterial dissection
- Thrombosis with leg ischemia.
- Embolization of thrombus atheroma or air (rare).
- Arteriovenous fistula formation. This is rare, but may occur if the femoral vein is situated underneath the artery rather than medial to it. Ultrasound is diagnostic and ultrasound-guided compression may cure the problem. Surgical repair may be needed for a large fistula.
- Femoral nerve trauma. This may happen during arterial access or hematoma compression, but is rare.
- Infection is extremely rare and may be related to multiple punctures or difficulties with maintaining a sterile technique (e.g., in a cardiac arrest situation).

Femoral access site complications are often related to the risk factors shown in Table 6.1.

Bleeding

Changes in PCI technique have greatly reduced complications at the femoral artery entry site:
- The use of smaller diameter guiding catheters where possible.
- The removal of the arterial sheath in the catheter lab.
- The immediate use of the Femostop arterial compression device after sheath removal in the catheter lab before the patient has returned to the ward.
- Anticoagulation with bivalirudin, which has been shown to reduce bleeding complications compared with unfractionated heparin.
- The world wide trend to radial access replacing femoral access; this is having a major impact on access site bleeding.

Table 6.1 Risk factors related to femoral artery entry site complications.

Patient	Procedure
Female gender	Femoral arterial puncture not central
Advanced age	Abbreviated compression time
Obesity, or very underweight patient	Sheath size. The larger sheath size the
Hypertension, vascular disease	higher risk of complications
Previous multiple procedures	Needle puncture of posterior wall of
Known clotting problems, anticoagulant	artery
administration, glycoprotein IIb/IIIa	Needle puncture too high: above
inhibitor administration,	inguinal ligament
thrombocytopenia	

Symptoms

Uncontrolled free bleeding from the femoral artery usually means that the vessel is lacerated and prolonged compression is needed. Overt bleeding sometimes causes hypotension, hypovolemia, local (abdominal) tenderness, back pain (retroperitoneal bleed), and groin hematoma. There may be a fall in hemoglobin as dilution occurs later.

Diagnosis and Treatment

Groin and abdominal ultrasound may be needed and occasionally an abdominal CT scan. Reverse anticoagulation, replace volume, local compression with a Femostop and even surgical repair may be required. Protamine 10 mg/1000 U heparin will reverse the unfractionated heparin. Bivalirudin cannot be reversed but has a short duration of action.

Avoid the Problem

Some patients are at a particularly greater risk of bleeding (see Table 6.1) and should be observed with extra care in the immediate post-PCI period. These include:

- Thin, underweight patients
- Hypertensive history
- Known previous bleeding problems
- Coagulation disorder, e.g., thrombocytopenia
- Those who have had a GPI administered
- Use of an 8F sheath for the procedure

It is important that the femoral artery puncture site should be below the inguinal ligament to avoid retroperitoneal bleeding, which may be hard to spot in the early stages. Patients at special risk should be mobilized later, and in particular patients receiving glycoprotein IIb/IIIa receptor inhibitors should remain in bed for the duration of their infusion. To limit the risk of femoral bleeding, the heparin dose should be ACT-controlled. Try to avoid removing the femoral sheath if the activated clotting time (ACT) is greater than 150 seconds.

Despite the excellence of the femoral artery closure devices, late hemorrhage can still occur. Patients are warned to avoid heavy lifting, bending, straining, running, etc., for a week after the procedure. In addition they are told to report immediately any sudden increase in pain or if they notice an enlarging lump in the groin.

Femoral Pseudoaneurysm (False Aneurysm)

An enlarging expansile tender lump over the femoral artery entry site is likely to be a false aneurysm or a hematoma. This occurs in less than 2% cases of femoral access patients. An ultrasound examination will make the diagnosis, and if it is a false aneurysm will identify its size and neck diameter. A false aneurysm is always increasingly painful, whereas a femoral artery hematoma, although unsightly, is uncomfortable but not exquisitely tender. Bed rest is

Table 6.2 Causes, symptoms, and complications of femoral pseudoaneurysm.

Causes	Symptoms	Complications
Female gender	Local pain	Rupture
Large sheath (>7F)	Swelling	Distal embolization
Low femoral puncture	Bruit	Necrosis
Inadequate compression	Hematoma	Infection
Diabetes, obesity	Local bleeding	

needed until the problem is sorted out. Causes, symptoms, and complications of femoral pseudoaneurysm are shown in Table 6.2.

Management

Most false aneurysms require some form of intervention; only the smallest, pea-size aneurysm may thrombose spontaneously.

Some clinicians start with ultrasound-guided compression, but others inject thrombin to obliterate the false aneurysm at diagnosis, believing that this is the most rapid and painless way to cure the problem. Rarely, surgical closure will be needed.

Ultrasound-Guided Compression

Ultrasound-guided compression, if attempted, should be done with the patient under local and/or i.v analgesia and sedation. Find the arterial pulse and locate the neck of the aneurysm. Position the probe over the neck. Continuous direct pressure over the neck of the aneurysm with the ultrasound probe for 30 minutes may close it off. Check the artery with ultrasound 24 hours after successful compression. The compression strategy can be painful, and both the patient and radiologist may prefer thrombin injection. It is quicker, less painful, and has a very high success rate.

Thrombin Injection

Injection of thrombin into the aneurysm under ultrasound guidance is very effective, particularly in heparinized patients. It is done with the patient under local analgesia, using a 19- to 22-gauge needle and 1000–5000 U of thrombin. Perform thrombin injection as shown in Figure 6.1.

The Ischemic Leg

Fortunately this is extremely rare. An ischemic leg may occur in arteriopathic patients with poor femoral vessels in whom sheath size is mismatched or when a closure device has been used inappropriately. A low cardiac output will compound the problem. Early surgical consultation is important. Femoral embolectomy or open surgical repair may be required. Signs, symptoms, and treatment of the ischemic leg are shown in Table 6.3.

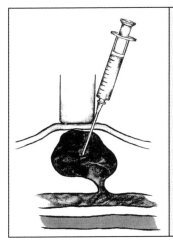

1. Locate the aneurysm with ultrasound.
2. Advance the needle under ultrasound guidance into the sac and inject thrombin.
3. If the flow in sac is still present, perform another injection.
4. After this, If the flow is only in the neck of the aneurysm withdraw the needle and check the artery after 24 hours.
5. The patient should stay in bed for 4–6 hours

Figure 6.1 Percutaneous thrombin injection with ultrasound control.

Table 6.3 Signs, symptoms, and treatment of acute extremity ischemia.

Signs and Symptoms: The 5 Ps	Treatment
Pain	Local lysis below puncture site
Pallor	Thrombus aspiration
Polar (cold)	Fogarty catheter embolectomy and open surgical repair
Paresthesiae	
Pulselessness	

Radial Access Site Problems

An Allen's test should be performed on all patients in whom radial artery access is planned, to ensure a patent ulnar artery in case of radial artery occlusion (see pp. 16–19).

Radial access site complications are rare, but the following may occur:
• Spasm, the main problem associated with radial artery access, is largely prevented by pretreatment with intra-arterial vasodilators and patient sedation.
• Bleeding and hematoma are usually easily controlled by local pressure.
• A compartment syndrome is rare, but is likely to need emergency surgical decompression (fasciotomy to relieve pressure, saving muscles and nerves). This may occur with unrecognized perforation. Common symptoms of compartmental compression include increasing pain, especially on passive stretching of the muscles in the involved compartment.
• Radial artery occlusion may occur and is usually symptomless, because of collateral flow from the ulnar artery.

Air Injection

Small volumes (tiny bubbles) of air injected usually have no adverse sequelae. Injections of larger volumes of air occur very occasionally – usually due to equipment failure such as angioplasty balloon rupture, or from air in a contrast-filled syringe. To avoid the latter, all bubbles should be removed from the syringe. It is also important to ensure that the guiding catheter is fully aspirated before injections are made, especially if small-caliber (5F) guide catheters are used.

Although air emboli are usually eliminated spontaneously, ischemia, arrhythmia, acute myocardial infarction, and hemodynamic instability may occur, and emergency procedures may be needed to resolve the problem.

Management
- 100% oxygen
- Attempt air aspiration and forceful saline intracoronary injections
- Full cardiopulmonary resuscitation (see p. 317).

No-Reflow/Slow-Reflow Phenomenon

- **Mechanism, 294**
- **Prevention, 295**
- **Management, 295**

This is uncommon in routine elective coronary intervention, but more common in primary PCI, saphenous vein graft PCI, or PCI of large (more than 4 mm) vessels – especially those vessels with bulky atheroma or thrombus. It may occur in up to 40% patients with percutaneous reperfusion after acute myocardial infarction.

By definition, no-flow or slow reflow is abnormal, inadequate tissue perfusion with no evidence of upstream mechanical epicardial arterial obstruction. Following balloon inflation the vessel is widely patent at the lesion site, but injected contrast is held up, creeping down the vessel slowly if at all. No-reflow can also be present in acute coronary syndromes.

Mechanism
The mechanism is poorly understood, but is due to microvascular obstruction. Studies in both animals and man suggest multiple contributing factors:
- *Coronary spasm.* This may be provoked by the guide wire or may be the result of trauma at the site of dilatation. Thromboxane and endothelin released from damaged cells also contribute.

• *Microemboli migrating distally.* These may be thrombus or plaque debris. It is a particular problem with right coronary rotablation, where temporary pacing is advisable.

• *Endothelial cell swelling.* Endothelial edema with bleb formation has been seen in experimental models and may be due to free radical release.

• *Platelet activation with platelet microemboli.* Vigorous antiplatelet therapy is essential.

• *White cell adherence to the endothelium.*

• *Collapse of the capillary bed* due to a drop in capillary perfusion pressure. It is important to avoid hypotension, and volume loading is necessary, especially if nitrates are used.

• *Reduced deformability of red cells* when hypoxic may contribute to peripheral sludging.

Prevention

In patients having primary PCI, pharmacological treatment with platelet inhibitors and anticoagulants is needed (see Chapter 4).

• Platelet inhibitors:
    – Aspirin 300–600 mg loading dose plus clopidogrel 600 mg loading dose orally.
    – Some use upstream glycoprotein IIb/IIIa inhibitors, e.g., intracoronary abciximab given as a 0.25 mg/kg bolus followed by infusion of 0.125 μg/kg per minute for 12–24 hours. However the combination of bivalirudin and clopidogrel may be equally effective, less costly, and safer.

• Nicorandil 12 mg IV prior to reperfusion

• Thrombus aspiration prior to balloon inflation. This appears to limit the occurrence and severity of slow or no-reflow.

• Unfractionated heparin or bivalirudin.

• Intracoronary nitroglycerin.

• Additional intracoronary agents (adenosine, verapamil) may be beneficial.

Management

Usually the phenomenon spontaneously reverts over minutes. However, persistent no-reflow implies abnormal tissue perfusion and increases the risk of arrhythmias, myocardial infarction, and mortality. Bradycardia may be provoked and usually settles with time and intravenous atropine (0.6 mg IV repeated). Temporary pacing is occasionally needed.

• Oxygen. Check pulse oximetry reading.

• Maintain ACT at 250–300 seconds.

• Control vasovagal reaction with atropine and fluids.

• Maintain systemic pressure with fluids and vasopressors and/or IABP if needed.

A combination of the following agents given via the intracoronary route plus volume loading may help restore brisk flow. Administration of drugs distally in the vascular bed through a low-profile catheter such as a Finecross ensures the medication is delivered to the site where it is needed.

- Nitrates 100–200 μg IC, up to four doses, to exclude coronary spasm.
- Abciximab 0.25 mg/kg bolus IC or IV, plus 10 μg/min 12 hour infusion IV after the procedure.
- Verapamil 50–200 μg IC up to 1000 μg bolus.
- Sodium nitroprusside 50–200 μg up to 1000 μg bolus.
- Adenosine up to 60 μg bolus IC, or 60 μg/kg/min for 3 hrs IV after the procedure.

Coronary Spasm

Coronary spasm is a common problem and not necessarily a cause for alarm. It is commonest in the proximal RCA, and may be due to stimulation from the guiding catheter at the ostium, the balloon itself, or the guide wire. Intracoronary nitrates are essential and regular doses may be needed. Occasionally, if spasm is persistent, the wire may need to be withdrawn. Spasm may cause:

- Underestimation of true vessel size.
- Misdiagnosis, where segmental spasm is mistaken for a real coronary lesion (see Pseudostenoses below).
- Poor distal flow, making it difficult to assess the distal vessel.
- Difficulty in advancing a balloon or stent.
- Hemodynamic problems, with angina and hypotension.

Prinzmetal angina is rare and is a combination of spontaneous coronary spasm usually with an atheromatous lesion. The combination may shut the vessel right down with marked ST elevation. These patients are particularly likely to develop spasm during PCI.

Pseudostenoses

Pseudostenoses may occur when a tortuous artery is straightened by a wire. They resolve when the wire is removed. To distinguish between pseudo- and real stenosis, partially withdrawing the wire so that flexible distal centimeters lie across the apparent lesions may allow the tortuous vessel to resume its shape and the pseudostenoses to disappear. If there is still doubt the wire may have to be withdrawn completely.

Coronary Perforation

- **Management of Perforation and Tamponade, 297**

Fortunately coronary perforation is a rare complication. It may be rapidly fatal unless diagnosed swiftly and treated urgently. It is usually due to:

- *Balloon oversizing.* Reference vessel (normal segment) diameter needs to be estimated or measured. This is usually done by "eyeballing," but IVUS or quantitative coronary angiography will give more exact diameters. Vein grafts may be particularly vulnerable with balloon oversizing or high-pressure inflation.

• *Wire tip perforation.* This is a problem especially with hydrophilic wires or very stiff wires. It is important to keep an eye on the wire tip during the PCI procedure as the wire may migrate with manipulation of the balloon or guide catheter.

• *Full Pressure Balloon inflation in a sub-intimal position and not in true lumen.* This is a potential problem in cases of chronic total occlusion. If there is uncertainty about the wire position, the balloon should not be inflated. However, in advanced chronic total occlusion (CTO) techniques (STAR, CART, reverse CART), low pressure balloon inflation within a false lumen is part of the procedure.

• *Balloon inflation at high pressure* in tough, calcified lesions.

• *Devices* can also cause perforation (excimer laser, Tornus catheter). A rotablator burr can cause perforation, especially during treatment of lesions on a bend.

The risk of perforation is higher in calcified, tortuous, and small vessels. For small vessels (e.g., septal channels), a very small balloon (<1.5 mm) under low pressure inflation (2–4 atm) is mandatory to avoid complications during CTO intervention. If the procedure carries a higher risk of perforation, glycoprotein IIb/IIIa inhibitors should be avoided to minimize the risk of bleeding.

The Ellis classification distinguishes three types of perforation (Figure 6.2). While type 1 perforation usually resolves without consequences or with minor symptoms, type 2 and 3 perforations are severe complications associated with hemodynamic instability and cardiac tamponade.

Management of Perforation and Tamponade

Early recognition is vital. Type 1 perforation is usually not a problem. With more significant perforation, intrapericardial bleeding occurs and the patient rapidly becomes symptomatic as tamponade develops. Chest pain and shortness of breath are common with clear lungs, jugular venous pressure elevation, pulsus paradoxus on the arterial pressure trace, tachycardia, and hypotension.

Emergency echocardiography is essential and shows the pericardial effusion with right atrial and right ventricular compression during diastole. Pericardial aspiration may be life-saving. Every catheterization laboratory must have an emergency pericardial aspiration tray containing the necessary equipment. The staff must know where this is kept.

Emergency noninvasive and invasive treatment:

• *Blood aspiration.* Following initial aspiration, continuous pericardial catheter drainage using an indwelling pigtail catheter is advisable. While the main therapeutic need is aspiration of blood, other measures may be necessary.

• *Replace volume.* Ensure volume replacement and administer inotropes if arterial pressure does not recover after aspiration.

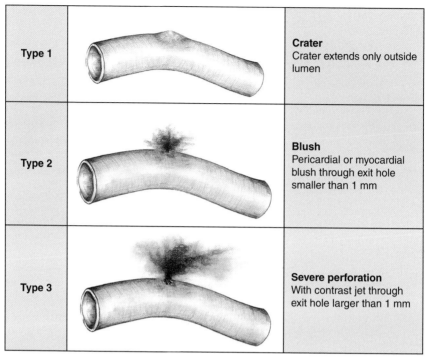

Type 1		**Crater** Crater extends only outside lumen
Type 2		**Blush** Pericardial or myocardial blush through exit hole smaller than 1 mm
Type 3		**Severe perforation** With contrast jet through exit hole larger than 1 mm

Figure 6.2 Ellis classification of perforation.

• *Reverse anticoagulation.* Discontinue heparin administration and reverse heparinization using protamine. Discontinue glycoprotein IIb/IIIa inhibitor administration. Wait if bivalirudin was given.

• *Manage bradycardia* using 0.5–1.0 mg atropine IV every 3 minutes up to 3 mg maximum dose.

• *Maintain blood pressure* using inotropic support.

• *Limit blood leakage* with an inflated balloon. The vessel itself can be managed by prolonged balloon inflation at or proximal to the perforation site. The balloon should be slightly oversized and deployed at low pressure (2–4 atm).

• *Seal with a covered stent.* A definitive treatment of a perforation is deployment of one or more JoStent PTFE-covered stents across the perforation site to seal it. These require high-pressure inflation.

• *Embolization.* This can be helpful particularly in side branches, small vessels, or distal perforation. Usually thrombin, microcoils, or Gelfoam are used.

• *Emergency cardiac surgery.* Perforation is now one of the few indications for urgent cardiac surgery during PCI. Ligation of the culprit vessel and distal grafting are usually needed.

Coronary Dissection

- **Left Main Dissection, 301**
  How to Avoid Left Main Dissection
  Left Main Dissection Management
- **Long Linear or Spiral Dissection, 301**
- **Dissection Management, 302**

Balloon angioplasty is a controlled dissection with necessary plaque fracture. A dissection flap is usually obvious on angiography and the flap can usually be welded back to the vessel wall with a stent. Sometimes dissections may be dangerous, extend down the vessel, and prove difficult to control. There are two caveats in diagnosis:

- A dissection flap may not be visible in a single plane and multiple angiographic projections may be needed to identify the problem. The possibility of a dissection flap should be considered in any case where distal flow is not as good as expected following balloon inflation or stenting.
- A final angiogram is recorded routinely following wire removal. This is to check for distal flow, which may be impeded by wire-induced spasm, but also for a hidden unexpected dissection flap which may have been held against the wall by the wire.

Various contributing risk factors are listed in Table 6.4.

The commonly used NHLBI (National Heart, Lung and Blood Institute) classification, designed before the stent era, describes types of dissection (Figure 6.3). Note that types C to F show persistence of contrast after it has cleared from the lumen.

There are a variety of dissections which can cause a problem. The two most important are left main dissections, and long linear dissections which need attention.

Table 6.4 Risk factors for coronary vessel dissection.

Lesion	Patient	Procedure
Long lesion	Acute myocardial infarction	Deep catheter engagement
Calcified lesion	Unstable angina	Excessive catheter manipulation
Tortuous lesion	Marfan's syndrome	Non-coaxial catheter
Eccentric lesion	Kawasaki's disease	Incorrectly sized catheter
Complex morphology	Aortic dissection	Balloon dilatation at a very high
	Cocaine	pressure
		Oversized balloon; balloon to
		artery ratio >1.2
		Slow, gradual balloon deflation

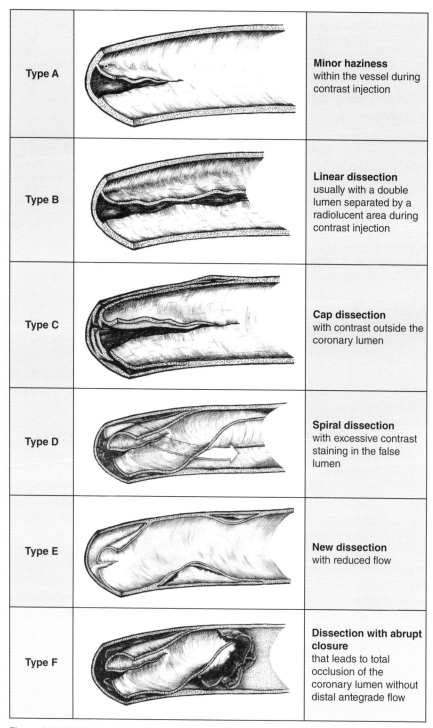

Type A	Minor haziness within the vessel during contrast injection
Type B	Linear dissection usually with a double lumen separated by a radiolucent area during contrast injection
Type C	Cap dissection with contrast outside the coronary lumen
Type D	Spiral dissection with excessive contrast staining in the false lumen
Type E	New dissection with reduced flow
Type F	Dissection with abrupt closure that leads to total occlusion of the coronary lumen without distal antegrade flow

Figure 6.3 NHLBI classification of dissection.

Table 6.5 Factors predictive of left main dissection.

Anatomy	Lesion	Procedure
Abnormal usually high takeoff	Ostial lesion	Excessive catheter manipulation
Sharp left main–LAD junction	Severe calcification	Noncoaxial catheter
	Severe stenosis	Deep catheter engagement

Left Main Dissection

A tiny dissection usually has no adverse consequences. A flow-limiting dissection is a relatively rare complication that may have severe consequences if not treated promptly. The patient may become symptomatic immediately, with chest pain, hypotension, and arrhythmias with ischemic ECG changes. Left main dissection is usually caused by the guiding catheter tip's being forced against the wall of the main stem during excessive manipulation. Injection of contrast through a guide that is not coaxial and against an arterial wall can cause or extend dissection. Other predictive factors for left main dissection are shown in Table 6.5.

This dissection may track retrogradely up into the aortic root or antegradely into the main stem bifurcation.

How to Avoid Left Main Dissection

The keys to avoiding left main coronary dissection are a slow and gentle approach to the vessel and ensuring a coaxial position within the main stem. If the guide or diagnostic catheter is not coaxial, and if gentle manipulation cannot achieve this, a change of guiding catheter should be considered.

An incorrectly undersized Judkins guide may be a problem with the tip forced up against the roof the main stem. Vigorous force with an Amplatz catheter in circumflex PCI may also force the tip against the roof of the main stem (Figure 6.4).

Left Main Dissection Management

A small extravasation into the wall of the left main coronary artery without much encroachment on the lumen can be watched. If there is flow limitation, the situation needs urgent stenting to restore hemodynamic stability. Not only is the main stem vessel rapidly narrowed by the flap, but the dissection may track up the aortic wall proximally or distally into the LAD and/or circumflex. If possible, both LAD and circumflex should be wired, but this may not be possible.

Long Linear or Spiral Dissection

This may occur in any vessel after balloon dilatation, but is most common in the right coronary artery. It is important to advance the guide wire to the distal vessel before balloon dilatation for this reason. Proximal stenting may seal off

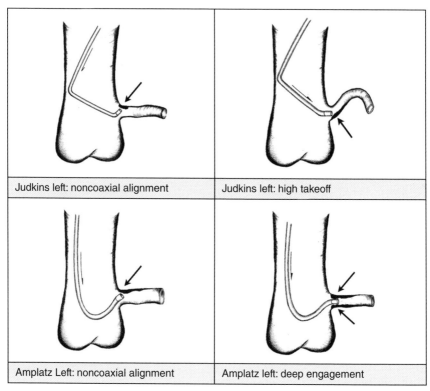

Judkins left: noncoaxial alignment	Judkins left: high takeoff
Amplatz Left: noncoaxial alignment	Amplatz left: deep engagement

Figure 6.4 Catheter-induced left main dissection (arrowed).

the entrance to the dissection, but more usually several stents are needed to sort the problem out.

Dissection Management
The management of dissection depends on which type of dissection has occurred.
• Most type A or B dissections can be left alone if they are not potentially flow limiting and will heal naturally.
• Flow-limiting type C to F dissections, however, are more complex and are associated with a higher mortality. Stenting is required. If the wire cannot cross the dissection into the distal vessel true lumen, or if for some other reason stent implantation is not possible, bypass surgery may be the only option, particularly if the vessel is larger than 2 mm. Once again it is important to ensure the wire is in the distal vessel prior to dilatation to safeguard against this problem. A distal wire position is critical in the presence of a complex dissection as it is in true lumen. It is very important that the wire is not inadvertently withdrawn when it is being wiped clean.

Stent Thrombosis

- **Definition, 303**
- **Risk Factors, 303**
  Do Drug-Eluting Stents Carry a Greater Thrombotic Risk?
  Procedural Factors
  Factors in Stent Design
  Relevance to Dual Antiplatelet Therapy
  Premature Discontinuation of DAPT
  Resistance to Antiplatelet Therapy
- **Management of Stent Thrombosis, 307**

Although stent thrombosis is relatively rare, it is a potentially catastrophic complication with a high chance of a large myocardial infarct or death. Improvements in stent design, polymer drug dose, antiplatelet treatment, and operative technique have reduced the stent thrombosis rate. Although uncommon, it remains an unpredictable and feared hazard.

Definition

This complication is categorized by level of certainty into definite, probable, and possible stent thrombosis and by time into early, late, and very late (Tables 6.6 and 6.7).

Risk Factors

Whereas acute or subacute stent thrombosis is usually related to lesion factors or procedural factors, late stent thrombosis is usually associated with inadequate stent endothelialization in response to the antiproliferative drug on the stent, to vessel wall inflammation in response to the polymer, to prematurely interrupted dual antiplatelet therapy (DAPT), or to new atheroma within the stent.

Table 6.6 Academic Research Consortium (ARC) classification of stent thrombosis by level of certainty.

Level of Certainty	Clinical Manifestation
Definite	In-stent total thrombotic occlusion (confirmed angiographically or pathologically) plus at least one of the following: • Acute ischemic symptoms • Ischemic ECG changes • Cardiac biomarker elevation
Probable	Any unexpected death within 30 days of stent implantation Any myocardial infarction related to acute ischemia (previously documented) in the implanted stent area without angiographic confirmation of stent thrombosis and in the absence of other obvious reason
Possible	Any unexpected death beyond 30 days of stent implantation

Table 6.7 ARC classification of stent thrombosis by time frame.

Type of Thrombosis	Time
Early	Acute: <24 hours
	Subacute: 24 hours – 30 days
Late	31 days – 1 year
Very late	After 1 year

Table 6.8 Risk factors for stent thrombosis.

Patient factors	Lesion factors	Stent factors	Procedure factors	Platelet factors
Diabetes mellitus	Lesion length	Polymer reaction	Inadequate stent expansion (malapposition)	Inadequate antiplatelet therapy
Renal failure	Lesion diameter	Drug reaction	Edge dissection	Resistance to antiplatelet agents
Low EF	Bifurcation lesion	In-stent restenosis	Other untreated stenosis in the vessel	Premature discontinuation of DAPT
Previous MI	Ostial lesion			
Hypersensitivity reaction	Thrombotic lesion			
Drug response				
Smoking				
Noncompliance with DAPT				

Following deployment the stent must endothelialize and become incorporated in the coronary artery wall. Persisting metal struts uncovered by functional endothelial cells are a risk factor for stent thrombosis. This is often caused by an inadequately implanted stent (malapposition) and can be made less likely by postdilatation with a noncompliant balloon at high pressure. In addition, other factors are known to increase the risk possibly by increasing platelet activation. Risk factors for stent thrombosis are shown in Table 6.8.

Do Drug-Eluting Stents Carry a Greater Thrombotic Risk?

It is generally agreed that DES, especially the first generation of DES, carry a slightly increased risk of thrombosis compared with bare metal stents. Studies suggest that the thrombosis rate for first-generation DES is possibly 0.6% per year for at least the first 4 years after implantation. The current generation of DES have a lower risk of stent thrombosis. The great advantage of reduction in restenosis and target vessel revascularization with DES outweighs the very slightly increased risk of stent thrombosis. DES are commonly used in complex procedures (unprotected, left main, bifurcation, CTO) and in high-risk patients (previous myocardial infarction, diabetes, renal failure). In both groups the risk of the procedure itself is higher than in simple PCI with a bare metal stent.

Procedural Factors
Whereas patient factors are often constant, procedural factors can be potentially eliminated. Any important residual dissection must be treated. The stent should be fully expanded over its entire length, usually with routine high-pressure postdilatation. Adequate antiplatelet therapy during and after the procedure significantly reduces the risk of stent thrombosis. If the patient requires surgery within 12 months, a bare metal stent is preferable to DES to avoid the risk of late stent thrombosis with premature discontinuation of DAPT in DES cases.

Factors in Stent Design
Changes in stent design are reducing the risk of stent thrombosis after DES. Struts are becoming thinner so it is easier for endothelial cells to cover them. The drug dose is less, so that there is less antiproliferative effect on endothelial cells. Some contemporary polymers, such as the fluoropolymer on the Xience stent, are associated with less allergy and inflammation than first-generation DES such as the Taxus or Cypher polymer. Clinical trials now show less stent thrombosis with the Xience stent than with the Taxus stent.

Relevance to Dual Antiplatelet Therapy
Stent thrombosis following bare metal stent deployment is rare after 30 days. DAPT (aspirin plus a thienopyridine) is therefore recommended for 1 month. However, current recommendations for DES are that DAPT should be continued for at least 1 year after DES implantation in view of the uncertainty of timing of adequate re-endothelialization.

Results from TYPHOON trial (2009) show that an extra year beyond the usual recommended 12 months of DAPT reduces the risk of very late stent thrombosis in patients with DES. Other trials provide conflicting data, and definite recommendations are unclear. The DAPT trial, which will randomize 20,000 patients, will provide important data on the value of DAPT beyond 1 year. A decision to prolong DAPT in high-risk patients is made individually based on risk profile.

Premature Discontinuation of DAPT
Compliance with DAPT, particularly during the first 6 months after PCI with a DES, is mandatory.

One recent study showed a 29% stent thrombosis rate in patients who discontinued their antiplatelet therapy early. It is essential that patients are warned before discharge of the risks of premature cessation. They should certainly not discontinue DAPT without discussion with their cardiologist, who can consider and discuss risks and benefits of this.

Resistance to Antiplatelet Therapy (see pp. 173–177)
Impaired response to conventional doses of antiplatelet therapy is becoming recognized as a contributing factor to stent thrombosis, but platelet responsiveness is not routinely tested for before PCI. Patients who survive a stent thrombosis should have their platelet function and clotting studied (see pp. 173–177). Patients in whom clopidogrel resistance is demonstrated should be switched to either ticlopidine or prasugrel. In some patients an increased dose of clopidogrel is effective.

Clopidogrel vs. Prasugrel
Prasugrel has been shown to be superior to clopidogrel in the TRITON-TIMI 38 trial in patients with acute coronary syndromes undergoing PCI and is an attractive alternative to clopidogrel. Nonfatal myocardial infarction was reduced in the prasugrel group but major bleeding was increased. The switch to prasugrel is a balance of risk of greater antiplatelet activity against a greater bleeding risk (see pp. 170–171).

Patients with DES Needing Surgery While on Antiplatelet Therapy
Patients who need to undergo surgery while receiving antiplatelet therapy require careful management. The procedural angiogram should be reviewed to assess the risk of thrombosis. For instance, a short, wide-caliber stent carries a low risk of thrombosis while a complex procedure in small-caliber vessels with multiple stents carries a high risk if DAPT is interrupted.
• Is the surgery really necessary or can it be delayed?
• If surgery is required and the surgeon is not happy to operate while the patient is receiving DAPT, clopidogrel should be stopped 7 days before surgery, and aspirin therapy continued. After surgery, clopidogrel administration can be resumed.
• It is important not to discontinue both antiplatelet drugs.
• Do not replace dual therapy with low-molecular-weight heparin as it is ineffective.
• If surgery is planned within 12 months in a PCI case, or if the patient might not be compliant with DAPT, use a bare metal stent rather than DES for PCI.
• Patients who develop gastrointestinal bleeding on dual therapy need endoscopy and possibly colonoscopy to determine the cause. If the cause is thought to be gastric erosions, a proton pump inhibitor, preferably pantoprazole 20–40 mg daily, should be given. Concerns that proton pump inhibitors decrease the effectiveness of clopidogrel have not been realized in clinical practice (see pp. 176–177).

Management of Stent Thrombosis

If presenting within 6 hours of symptom onset, patients should have a primary PCI (see pp. 134–149). The procedure may be difficult, but having reopened and fully expanded the original stent, an assessment of whether another stent is needed will be made. If primary PCI is not available, thrombolytic therapy can be effective, especially if administered early.

Restenosis

- **A Biochemically Driven Healing Process, 307**
- **Bare Metal Stents, 308**
- **Drug-Eluting Stents, 308**
- **Pattern of In-Stent Restenosis, 308**
- **Treatment of Restenotic Lesions, 310**

In the DES era restenosis is no longer the Achilles heel of PCI as it was in the balloon angioplasty and bare metal stent era. Restenosis after balloon angioplasty is due to negative remodeling (vessel shrinkage and recoil). Bare metal stents prevent vessel recoil but stimulate an increased healing intimal hyperplastic response that causes restenosis. The antiproliferative drug of a DES limits the intimal hyperplastic response, hence limiting restenosis.

A Biochemically Driven Healing Process

Restenosis is caused by smooth muscle cells in the media of the arterial wall proliferating and migrating into the subintimal layer, together with intimal hyperplasia. It is a healing process in response to trauma, but unfortunately the process becomes exaggerated and may cause excessive luminal narrowing. Histologically, the restenotic segment is packed with smooth muscle cells and not lipid, and is completely different from the original atheromatous lipid-laden plaque. It occurs most commonly in the first 3 months following a PCI procedure.

In the normal vessel, the fully differentiated smooth muscle cell has a low proliferation rate, and the intact endothelium secretes inhibitory factors (e.g., prostacyclin, nitric oxide, heparin sulfate). Endothelial denudation, rupture of the internal elastic lamina, and medial stretch at angioplasty result in loss of these inhibitory factors and release of many different growth factors from smooth muscle cells, endothelial cells, and platelets, which are attracted to the area of denuded endothelium. The media becomes exposed to plasma mitogens. Stress-activated protein kinase (SAPK) is upregulated. Matrix degeneration by matrix metalloproteinases facilitates smooth muscle cell migration. Finally, the healing process is completed by upregulation of vascular endothelial growth factor (VEGF) with regrowth of the endothelium over the new smooth muscle cell mass. Factors increasing the risk of restenosis are listed in Table 6.9.

Table 6.9 Factors increasing risk of restenosis.

Patient	Lesion	Procedure	Device
Diagnosis	Ostial lesion	High-pressure inflation	Long stent
Diabetes	Long lesion	Inadequate initial dilatation	Drug carrier
Allergies	Proximal LAD lesion	Gap between adjacent	Drug itself
Smoking	Small vessel	stents	
Genetic	Vein graft lesion	Balloon-only PCI	
ACE polymorphism		Complex dissection	
		Stent malapposition	

Bare Metal Stents

The BENESTENT randomized trial was the first along with the STRESS trial to show the reduction in restenosis with the use of a bare metal stent compared with balloon-only angioplasty. The simple lesions treated have become known as "Benestent type" lesions, representing a discrete stenosis in a vessel 3.0 mm in diameter or more and less than 15 mm in length. The use of a bare metal stent reduced the angiographic restenosis rate from 32% to 22% at 7 months.

Drug-Eluting Stents

Many studies have shown that DES reduce the incidence of in-stent restenosis still further. The RAVEL trial was one of the first trials to show the reduction of restenosis when DES were used. The restenosis rate in nondiabetic patients was reduced from 36% (bare metal stent) to 0% (DES). Clinical restenosis after DES is rarely seen except in diabetic patients.

Pattern of In-Stent Restenosis

There are various angiographic patterns of in-stent restenosis, depending on the length (focal restenosis) and position relative to the previously implanted stent (Figure 6.5). Focal restenosis is rare, relatively easy to treat, and carries a good prognosis. Diffuse restenosis, however, is more frequent and remains difficult to treat, with a worse prognosis. Restenosis after DES implantation is usually discrete.

There are a few important points which may help prevent in-stent restenosis:

- Focus on good lesion preparation. Use debulking if necessary.
- Stent length matters – the shorter the stent, the better.
- Minimize stent overlap: only at stent junctions.
- Avoid stent oversizing.
- Avoid very high postdilatation inflation pressures (>20 atm).

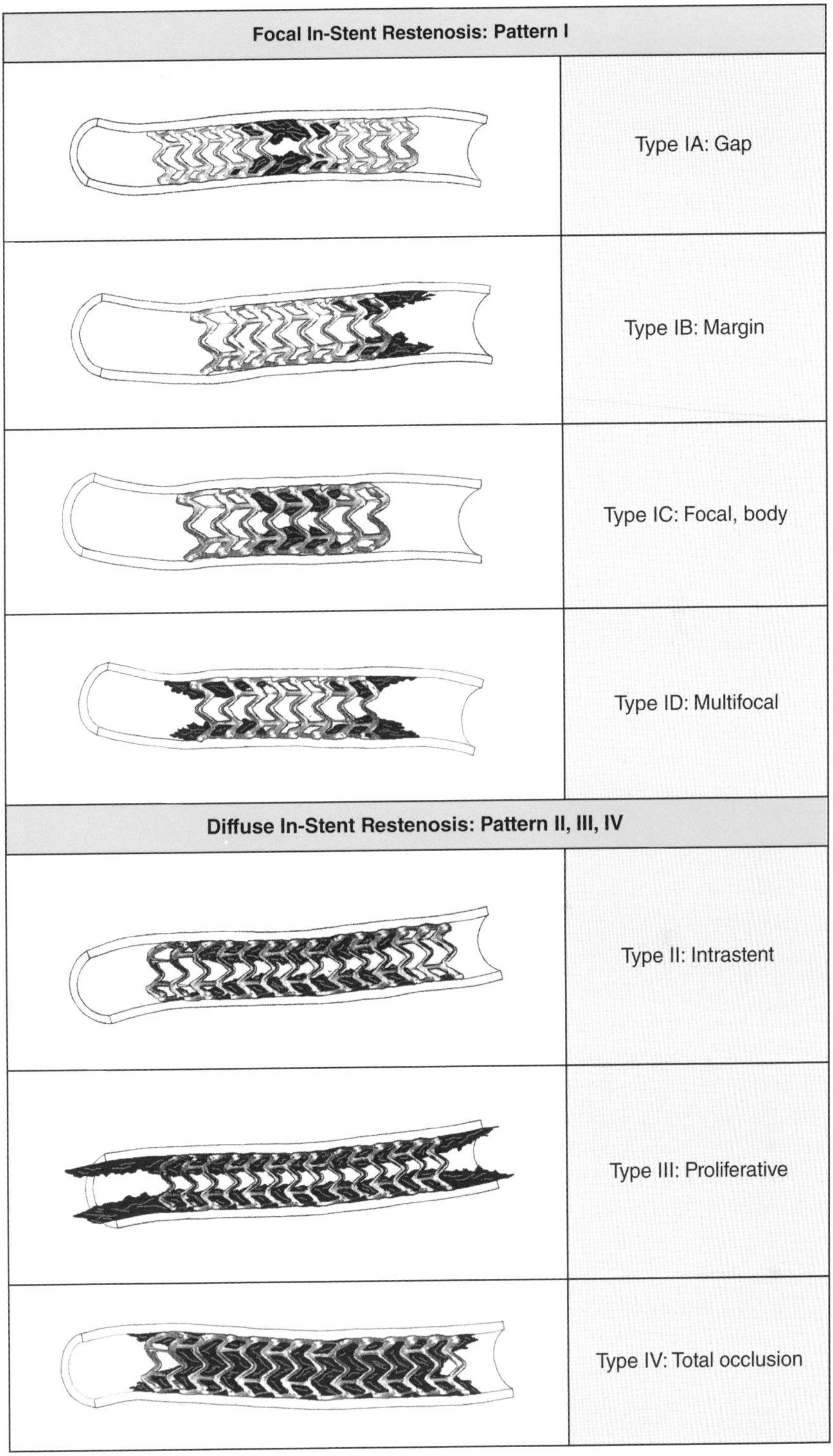

Focal In-Stent Restenosis: Pattern I	
	Type IA: Gap
	Type IB: Margin
	Type IC: Focal, body
	Type ID: Multifocal
Diffuse In-Stent Restenosis: Pattern II, III, IV	
	Type II: Intrastent
	Type III: Proliferative
	Type IV: Total occlusion

Figure 6.5 Angiographic patterns of focal and diffuse in-stent restenosis.

- Use abciximab in diabetic patients.
- Stent only significant flow-limiting lesions (FFR <0.8).

Treatment of Restenotic Lesions

Predilatation of a restenotic lesion can be difficult as the smooth surface of the lesion allows the balloon to slip out of position ("melon seeding"). A longer balloon may be needed to deal with this.

Sometimes a cutting balloon will facilitate adequate dilatation of the stenotic tissue and stent.

- *Short segments* of restenosis (<15 mm), whether in the stent or adjacent, can be managed by deployment of a new DES. A new DES, slightly longer than the original and 0.5 mm larger in diameter, is used to treat restenosis ("sandwich stenting"). Inadequate stent expansion is a predisposing cause for restenosis, so it is important to ensure that the original stent is adequately expanded. IVUS can be helpful. If the original stent was underexpanded, dilatation with a larger noncompliant balloon at high pressure (e.g., 20 atm) may correct this problem.
- *Long segments* of restenosis are a major problem. The choices are: continuing medical treatment, several long DES, drug-eluting balloons, or bypass surgery.
  - *Drug-eluting balloons* are showing promise in the treatment of in-stent restenosis.
  - *Brachytherapy*, which held so much hope for these long restenotic segments, has not fulfilled its promise and has been largely abandoned.

Stent Loss

- **Loop Snare, 311**
- **Two-Wire Technique, 311**
- **Balloon Technique, 311**

Stent dislodgment from the delivery balloon usually occurs in severely calcified or angulated lesions. Although stent loss is a very rare complication, it is associated with increased risk of further complications. Stent loss is more frequent in cases of direct stenting than in cases in which the lesion is prepared and predilated.

It is possible to deal with the situation by crushing the lost stent and covering it with another stent without attempting retrieval, but in the majority of cases the lost stent can be successfully retrieved using a variety of retrieval devices and techniques. Sometimes it is possible to pass a small, very-low-profile balloon through the dislodged stent, then progressively dilate and deploy it. This is easier if the guide wire is still in situ through the stent (see "Two-Wire Technique" and "Balloon Technique" below). Some retrieval devices, such as biliary forceps, basket, or Cook retained fragment retriever, are quite bulky and carry a high risk of dissection and perforation. The most popular techniques are described below.

Loop Snare

This commonly used retrieval device consists of a plastic catheter with a movable nitinol looped wire inside. The loop opens at a 90° angle from the delivery catheter and facilitates stent capture and retrieval. If the loop device is not available, it is possible to extemporize using a 5F multipurpose guiding catheter with a looped guide wire inside. To make this snare, pass the wire through the 5F catheter, and once the tip exits from the distal end, the wire can be looped and reinserted into the catheter. To capture a lost stent, advance a loop snare into the vessel, place it around the lost stent, tighten, and withdraw the entire system.

Two-Wire Technique

This technique is best for retrieval of a stent which has slipped off the delivery balloon, but remains on the guide wire. Advance a second wire from the stent lumen through the struts to lie outside the stent, twist both wires several times to capture the dislodged stent, then withdraw the trapped stent.

Balloon Technique

A lost stent can be also retrieved using a small balloon which is advanced through the lost stent and inflated distally at low pressure. The inflated balloon should then be withdrawn, pulling the stent back into the guiding catheter. This technique, once again, can only be used when the guide wire lies within the lost stent.

Hypotension

Artifactual Hypotension

Artifactual hypotension can be caused by several simple problems:

A partly open rotating hemostatic valve or a poor connection between tubes. Connections need to be checked.

Guide or diagnostic catheter-induced pressure damping can be due to deep catheter engagement, especially if there is ostial stenosis. This can be solved by disengaging the catheter and the pressure will recover.

Catheter kinking will also cause pressure damping. X-ray the entire catheter. If it is kinked, attempt to untwist it with the aid of a guide wire. Do not pull a kinked guide out of the artery as this will tear the entry site.

Air or thrombus within the catheter. Always aspirate a catheter recording a damped pressure. If there is doubt the catheter must be changed.

True Hypotension

Vasovagal reaction. This is common and often associated with "hot" feelings and nausea. It may be a contrast reaction (see above) or due to patient pain or fear. There is hypotension with inappropriate bradycardia. Treat with intravenous atropine and normal saline. Right ventricular pacing and intravenous analgesia may be needed if recovery is not brisk. The hypotension associated

with a prolonged vagal reaction may predispose to vessel occlusion. *Myocardial ischemia and coronary occlusion.* There may be ECG changes to support the diagnosis. Angiography will determine which vessel is responsible. *Arrhythmia.* This is readily apparent from the monitored ECG.
Tamponade. Usually occurs in the context of vessel rupture or during procedures such as trans-septal studies. Echocardiography is needed urgently to make the diagnosis and guide drainage (see above).
Retroperitoneal bleeding or other blood loss. Usually blood loss is apparent, but retroperitoneal bleeding is concealed and should be considered if other explanations for hypotension are not present. Abdominal ultrasound in the lab or subsequent CT scanning may be needed.
Contrast reactions. A contrast reaction such as an anaphylactoid reaction can be devastating and require emergency resuscitation. It may be associated with other manifestations such as laryngeal edema. Treatment is described above.

Hypoglycemia

Profound hypoglycemia can occur especially in diabetic patients, and should be considered for unexplained change in consciousness, sweating, and sometimes hypotension. Physical responses to hypoglycemia may be blunted by beta-blockade. Blood sugars should be checked during the procedure in diabetic patients.

Contrast-Induced Nephropathy

Severe renal dysfunction with a creatinine clearance below 30 ml/min in patients undergoing PCI or bypass surgery is known to be independently associated with an increased rate of adverse events and mortality.
   Renal failure may occur after PCI, most frequently as a result of the following:
- Pre-existing renal impairment
- Dehydration
- Prolonged hypotension
- Excess contrast dosing

Renal insufficiency accelerates the course of coronary disease, and pre-existing renal disease is the most important risk factor for contrast-induced nephropathy (CIN) following coronary intervention. Patients at higher risk of CIN are those with diabetes, hypertension, and congestive cardiac failure.

Inevitably, some high-risk patients may develop postprocedural contrast nephropathy. CIN is one of the most important independent predictors of poor outcomes and increases morbidity and mortality. The mechanism is similar to that in acute tubular necrosis. After contrast administration, glomerular filtration rate (GFR) drops, causing medullary ischemia. In addition, contrast molecules are toxic and may cause damage to renal tubular cells. Hypersensitivity reactions may also occur, causing nausea and vomiting, urticaria, hypotension, or anaphylaxis.

Recognizing Contrast-Induced Nephropathy

A standard definition of CIN has not been established. However, this complication becomes apparent when new renal dysfunction occurs after contrast in the absence of other obvious causes. Indicators which help in the recognition of CIN include the following:

- Serum creatinine level rises by more than 25% from baseline.
- Absolute creatinine rises by more than 0.5 mg/dl from baseline.
- GFR rises more than 25% from baseline.
- Serum creatinine increases within 24 hours after the procedure, with creatinine peak 5–7 days later and normalization 7–10 days later.
- Oliguria, anuria.

Assessing Renal Function

The glomerular filtration rate and the Cockcroft–Gault equation are simple methods by which to assess renal function. They should be used before interventional procedures in all patients with known renal dysfunction.

- *Glomerular filtration rate* (GFR) measures renal excretory function. Normal values for GFR are 120 ± 25 ml/min (men 5 ml higher than women). In general, values above 90 ml/min are normal for all patients. To avoid gender differences, the result may be standardized for average surface area (i.e., per 1.73 m^2). The best validated method to obtain an estimate of GFR (eGFR) is the MDRD (Modification of Diet in Renal Disease Study Group) formula:

$$eGFR \text{ in } ml/min/1.73 \text{ m}^2 = 186 \times (\text{serum creatinine in } mg/dl)^{-1.154}$$
$$\times (\text{age in years})^{-0.203} \times (0.742 \text{ if female})$$
$$\times (1.212 \text{ if African American})$$

If creatinine has been measured in μmol/l substitute the number 32788 for 186. The formula applies to patients aged >18.

• *The Cockcroft–Gault equation* uses serum creatinine, age, and weight to estimate creatinine clearance (CrCl) in milliliters per minute, which in turn gives an estimate of GFR (eGFR). It avoids the need for a 24 hour urine collection.

Creatinine clearance in ml/min

$$= \frac{(140 - \text{age}) \times \text{body weight (kg)} \times (0.85 \text{ if female})}{\text{serum creatinine (mg/dl)} \times 72}$$

If serum creatinine is measured in μmol/l, the constant in the numerator is 1.04 for females and 1.23 for males. Omit the number 72 in the denominator.

Risk Factors

Patients with renal insufficiency (eGFR < 60 ml/min), diabetes, or dehydration are particularly vulnerable to CIN and require a preprocedural check and hydration. In high-risk patients the use of a low-osmolar contrast at minimum volume is recommended. Note, however, that iso-osmolar contrast does not decrease rates of CIN compared with low-osmolar contrast media. Risk factors for CIN are listed in Table 6.10.

Risk Assessment

The potential risk of CIN can be assessed before the procedure using a simple risk score. The score is based on factors related to both patient and procedure. The higher the score, the higher the risk that the patient will develop CIN after the procedure (see Tables 6.11 and 6.12).

Prevention of CIN

The following protocol is advised for any patient with a serum creatinine concentration above 135 μmol/l:

Table 6.10 Patient and procedural risk factors for contrast-induced nephropathy.

Patient-Related Risk Factors	Procedure-Related Risk Factors
Renal insufficiency, renal transplant	High contrast volume
Diabetes mellitus	High contrast osmolality
Age >75 years	Multiple contrast injections within 72 hours
Congestive heart failure (NYHA 3/4)	Use of IABP
Impaired left ventricular function	Diuretics
Acute MI/previous MI	Nephrotoxic agents (nonsteroidal
Atherosclerosis	anti-inflammatory agents, antibiotics)
Anemia	Angiotensin converting enzyme inhibitors
Hypotension (SBP < 80 mmHg)	

IABP, intra-aortic balloon pump; MI, myocardial infarction; NYHA, New York Heart Association class; SBP, systolic blood pressure.

Table 6.11 CIN risk score based on patient risk factors (adapted from Roxana Mehran).

Patient-Related Risk Factors	Integer Score
Hypertension	5
IABP	5
Congestive heart failure	5
Age >75 years	4
Anemia	3
Diabetes mellitus	3
Contrast media volume	1 for each 100 ml
Serum creatinine >1.5 mg/dl	4
or	2 for eGFR 40–60
eGFR < 60 ml/min/1.73 m^2	4 for eGFR 20–40
	6 for eGFR <20

Table 6.12 Interpretation of CIN risk score (adapted from Roxana Mehran).

Risk Score	Risk of CIN	Risk of Dialysis
≤5	7.5%	0.04%
6–10	14.0%	0.12%
11–16	26.1%	1.09%
≥16	57.3%	12.6%

• Assess the risk, carefully looking for chronic renal impairment, left ventricular function, etc.
• Stop metformin, diuretics and nonsteroidal anti-inflammatory agents 48 hours prior to the procedure, and restart at 48 hours after the procedure if renal function is satisfactory.
• Hydration is essential. Start fluid administration with normal saline (1 ml/ kg body weight per hour) 12 hours before the procedure.
• Put diabetic and at-risk patients first on the catheter list to maximize hydration.
• Keep contrast volume to less than 3 ml/kg.
• Use low or iso-osmolar contrast.
• Take a renal film at the end of the procedure to check for renal size and function and to exclude obstruction.
• Continue hydration for 12 hours after the procedure.
• Check on overall renal function; do not rely only on serum creatinine levels.
• Check creatinine level (12–72 hours after procedure). It usually increases within 24 hours after the procedure in patients with renal impairment.

- Check the GFR, which depends on age, gender, and body mass index; GFR falls with age.
- In very high-risk patients, consider continuous veno-venous hemofiltration (CVVH). Start this early rather than waiting days for renal function to deteriorate.

Other Preventive Technology

N-Acetylcysteine (NAC). The evidence that NAC is beneficial is not strong and is debatable, based largely on meta-analysis of heterogeneous studies. NAC is a vasodilator and an antioxidant that is rapidly absorbed and converted in the liver to cysteine. Dose is 600 mg PO twice daily the day before and on the day of the procedure. Some studies continued 600 mg twice daily for 2 days after the procedure. One study using NAC in primary angioplasty found 1200 mg twice daily better than 600 mg twice daily in prevention of contrast nephropathy. An intravenous preparation is also available: An NAC ampoule of 2 g is diluted to 10 ml with 50 ml 5% dextrose or 0.9% NaCl given over 15–30 minutes (IV dose is 600 mg = 3.0 ml of this solution).

Sodium bicarbonate. Sodium bicarbonate used with NAC and rehydration seemed to be better than just using NAC with rehydration in the REMEDIAL trial. It is not used routinely, and good hydration prior to the procedure is the most important factor in prevention.

Dose of sodium bicarbonate: Use 1.26% sodium bicarbonate = 150 mmol/litre
Before the catheter: 3 mls/kg/hour sodium bicarbonate for 1 hour
After the catheter: 1 ml/kg/hour sodium bicarbonate for 6 hours

RenalGuard is a new device under investigation that is designed to create and maintain high urine output, prevent contrast agents from clogging renal tubules, and limit exposure to toxins in the kidneys. Fluid replacement is matched automatically to reduce side effects associated with over- or underhydration.

Other drugs. There is no unequivocal evidence that administration of any available agent is beneficial. The majority of agents previously used in therapy for CIN prevention, such as dopamine, mannitol, furosemide, or calcium channel blockers, either show no benefit or cause harm.

Targeted renal therapy. This approach is based on the direct delivery of thera-peutic agents to the kidney through the renal arteries. Targeted renal therapy increases local drug concentration and helps avoid side effects due to first-pass drug elimination by the liver.

Therapeutic hypothermia. Mild hypothermia (cooling down to 33–34 °C) has been proven to reduce metabolic demand by preserving cellular ATP and maintaining mitochondrial integrity. It has potential to protect against acute renal failure.

Anticoagulants and Antiplatelet Agents in Renal Failure

In patients with NSTEMI, diabetes or chronic kidney disease (CrCl < 30 ml/min), anticoagulants should be administered carefully. Heparin should be given under ACT monitoring and bivalirudin dose reduced to 1.0 mg/kg per hour. Abciximab can be given in the standard dose but eptifibatide is contraindicated. Fondaparinux is also contraindicated if CrCl is below 20 ml/min. Clopidogrel may be used carefully but prasugrel should not be used.

Trials

CARE
In this trial 468 high risk patients with pre-existing renal disease were assigned to iopamidol-370 vs. iodixanol-320. The study compared the incidence of CIN when the two contrast agents were used. Primary end points related to a serum creatinine concentration more than 0.5 mg/dl above baseline 45–120 hours after administration. The study showed that there was no statistical difference between the two agents, but that iopamidol recipients had a slightly smaller mean increase in serum creatinine.

REMEDIAL
In this study 393 patients with eGFR below 40 ml/min were randomized to receive either saline plus N-acetylcysteine (NAC) or bicarbonate plus NAC or saline plus ascorbic acid plus NAC. The study demonstrated that the strategy of volume supplementation by sodium bicarbonate plus NAC seemed to be superior to the combination of normal saline with NAC alone or with the addition of ascorbic acid in preventing CIN in patients at medium to high risk.

New ST Elevation or Marked ST Depression

New ST elevation or marked ST depression may represent potential myocardial infarction. This is due to acute coronary occlusion from acute dissection or thrombus or both. It can also be associated with prolonged no-reflow or loss of a major side branch. Stenting has lowered the acute referral rate for coronary bypass surgery dramatically over the last few years. The risk of a new Q wave infarct during PCI is very low.

Cardiac Arrest

Once cardiac arrest occurs there are major difficulties as external cardiac massage interferes with fluoroscopy. The survival of the patient will depend on the cause, e.g., coronary arterial occlusion, and treatment of this. At the same time the anesthetic and other cardiac personnel must help deal with the resuscitation.

A few important issues associated with CPR quality should be emphasized:
- Compress the chest hard and fast, that is, at least 100/min, allowing complete chest recoil.
- Minimize interruptions in compression.
- Avoid excessive ventilation.
- Change the compressor every 2 minutes.

- Maintain a 30:2 compression:ventilation ratio.
- Attempt to improve CPR quality if diastolic pressure is below 20mmHg.
- Always check the rhythm on the monitor along with the pulses – treat the patient, not the monitor.

In addition:

- In cardiac arrest (ventricular fibrillation, VF/pulseless ventricular tachycardia, VT), give an immediate single-shock defibrillation 360J (monophasic) or 120–200J (biphasic) and immediately continue CPR.
- Continue CPR with 30:2 compression:ventilation ratio and 8–10 breaths/min. Good compression is much more important than exact timing of ventilation.
- Place electrodes (pads) on the right upper chest and back, also in patients with ICD or pacemaker (see p. 138).
- Give 1mg epinephrine IV every 3–5 minutes.
- Give amiodarone; first dose 300mg bolus, second dose 150mg for refractory VF/VT.
- Continue CPR and monitor CPR quality for 2 minutes.
- Observe pulse, blood pressure, and continuous waveform capnography to monitor correct placement of an endotracheal tube.
- Check rhythm again.
- In case of VF/pulseless VT give another DC shock and continue CPR as above.
- In case of stable monomorphic VT, perform waveform synchronized cardioversion with shocks at initial energies of 100J. If there is no response to the first shock, increase the dose of energy and perform shock again.
- For stable but refractory VT try RV overdrive pacing.
- In case of pulseless electrical activity (PEA), avoid atropine administration. Atropine is no longer recommended.
- In case of symptomatic or unstable bradycardia establish RV pacing. Chronotropic drugs may be an alternative.
- In case of regular monomorphic wide-complex tachycardia, give adenosine as a diagnostic agent.

Do not give adenosine in irregular wide-complex tachycardia. This may cause degeneration of the rhythm to VF.

- Treat underlying reversible causes listed in Table 6.13.
- Once the circulation is restored, monitor arterial oxyhemoglobin saturation and maintain saturation above 94%.

Table 6.13 Reversible causes of cardiac arrest.

The 5 Hs	The 5 Ts
Hypovolemia	Tension pneumothorax
Hypoxia	Tamponade, cardiac
Hydrogen ion (acidosis)	Toxins
Hypo-/ hyperkalemia	Thrombosis (pulmonary)
Hypothermia	Thrombosis (coronary)

Emergency CABG

The introduction of stents has resulted in a sharp fall in the need for emergency CABG. All PCI units should have access to urgent cardiac surgery with special arrangements in place for "offsite" units. The aim for offsite units is for the patient to be on bypass within 1 hour of the emergency call. Patients transferred for emergency surgery are inevitably at high risk. The reasons for emergency transfer are situations in which the interventionist is unable to repair or remedy the problem, e.g.:
• Long linear dissection
• Coronary perforation
• Unstable angina with a very tight stenosis crossed by a wire but which cannot be crossed by even the smallest balloon, and where rotablation is not an option. In this situation transfer the patient with the wire in situ across the lesion.
• Abrupt vessel closure (either target or adjacent vessel)
• Left main stem dissection
    In high-risk PCI cases the coronary anatomy should be discussed with the surgeon preoperatively. It may be felt that there is no suitable surgical option, and this situation must be discussed with the patient.

Death

In the consent form the patient should be advised that there is a very small risk of death (<1/1000). PCI mortality risk is higher in patients with acute myocardial infarction, cardiogenic shock, impaired left ventricular function, or additional critical aortic stenosis.

Key Learning Points

• Complication rates have fallen sharply with improved technology.
• Femoral access complications are more common than radial access ones.
• Many complications are avoidable with good pre-PCI preparation and careful strategy selection.
• Coronary perforation needs quick, skilled intervention and a surgical opinion at the outset.
• The no-reflow phenomenon is usually reversible.
• Not all the factors related to stent thrombosis are modifiable.
• The optimal length of a dual antiplatelet therapy course after DES placement remains uncertain.
• Preprocedural renal insufficiency is the most important risk factor for contrast-induced nephropathy.
• Preprocedural hydration is the best way of preventing contrast-induced nephropathy.
• Postprocedural monitoring of renal function is essential.

7 | Intracoronary Imaging

Intravascular Ultrasonography

Essential Angioplasty, First Edition. E. von Schmilowski, R. H. Swanton.
© 2012 John Wiley & Sons, Ltd. Published 2012 by John Wiley & Sons, Ltd.

Introduction

Intravascular ultrasonography (IVUS)-guided intervention is different from standard angiography. It gives us detailed information about lesion morphology and allows precise and direct visualization of the vessel wall, atherosclerotic plaque, and coronary lumen. It plays an important role in understanding the pathophysiology of the coronary artery plaque and the mechanisms leading to restenosis and stent thrombosis.

Unfortunately, angiographic assessment of a lesion is not precise, and in many cases the severity of coronary artery disease may be underestimated due to positive remodeling. This is a part of the atheromatous process within coronary arteries. In some cases foreshortening and overlapping side branches may influence interpretation, and assessment is particularly difficult in ostial and bifurcation lesions. For these reasons, IVUS is used, particularly before complex angioplasty as well as after the procedure to check stent expansion and apposition.

Angiography provides a general estimation of the vessel (vessel size, lesion length, ostial lesion location, etc.), but shows only the luminal contour. IVUS, on the other hand, gives us detailed anatomical information on the vessel and is also used to make precise measurements. It can also provide information on the epicardial coronary artery flow as well as the plaque composition. Advantages and limitations of IVUS are listed in Table 7.1.

There is no doubt that IVUS can be clinically useful in individual patients; however, a clear contribution to better clinical outcomes has not been shown except in left main PCI. Therefore its routine use in current practice is still limited.

Equipment and Technique

Image quality is described by spatial and contrast resolution and is related to ultrasound frequency. This has improved over the last few years and in current devices is 30–50 MHz, which allows precise plaque characterization. The IVUS system consists of three components: a specially designed catheter with a minimized ultrasound probe, a pullback device, and a console that is responsible for cross-sectional images. The standard catheter size is from 2.6F to 3.5F and is compatible with a 6F guiding catheter. The images are generated by passing an electrical current through a piezoelectric crystal

Table 7.1 Advantages and limitations of intravascular ultrasonography.

Advantages	Limitations
Real-time high-resolution images	Poor image quality
Full visualization of the vessel wall	Image distortion
Assessment of total vessel lumen and diameter	Artifacts
Assessment of lesion length and severity	Overestimation of lumen area
Assessment of complex lesions: intermediate lesion, ostial lesions, bifurcation lesions, haziness, dissection	Results depend on cardiac cycle (max. lumen area should be measured in mid-systole)
Assessment of unusual lesion morphology: aneurysm, plaque rupture	Difficulties in differentiating different tissue components (similar composition)
Plaque composition and plaque burden	Difficulties in assessing thrombus
Stent size and length	Poor assessment of plaque composition (except calcium)
Residual disease	Poor assessment of vulnerable plaque
Assessment of stent apposition	Does not provide histological information
Assessment of remodeling	Does not provide information about entire vessel anatomy
Mechanism and causes of restenosis	Unable to predict late events
Safe technique with very low risk of spasm, dissection or vessel closure	Prolongs procedure time

which produces high-frequency ultrasound waves that are reflected by tissue. Part of the ultrasound energy returns to the transducer, creating an electrical impulse which is transformed into an image. Gradual withdrawal of the ultrasound probe catheter can be either manual or motorized. The motorized device withdraws the catheter at a constant speed, usually 0.5 mm/s. Although pulling the probe back manually allows stopping at any point to focus on a specific area, the motorized device provides a smoother and more reliable movement.

Intracoronary glyceryl trinitrate (GTN) and heparin are administered before advancing the IVUS catheter. The imaging probe is advanced over the wire distal to the area of interest, the pullback device used to withdraw the catheter, and the images are recorded.

The procedure step by step:
• First decide what type of lesion you need to image (ostial lesion, left main, saphenous vein graft).
• Administer intracoronary GTN 100–200 μg.
• Use a 40 MHz IVUS catheter probe.
• Advance the probe 100 mm beyond the lesion.
• Use automated pullback at 0.5 mm/s until a point of 10 mm proximal to the lesion or the vessel ostium is reached.

• Assess lesion severity and morphology, including possible calcification, thrombus, or in-stent restenosis.
• Measure vessel size, luminal diameter, and lesion length.
• Assess the final result and possible complications.

Image Artifacts

Artifacts may affect the IVUS image and can lead to misinterpretation. One of the common artifacts visible on the screen is a narrow acoustic shadow caused by the guide wire. Other artifacts, visible as bright halos of various thickness surrounding the catheter, are caused oscillations of the transducer; these usually obscure the area close to the catheter, making it impossible to image. Very common multiple reflections or signal dropout are caused by calcium (IVUS energy is reflected by calcium).

Another problem is blood speckle, which is the ultrasound reflection from aggregated blood cells. These may interfere with lumen visualization and cause difficulties in differentiating the lumen from tissue, particularly in tight lesions or within a dissection. A saline flush helps clear the lumen and tissue border detection.

Nonuniform rotational distortion (NURD) can usually be recognized when the rotating transducer inside the catheter is exposed to frictional forces, e.g., in tortuous lesions, when the catheter is bent or the hemostatic valve is too tight. In such situations some segments of the images are stretched or compacted. Sharp movements of the drive cable of the mechanical catheter cause cyclical oscillations and result in image distortion. Usually catheter manipulation eliminates these artifacts. An unstable catheter position may result in motion artifacts and image deformation.

Measurements

Several definitions should be considered in assessing the vessel and a lesion. First, there is a difference between a lesion and a stenosis. Whereas a lesion is an accumulation of atherosclerotic plaque a stenosis means a lesion that compromises at least 50% of the luminal cross-sectional area (CSA) compared with a reference segment of lumen defined in advance. The reference lumen refers to the site with the largest lumen proximal or distal to a stenosis but within the same segment. Lesions and stenoses often need a number of image slices, particularly if one is dealing with diffuse disease. Over 90% of angiographically normal arteries have identifiable atheromatous lesions on IVUS.

All measurements should be performed in relation to the center of the lumen (not to the IVUS catheter) from two borders of the vessel wall: the luminal border and the external elastic membrane (Figure 7.1). The innermost layer of the vessel wall is the intima. Normally the intima is up to two layers of cells thick, but it is significantly thicker with the presence of atheroma. Outside the intima is the internal elastic lamina and then the media, which is composed of smooth muscle cells and elastin ensuring vascular tone. Finally,

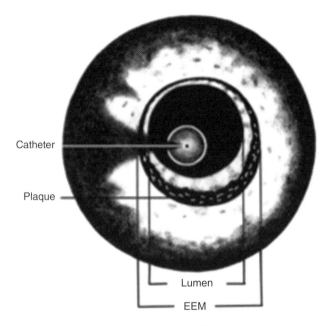

Figure 7.1 Schematic intravascular ultrasound image. EEM, external elastic membrane.

Table 7.2 Layers of the vessel wall seen on IVUS.

Inner layer	Middle layer	Outer layer
Intima	Media	Adventitia
Atheroma	(less echogenic than intima)	Periadventitial tissue
External elastic membrane		

outside this is the adventitia, which consists of multiple layers of connective tissue, scattered elastin plus vasa vasorum and serves as additional vessel support and vessel wall nutrition (Table 7.2).

The catheter positioned inside the vessel is surrounded by the lumen, vessel wall, and other structures such as side branches, veins, or pericardium. Note that a catheter should not be positioned obliquely, but parallel to the vessel long axis, and measurements should be done at the leading edge not at the trailing edge.

Vessel size and lesion length should be measured first in order to choose the stent size and length. Then lesion morphology is assessed. It has been shown that minimum luminal area (MLA) is a predictor of coronary flow reserve, fractional flow reserve, and perfusion scan results. Note that a flow-limiting stenosis can be recognized with IVUS if the MLA is smaller than $4.0\,mm^2$ in a proximal epicardial artery. This, however, does not apply to left main (stenosis if MLA <6.0 mm^2) and saphenous vein graft lesions.

Lumen and EEM Measurement

The lumen should be measured using the interface between the lumen and the leading edge of the intima. First the luminal border needs to be determined, then the further measurements can be derived, such as luminal cross-sectional area (CSA, the area bounded by the luminal border), minimum and maximum lumen diameters (the shortest and the longest diameters through the center of the lumen), lumen eccentricity, and luminal area stenosis. The external elastic membrane (EEM) is defined as the interface border between the media and the adventitia. The EEM should be measured in a relatively straight vessel, avoiding large side branches, stents, or heavy calcification, which usually cause shadowing and lead to misinterpretation. It is important to measure EEM CSA, which is the area bounded by the EEM border, as well as the minimum and maximum EEM diameters, which are the shortest and the longest diameters through the center of the EEM.

Atheroma and Calcium Measurements

It is very difficult to determine the area of true atheroma due to poor delineation of the internal elastic membrane. Therefore all measurements should include both the plaque and the media.

• *Plaque cross-sectional area.* This area is measured by subtracting the luminal area from the EEM area in order to obtain plaque cross-sectional area.

• *Minimal and maximal plaque thickness.* the largest and the shortest distances from the intimal leading edge to the border of EEM.

• *Plaque and media eccentricity.* This shows whether abnormal intimal thickening is present throughout the 360° arterial circumference.

• *Plaque burden.* This is the area inside the EEM occupied by atheroma despite the lumen compromise.

• *Plaque eccentricity.*

• *Calcium* is well imaged in IVUS and appears as bright echoes, often causing acoustic shadows according to location and distribution. Acoustic shadowing is either superficial or deep in relation to the plaque.

Stent Measurement

Stent struts are highly reflective and easy to visualize (as echogenic points around the vessel). This allows assessment of stent expansion and stent apposition against the vessel wall as well as stent CSA and stent diameter. To determine stent size, proximal and distal reference sites of the vessel have to be measured. These can be obtained using the largest lumen proximal or distal to a stenosis but within the same segment and within 10 mm of the stenosis with no large side branches. It has been shown that stent implantation with IVUS guidance, particularly in certain lesion subsets (ostial lesion, left main stem, small vessels), has a lower rate of in-stent restenosis than those deployed without IVUS guidance.

Remodeling

The term "remodeling" refers to an increase or decrease in the EEM area during the atherosclerotic process. Positive remodeling occurs when the EEM area increases during atheroma development and negative remodeling when it decreases. Remodeling index is used to describe the direction of the process: index >1.0 describes positive remodeling (the lesion EEM area is greater than the reference EEM area) whereas index <1.0 indicates negative remodeling.

Interpretation

To facilitate image interpretation it is best to become familiar with certain landmarks, e.g., side branches, and with differences in the acoustic signal (echogenic and echolucent structures), listed in Table 7.3.

Echogenic structures are visible on the ultrasound display, whereas echolucent structures are seen as black space. Differences in echogenic properties are due to different amounts of collagen and elastin. Collagen, for example, has much higher reflectance than smooth muscle. It is also important to make sure that the catheter has been positioned properly in order to avoid image quantification errors. Catheter angulation can affect apparent vessel geometry, particularly in large vessels.

Plaque Morphology

Calcific Plaque

This is the most easily recognizable type of plaque on IVUS as in most cases it is seen as an intensely bright reflection. However, this is not an absolute rule. Similar bright reflections may also occur in dense fibrous tissue. If the plaque characteristics are not clear, it is best to describe it as a fibrocalcific plaque. Calcific plaques are seen in the majority of lesions assessed by IVUS.

Fibrotic Plaque

Fibrotic plaque is usually seen as a bright echogenic area similar to the adventitia. Only very dense fibrotic lesions may be confused with calcium; normally fibrotic plaques are less intense than calcific plaques but brighter than smooth muscles or lipid tissue.

Table 7.3 Image interpretation based on echogenicity.

Echogenic Atheroma	Reduced Echogenicity	Echolucent/Soft Atheroma
Blood vessel wall inner lining	Necrotic zone within a plaque	Blood itself
Calcific plaque	Intramural hemorrhage	Healthy tissue
Fibrocalcific plaque	Thrombus	High lipid concentration
Dense fibrotic plaque	Fibrotic plaque	Minimal collagen and elastin
		Intimal hyperplasia

Lipid Plaque

Lipid plaque on IVUS has a soft gray appearance with varying intensity. Usually, radiolucent areas inside fibrous plaque reflect lipid deposits. Sometimes, however, shadowing from a densely fibrotic plaque can be misinterpreted as lipid.

Blood

In still images, blood speckle may have a pattern similar to atheromatous plaque. Sometimes blood stagnating proximal to a stenotic segment may cause a similar effect. The best way to recognize the real pattern is to clear the lumen with a saline flush. It should be noted that the blood speckle pattern changes constantly with systolic and diastolic blood flow and is more echogenic in systole.

Challenging and Unusual Situations

Aneurysm and Pseudoaneurysm

Very often an aneurysm recognized on angiography is in fact a pseudoaneurysm or not an aneurysm at all when analyzed by IVUS. To differentiate a true aneurysm from a false aneurysm, search for the media (Table 7.4). In a true aneurysm the lesion includes all layers of the vessel wall with an EEM. The media is thin and expanded but fully surrounds the boundary of the aneurysm. The pseudoaneurysm has only one layer of the vessel, which is the adventitia; the media has ruptured.

Angiographic Filling Defects and Hazy Lesions

Usually, a filling defect seen on angiography relates to the presence of thrombus. However, sometimes it may also be a calcified lesion, particularly in the main stem. Hazy lesions, which are relatively often observed on angiography, usually correspond with thrombus, calcification, dissection, or positive remodeling.

The most common reason of a persistent haziness either proximal or distal to a stent which has just been deployed is stent edge dissection. This usually occurs from high-pressure deployment and seems not to influence long-term prognosis. IVUS is a helpful tool in these situations as it prevents unnecessary additional stent implantation.

Table 7.4 Differences between aneurysm and pseudoaneurysm on IVUS.

	Aneurysm	Pseudoaneurysm
Number of layers of the vessel wall	All layers	One layer – adventitia
The media	Fully covered	Ruptured

Dissection

Dissection can be detected on IVUS as an accumulation of blood limited to the intima or extending into the media or through the EEM. If blood is limited to the media space, displacing the internal elastic membrane inwards and the EEM outwards, this indicates an intramural hematoma. Intramural hematoma is usually caused by intimal fracture of a plaque or by mechanical injury during intervention, e.g., from use of a stiff wire. It is associated with adverse clinical vascular outcomes, and an IVUS-guided procedure is always helpful.

IVUS-Guided PCI

IVUS has greatly contributed to our understanding of the coronary atherosclerotic process and lesion assessment. It helps in the decision of which lesion should be treated and which not. It helps the determination of stent selection. It can also confirm complete stent apposition and exclude edge dissection. These factors are important predictors of early and late complications.

Although IVUS is not used routinely in PCI, in some cases such as complex PCIs, in patients with diabetes, low ejection fraction, thrombotic lesions, or in left main stenting, an IVUS-guided procedure should be always considered.

Acute Coronary Syndromes

Plaque Burden

There is a correlation between the development of an acute coronary syndrome and plaque burden. The majority of plaque volume resides in nonstenotic segments, and it has been well established that vulnerable and ruptured plaques arise from these nonstenotic segments. Hence, plaque burden measurements may suggest the presence of vulnerable plaque. Plaque burden is calculated as plaque area/external elastic lamina area x 100.

Attention should also be paid to minimal lumen area (MLA) and the presence of thrombus. These are important predictors of an acute coronary syndrome. Finally, calcium density may help differentiate stable from unstable angina. In unstable lesions calcification is less severe, whereas in stable angina it is more dense (Table 7.5).

Plaque Rupture

Ruptured plaques causing acute coronary syndrome are eccentric and show a large vessel area and large vessel lumen with obvious signs of positive remodeling (Table 7.5). There is often an empty space within the plaque due to embolization of atherosclerotic material which in time becomes the site of thrombus. However, thrombus is present in only half of the lesions with ruptured plaque. Therefore it is likely that clinical symptoms depend on the original stenosis or on the presence of thrombus, not on plaque rupture.

Table 7.5 Presence of positive and negative remodeling and calcification on IVUS in patients with acute coronary syndrome and stable angina.

	Acute Coronary Syndrome/ Myocardial Infarction	Stable Angina
Positive remodeling (increase of EEM)	+++	+
Negative remodeling (decrease of EEM)	+	+++
Calcification	Very small deposit or no calcification	Extensive

Plaque rupture is often associated with complex lesion morphology confirmed on angiography. This has been proven in patients who underwent angiography less than one week before an acute myocardial infarction.

Ruptured plaque can be recognized when three out of five following criteria are met:

- Lesion EEM >14.3 mm^2
- Reference lumen area >8.1 mm^2
- Maximum lesion plaque thickness >1.6 mm^2
- Lesion plaque burden >0.63
- Remodeling index >0.87

Acute Myocardial infarction

Culprit plaques have certain markers of instability such as thrombus, positive remodeling, or large plaque mass. This may suggest that the vascular event in patients with acute myocardial infarction is determined by lesion morphology. The most common lesion characteristics in patients with acute infarct are the following:

- Dissection
- Echolucent area
- Low echogenic thrombus
- Brightly speckled material

The majority of acute myocardial infarctions can be recognized and confirmed on standard angiography as complex lesions with thrombus formation and ruptured plaque with a significant narrowing or total occlusion. On real-time IVUS, thrombus appears as a sparkling pattern, and it may not be easily recognizable or may be misinterpreted as vessel dissection. Thrombus has often a lobular shape and presents with microchannels with echodensity less than 50% of the surrounding adventitia and deep calcification. It may also appear after stent implantation.

In some patients, however, despite clinical symptoms and ECG changes, coronary arteries remain normal on angiography. In these situations IVUS guidance should be used to confirm the diagnosis, which may include coronary spasm, dissection, or ruptured plaque not seen on angiography.

Stable Angina

In patients with stable angina and single-vessel disease, fibrocalcific plaque is associated with negative remodeling (Table 7.5). Positive remodeling before angioplasty is associated with a higher rate of postprocedural major adverse cardiac events, target lesion restenosis, and in-stent restenosis.

IVUS in Specific Subsets of Lesions

It has been questioned whether the routine use of IVUS guidance in the implantation of drug-eluting stents (DES) has any significant benefits in terms of modification of interventional strategy or outcomes. There is evidence, however, that in complex PCIs (left main stenting, bifurcation lesions, ostial lesions, heavily calcified lesions, saphenous vein graft lesions, or diffuse in-stent restenosis) IVUS guidance may be of value. It allows a better understanding of the nature of the disease which leads to a more tailored and focused treatment and a better result.

Proximal Epicardial Artery

It may be difficult to decide whether or not to intervene in an intermediate coronary lesion with a stenosis between 40% and 70%. Compared with IVUS, angiography underestimates lumen diameter, and either IVUS or fractional flow reserve (FFR) should be performed to assess the lesion further. It has been established that a lesion causing a minimum CSA less than $4.0\,mm^2$ and a percentage area of stenosis greater than 60–70% in a proximal epicardial artery is a flow-limiting, significant stenosis. There is a strong correlation between minimum CSA and FFR for detecting ischemia: CSA cutoff below $4.0\,mm^2$ is significantly related to FFR below 0.75. This does not apply to the left main (see below).

Left Main Stem

Angiographic visualization of the left main is often difficult and unreliable due to its anatomy. The left main has the greatest angiographic variability of all coronary segments, the ostial view may not be clear due to contrast injection, the left main body may be too short to be assessed precisely, and the distal portion of the left main may be hidden by the bifurcation or vessel overlap. In this context IVUS is useful, particularly if the angiographic view is unclear.

IVUS-guided left main stenting reduced long-term mortality compared to non-IVUS-guided procedures in the MAIN-COMPARE registry (see p. 201), and many interventionists use it routinely in this type of procedure.

In imaging the left main coronary artery it is important to place the guide wire and the IVUS catheter distally beyond the bifurcation (in most cases into the left anterior descending artery) to ensure the most coaxial alignment with the left main. An oblique image (non-coaxial alignment) can result in overestimation of the left main lumen CSA. Note that the significance of left main stenosis is based on lumen dimension, not on plaque burden.

Left main stenosis is considered hemodynamically significant if the luminal CSA is less than $6.0\,mm^2$ as a cutoff value for revascularization, or minimum luminal diameter (MLD) is less than 3.0 mm and luminal diameter stenosis on IVUS is less than 50% of the reference diameter. Interpretation in patients with a CSA between 6.0 and $7.5\,mm^2$ should take into account clinical history, stress test, or FFR result.

Ideally the IVUS criteria should correlate with FFR which for left main stenosis is less than 0.75. Studies have also reported that the MLD is an independent risk factor for major adverse cardiovascular events. Generally a stenosis area greater than 50% requires revascularization.

The luminal CSA is the sum of the luminal areas of the two daughter vessels (that is, the left anterior descending and left circumflex arteries, and each of them should be $>4.0\,mm^2$), which is 150% of the parent left main.

Bifurcation Lesion
Most bifurcation lesions should be assessed by IVUS for optimal visualization of both branches. Side branch visualization is important, as the presence of a side branch lesion increases the risk of side branch occlusion and myocardial infarction. Bifurcation lesions show specific hemodynamic characteristics which result in potential early and eccentric plaque development (see p. 207). The proximal segment of the side branch can be visualized during pullback through the main vessel, although in some cases, e.g., in ostial branch involvement, this can be difficult.

Ostial Lesion
Ostial lesions are challenging. They are often severely calcified, requiring effective predilatation and good visualization. Many experienced operators use IVUS routinely when dealing with these lesions. The main advantage of IVUS is that it allows differentiation between true ostial lesions, which can be recognized when the MLA and the maximum plaque burden are located at the ostium, and the near-ostial lesion, where a proximal reference segment can be identified. With the aorto-ostial lesion, it is important to withdraw the guiding catheter slightly into the aorta in order to recognize the true aorto-ostial lesion. If the guiding catheter is placed in the vessel lumen, the ostial lesion may be missed and misinterpreted as a calcified lesion. The IVUS transducer should be coaxial to the ostium of the vessel to ensure reliable measurements.

Calcified Lesions
Heavily calcified lesions carry a higher risk of complications because they have higher rates of stent underexpansion, stent thrombosis, and in-stent restenosis. Severe calcification may result in inadequate dilatation. The worst situation is an underexpanded stent in a calcified lesion with a high risk of stent thrombosis; these lesions always require preparation and probable rotablation before stenting.

Saphenous Vein Grafts
Usually vein graft plaques are diffuse and concentric; often they are bulky and friable with just mild calcification. The procedure carries a higher risk of distal embolization, myocardial infarction, and late cardiac events than PCI of a native vessel. Moreover, vein graft remodeling and plaque development may be underestimated on angiography. In general, a saphenous vein graft lesion requires direct and undersized stenting that is less than 90% of the reference lumen (see Figure 5.32). Adequate stent apposition is crucial as lack of apposition is associated with adverse events. Whereas IVUS is very useful in postprocedural assessment of stent apposition, preprocedural use of IVUS is not recommended, particularly in severely degenerate grafts with the risk of dislodging friable atheroma and distal embolization.

In-Stent Restenosis and Edge Problems
Whereas restenosis after balloon angioplasty is caused in part by by geometric remodeling and recoil, in-stent restenosis is driven by intimal hyperplasia or by intimal hyperplasia and negative remodeling (decreased EEM), e.g., edge restenosis. Sometimes underexpansion may also be misinterpreted as in-stent restenosis. Ostial lesions are particularly prone to in-stent restenosis as even minimal intimal hyperplasia covering stent underexpansion can cause restenosis. There is strong evidence that late lumen loss within a stent correlates with tissue growth more than with stent recoil.

Assessment of the Restenotic Lesion
To assess the restenotic lesion you need to identify the image slice with the smallest luminal area at follow-up and compare it with the same image slice before and after intervention. The larger the minimum stent area (MSA) after deployment and post-dilatation, the lower the rate of restenosis. The smallest acceptable MSA is from 6.5 to $7.5\,mm^2$. In some cases, however, such as in small vessels or in patients with diabetes, it may not be possible to achieve this. Stents with an MSA of less than $5.5\,mm^2$ and that are over $40\,mm$ in length are at higher risk of in-stent restenosis.

To assess the restenotic lesion, proceed as follows:
• Assess the length and size of the vessel.
• Select the stent length based on a measurement of the distance between proximal and distal reference sites.
• Always use motorized pullback.

- Select the stent size based on measurement of the reference lumen dimensions.
- Ensure full stent apposition.

Complete lesion coverage and adequate stent expansion without gaps between stents are very important in treatment of in-stent restenosis. In focal in-stent restenosis that is less than 10–20 mm in length, high-pressure balloon dilatation followed by an IVUS check is a reasonable initial treatment option. Alternatively, a sandwich stent (implantation of a second drug-eluting stent) may be effective. It is also useful to use a sandwich stent to cover overlapping stents if there is focal restenosis at the overlap due to delayed endothelialization in the overlapped area. Diffuse in-stent restenosis from dense intimal hyperplasia, longer than 20 mm on IVUS, can be treated with a drug-eluting balloon. In some cases surgery is the only alternative (see also pp. 307–310).

Edge Restenosis

This is usually defined as 50% decrease in edge lumen CSA and is determined by plaque burden at the edge of the stent during implantation, stent area at the edge of the stent, and in-stent intimal hyperplasia. The best way to assess edge restenosis is to select a segment from the stent edge that is longer than 5 mm and to analyze every millimeter step by step.

Stent Underexpansion

The result of stent deployment is determined by optimal stent expansion (a minimal stent area greater than 70% of the CSA of the postdilating balloon) and full stent apposition without mechanical complications. Correct implantation technique (that is, media to media) is an IVUS principle that minimizes the risk of underexpansion and malapposition.

It is likely that properties of the atherosclerotic vessel wall such as plaques of calcium may be responsible for suboptimal stent expansion, but in most cases stent underexpansion is simply due to undersizing the stent. Often poor angiographic visualization, particularly of tight lesions, may lead to lesion underestimation even after GTN injection. Visualization of distal segments may also be difficult due to limited antegrade flow and competitive flow from collaterals. To avoid this, most tight stenoses should be predilated. In all IVUS-guided procedures, postdilatation with a noncompliant balloon is very important.

DES underexpansion is an important predictor of stent thrombosis and stent failure. This can be recognized in IVUS if MSA is less than $5\,\mathrm{mm}^2$ and less than 80% of the mean reference lumen. Outcome with the smallest MSA depends on the amount of neointimal hyperplasia and its suppression. Greater amounts of neointima mean less suppression requiring a larger MSA to minimize the risk of in-stent restenosis. Recent studies show that the optimal MSA after left main stenting is $8.7\,\mathrm{mm}^2$.

Stent Malapposition and Stent Thrombosis

The traditional criteria for optimal stent expansion have been reported in the MUSIC study (Multicenter Ultrasound Stenting in Coronaries) as final stent MSA greater than 80% of the reference CSA (or MSA greater than 90% if reference CSA area is smaller than $9\,mm^2$). IVUS predictors of very late stent thrombosis are related to stent expansion and stent malapposition.

Nevertheless, there is no evidence that either acute or late stent malapposition increase adverse cardiac events or stent thrombosis. It is likely, however, that large wall gaps between a stent and a vessel may increase the risk of stent thrombosis, due to delayed healing, inflammation, or hypersensitivity. Likewise, incomplete stent expansion with smaller minimum stent area after stent implantation may be related to the further in-stent restenosis and stent thrombosis.

Late stent malapposition, also called late acquired incomplete stent apposition, is more common and is likely to occur in complete total occlusion (CTO) lesions and after primary PCI in patients with acute myocardial infarction. Late malapposition in acute myocardial infarction is probably associated with positive remodeling. Incomplete stent apposition can be avoided by high-pressure postdilatation with a noncompliant balloon.

Complications of IVUS

IVUS is considered a safe procedure. Complications are extremely rare, but may occur particularly in patients with acute myocardial infarction or unstable angina. These include coronary spasm, dissection, thrombosis, and acute occlusion.

Trials

AVIO

In this study, 142 patients in each arm were randomized to IVUS-guided and angiography-guided stent implantation. IVUS-guided PCI resulted in a larger minimum lumen diameter than did angiography-guided stent implantation. Clinically, however, at 30 days and at 9 months there was no significant difference in the combined end point of myocardial infarction, target lesion revascularization, target vessel revascularization, and cardiac death. All patients presented with complex lesions, such as long lesions (>28 mm), CTOs, bifurcation lesions, small vessel lesions, or multiple lesions requiring four or more stents. Patients who underwent stent implantation guided by IVUS had a significantly greater postprocedure in-lesion minimum lumen diameter as evaluated by coronary angiography. This trial also established definite criteria for optimal stent expansion.

PROSPECT

This study randomized 700 patients with acute coronary syndrome, either STEMI within 24 hours (30.3%), NSTEMI (65.6%), or unstable angina with ECG changes (4.2%), who underwent successful PCI in one or two major coronary arteries. Quantitative coronary angiography of the entire coronary tree, IVUS, and virtual histology were performed.

Over 3.4 years' follow-up, the culprit and nonculprit lesions demonstrated similar levels of major adverse cardiac events (a composite of cardiac death, cardiac arrest, myocardial infarction, unstable angina, and increasing angina). Half of the events occurred within 1 year and half between 1 and 3 years.

The nonculprit lesions were not linked to any cases of cardiac death but were most commonly associated with increasing angina (8.5%), unstable angina (3.3%), and myocardial infarction (1.0%).

Key Learning Points

- IVUS allows visualization of the vessel wall, atherosclerotic plaque, and coronary lumen.
- A luminal area of less than $4.0\,mm^2$ in a proximal epicardial artery is a flow-limiting stenosis (except lesions in the left main and saphenous vein grafts).
- IVUS guidance is recommended in PCI of left main or complex bifurcation lesions.
- Significant left main stenosis can be recognized if absolute luminal CSA is less than $6.0\,mm^2$ or MLD is less than 3.0 mm.
- IVUS is important in understanding DES failure.
- DES underexpansion leads to restenosis, particularly in high-risk patients.

Virtual Histology

Virtual histology allows detection of a vulnerable plaque and is a predictor of acute coronary events. This technology uses amplitude and frequency analyses of the IVUS signal to differentiate types of vulnerable plaque (Table 7.6). There are four types of tissue component correlating with the radiofrequency data.

- *Fibrous tissue*, visible as a dark green area. This consists of collagen fibers packed tightly with no signs of intrafiber lipid areas or macrophage infiltration. This type of plaque is often present in patients with diabetes or in the elderly.
- *Fibrolipid tissue*, visible as a yellow/light green area with bundles of loosely distributed collagen fibers and some lipid. This is a cellular rather than necrotic area with no cholesterol clefts. Macrophage infiltration may also occur.
- *Necrotic core*, represented as a red color in virtual histology, consists of a mixture of lipids plus a necrotic core with some foam cells and necrotic lymphocytes. This necrotic region has cholesterol clefts and calcification. Collagen is not visible.
- *Dense calcium*, visible as a white focal area with some calcium crystals at borders. The main cause of calcium is inflammation and intramural hemorrhage.

Table 7.6 Type of vulnerable plaques in virtual histology.

Type of Plaque	Tissue Characteristic	Color on Virtual Histology	Risk of Rupture
Adaptive intimal thickening	*Fibrous tissue* Collagen fibers	Green	Low
Pathological intimal thickening	*Fibrolipid tissue* Mostly fibrotic with some lipid, necrotic and calcium deposits	Green with some minor yellow, red, and white spots	Low/middle
Pathological intimal thickening	*Lipid/necrotic tissue* Mostly fiber and lipid deposits with necrotic core infiltrated with calcium	Green with red core inside. White spots inside red area	High
Pathological intimal thickening	*Dense calcium*	White focal area	Very high

Vulnerable plaque characteristics in elderly patients are different from those in a younger population. In patients aged over 65 years the majority of plaques are fibrous or lipid (mostly red and white with some minor green areas). In younger patients, fibrolipid plaques are dominant (mostly green with some red areas).

Stable lesions are very easy to recognize. These are mostly green with some minor yellow or red areas. Virtual histology helps identify thin cap fibroatheroma (TCFA) which represents vulnerable plaque.

Fractional Flow Reserve (FFR)

This technique is used prior to coronary angioplasty to determine the functional significance of a lesion. FFR describes the ratio of hyperemic flow in the stenotic vessel to normal hyperemic flow. In other words, FFR is an expression of the extent to which maximum myocardial flow in the stenotic territory is limited by the epicardial stenosis.

The technique involves passing a pressure-wire (with a transducer at its tip) across the lesion and measuring the pressure distal to the stenosis and the pressure proximal to the stenosis using the coronary ostial pressure (from the guiding catheter) as the prestenotic pressure. Alternatively the measurements can be made after wire withdrawal (Figure 7.2). Maximal hyperemia is important in calculating FFR and is best obtained by

(a)

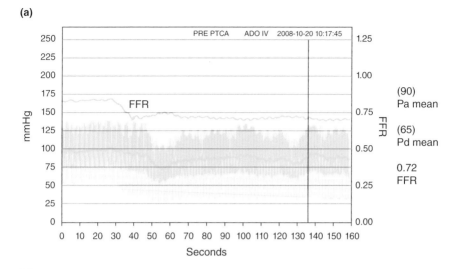

(b)

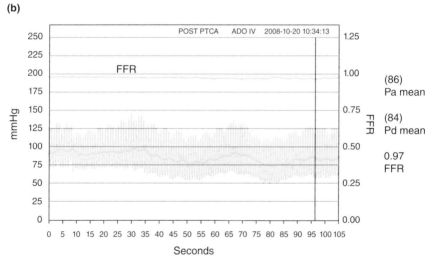

Figure 7.2 FFR measurements in a man with an LAD stenosis. (a) Before stenting. FFR is 0.72. (b) After stenting FFR has returned to normal: 0.97. Pa: arterial pressure proximal to the stenosis (measured at catheter tip); Pd: arterial pressure distal to the stenosis (measured at wire tip).

administration of bolus of adenosine (IV or IC). In patients with no inducible ischemia (FFR 1.0–0.80), medical treatment is recommended. FFR of 0.80–0.75 indicates a so-called gray zone, and FFR below 0.75 suggests inducible ischemia.

Although both IVUS and FFR play an important role in the assessment of ambiguous lesions and in risk stratification, they are suited to different conditions and answer different questions. While IVUS is helpful in assessing vessel size and wall composition, FFR is useful for the assessment of the significance of a stenosis. In general, IVUS should be used when a decision has been made to treat the lesion and FFR when the lesion significance needs to be assessed and an unnecessary procedure avoided.

FFR is useful not only in determining whether PCI of a specific coronary lesion should be performed or not, but is also helpful as an alternative to noninvasive functional testing. It is reasonable to use FFR to assess the effect of an intermediate coronary stenosis with 30–70% luminal narrowing in symptomatic patients. However, routine use of FFR in patients with angina and a positive stress test is not required. Sometimes angiography is not precise, and a seemingly mild stenosis seen on angiography may in fact be hemodynamically significant. A functional examination with FFR should be considered in the following situations:
• If there is doubt on angiography whether a moderate stenosis is functionally significant in a symptomatic patient
• If IVUS is positive but noninvasive tests are negative
• If the target lesion is short and moderate at quantitative coronary angiography
• In an ostial lesion with unusual anatomy

In patients with acute coronary syndromes FFR should not be performed during or soon after an acute myocardial infarction. During the acute phase of acute myocardial infarction FFR does not provide reliable information about the infarct-related artery, but it can be useful in assessment of the contralateral artery. One month after a myocardial infarction, however, FFR greater than 0.80 excludes the presence of residual ischemia.

Trials

FAME

In this study, 1000 patients with multivessel disease were randomized to either routine angiography-guided PCI (PCI of all lesions >50%) or FFR-guided PCI with stenting only in those lesions with FFR less than 0.80. Clinical outcomes were compared at 1 year. FFR guidance in multivessel disease reduced the rate of the composite end point at 1 year by 30% and reduced mortality and myocardial infarction at 1 year by 35%. This study shows that FFR-guided PCI is associated with a lower incidence of major adverse cardiac events compared with angiography-guided PCI in patients with multivessel disease.

DEFER

In the DEFER study 235 patients with intermediate single vessel disease were studied with FFR. Patients in whom the FFR was greater than 0.75 were randomized to stenting or deferral. If the FFR was less than 0.75 stenting was undertaken. Deferring intervention if the FFR was greater than 0.75 was a safe strategy, with death or myocardial infarction related to the index stenosis less than 1%/year.

Key Learning Points

- FFR determines whether PCI of a specific coronary lesion should be performed or not.
- FFR is an alternative to noninvasive functional testing.
- If the FFR is greater than 0.75 it is safe to leave the lesion alone.
- FFR below 0.75 suggests inducible ischemia.
- FFR should not be performed during or soon after acute myocardial infarction.
- During the acute phase of myocardial infarction FFR does not provide reliable information about the infarct-related artery.

Optical Coherence Tomography

- **Preprocedural Assessment, 340**
  Lumen Area
  Plaque Composition
- **Stent Failure, 340**
  In-Stent Restenosis
  Stent Thrombosis
- **Stent Apposition, 342**
- **Thrombus, 343**
- **Vessel Injury, 343**
- **Unusual Structures, 343**
- **Complex Lesions, 343**
  Bifurcation Lesions
  CTO Lesions

Although standard coronary angiography provides excellent imaging during interventional procedures, it does not provide information on the interaction between the stent and the vessel wall. Angiography is really "lumenography" and there are problems with edge detection and definition with overlapping shadows. Angiography also has limited prognostic relevance in terms of stent failure or cardiac events. The development of new technologies including optical coherence tomography (OCT) has opened new possibilities for the assessment of the short- and long-term outcomes of stent implantation. The high-resolution and high-quality images of the coronary arteries provided by OCT in vivo allow precise lesion assessment including lumen dimensions and plaque composition. This technique also provides valuable information about mechanisms responsible for stent thrombosis or in-stent restenosis. Moreover, OCT is capable of assessing long coronary segments using only small amounts of contrast. It is likely that OCT will be used with increasing frequency, not only for optimizing stent implantation, but also for preventing complications such as in-stent restenosis, stent thrombosis, or intra-stent and edge dissection. Figure 7.3 shows schematic OCT images.

Preprocedural Assessment

Lumen Area
OCT gives us information about lumen dimensions and plaque composition. Luminal area describes the severity of the stenotic lesion and allows precise area measurements. The great advantage of OCT images is the very clear delineation of the lumen–intima interface, which ensures good reproducibility of area measurement.

Plaque Composition
Information about plaque composition is a very important part of preprocedural assessment which can influence treatment strategy. Firstly, a severely calcified lesion needs careful lesion preparation for optimal stent expansion. Second, it has been shown that lipid composition of the plaque is associated with increased risk of the no-reflow phenomenon. Finally, culprit plaque such as ruptured fibrous cap with thrombus, which are well imaged in OCT, are related to acute coronary syndromes and may influence the interventional procedure. As with virtual histology thin cap fibroatheroma (TCFA) can be identified.

Types of plaque composition assessed by OCT:
- *Fibrous plaque*, usually homogenous, easily visible, with rich signal and well-defined borders.
- *Lipid-rich plaque*, which is often diffuse and thinner than fibrous plaque, with poor borders and poor signal.
- *Fibrocalcific plaque*, which despite poor signal is easy recognizable because of its sharply defined borders.

Stent Failure
In OCT stent failure means in-stent restenosis, stent strut fracture and stent thrombosis. OCT has a greater resolution than IVUS and allows the detection of tissue coverage in DES, and even minimal malapposition or very small edge dissection.

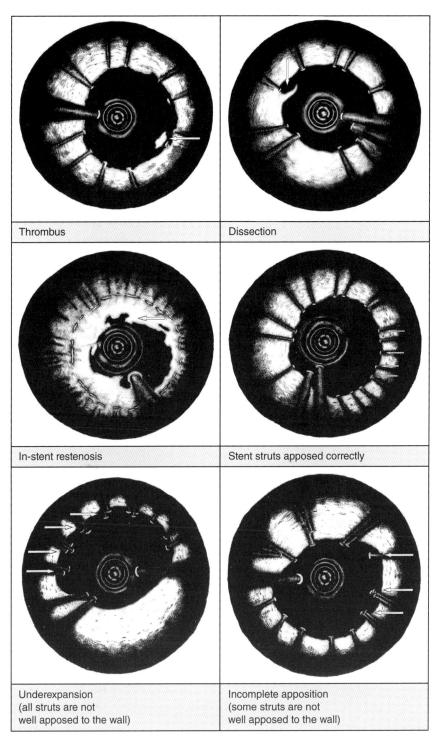

Figure 7.3 Schematic optical coherence tomographic images.

In-Stent Restenosis

Although the introduction of DES has significantly reduced the risk of in-stent restenosis, the problem persists. OCT can be a useful tool in the identification of the mechanism and the choice of optimal treatment. Predictors of restenosis using OCT are:

- Inadequate stent expansion
- Gaps between stents
- Incomplete lesion coverage
- Stent fracture or irregular distribution of stent struts
- Stent apposition
- Severe vessel damage due to high-pressure deployment
- Severity and extension of neointimal proliferation in patients with previously implanted stents

Stent Thrombosis

Stent thrombosis remains one of the major problems in interventional cardiology, and although relatively rare, the consequences are serious. The OCT technique provides insight into the vascular healing process after PCI. Stent underexpansion or malapposition may lead to subacute stent thrombosis. Late stent thrombosis, however, is strongly related to delayed endothelialization on the surface of the stent.

DES have proved of significant benefit in preventing in-stent restenosis, mostly by inhibiting neointimal proliferation. An obvious sign of this process is tissue coverage, which is well seen in OCT as tiny layers of tissue covering stent struts. The great resolution of OCT enables visualization of each strut, allowing determination of whether they are covered adequately or not. In primary PCI in patients with acute myocardial infarction struts frequently remain uncovered and this may be related to plaque composition. Information about stent coverage is helpful in guiding future treatment, and may influence recommendations regarding the duration of dual antiplatelet therapy. More trial data is needed in the value of OCT in guiding long-term therapy.

Stent Apposition

There is no doubt that OCT is better than IVUS for assessing the adequacy of stent apposition to the vessel wall. Poor apposition contributes to stent thrombosis. Most malapposed struts are located in areas of stent overlap and in heavy calcified lesions. It seems that strut thickness and cell design as well as lesion characteristics (for example, long, calcified lesions) are associated with a higher risk of stent malapposition. OCT helps assess plaque morphology and influences the choice of treatment. However, there is no evidence yet that the use of OCT influences clinical outcomes.

Thrombus

Thrombus is usually visible as a structure (with its associated shadow) protruding into the vessel lumen, sometimes attached to the stent strut. The excellent resolution of OCT allows the detection of even small intracoronary thrombi attached to stent struts. Thrombus formation is more likely to occur within long stents, uncovered struts, and in asymmetric stent expansion. However, the detection of these small thrombi is not associated with thrombotic clinical events.

Vessel Injury

Although vessel integrity is important in the prevention of thrombus formation, there is no clinical evidence that the necrotic core which can be found between the stent struts in OCT is associated with stent thrombosis or other long-term complications.

Unusual Structures

In occasional cases coronary angiography shows unclear images which may cause doubt as to whether to proceed further or to leave the lesion untreated. It is important to clarify the reason for these images to avoid unnecessary intervention. Hazy lesions at the edge of the stent are commonly associated with edge dissection, thrombus, or uncovered plaque. Ambiguous images inside the stent often correspond with intracoronary thrombus or intrastent dissection. In general, however, hazy lesions are not associated with a risk of further clinical events.

Complex Lesions

Bifurcation Lesions

Bifurcation lesions remain one of the most difficult subsets of lesions, with a higher rate of stent failure. Although DES have reduced the risk of restenosis, there are still concerns with bifurcation lesions. The most common problems are malapposition in the ostium of the side branch and delayed endothelialization in the malapposed or overlapping struts. Both malapposition and delayed endothelialization increase the risk of stent thrombosis and can be detected with OCT. Stent failure may also be related to atherosclerotic plaque characteristics, which can also be identified with OCT.

CTO Lesions

Despite advances in CTO-dedicated equipment, chronically occluded lesions are still technically demanding, and the procedural success rate is lower than in other lesions. OCT cross-sectional images of occluded arteries give good images of the the vessels and help guide procedures with minimal risk. OCT can also identify microchannels and help crossing the cap of the occlusion. Microchannels can be detected with OCT as it can differentiate between the occluded lumen and the various layers of the vessel wall. OCT can help guide the procedure with information about occluded plaque composition, recognition of a true lumen, and differentiation from a false lumen.

Key Learning Points

- Optical coherence tomography provides high-resolution and high-quality images of the coronary arteries.
- Optical coherence tomography allows precise lesion assessment: lumen dimension and plaque composition.
- Optical coherence tomography helps in the assessment of stent failure (in-stent restenosis, stent fracture and stent thrombosis).
- Underexpansion is recognized when all struts are not well apposed to the wall.
- Incomplete apposition is recognized if some struts are not well apposed to the wall.

List of Trials and Studies

ABSORB
ACCELL-AMI
ACCELL-RESISTANCE
ACME
ACUITY
ARRIVE SVG
ASSENT IV
AVIO
BARI 1
BARI 2
BARI 2D
BBC ONE
BENESTENT
BRANCH
BRAVE-3
CABRI
CACTUS
CARDIa
CARE
CARESS-IN-AMI
CAVEAT II
CHAMPION
CLASSICS
COGENT
COURAGE
CREDO
CURE
DIABETES
DIVERGE
EMERALD
EMERALD AIMI
ENDEAVOR IV

Essential Angioplasty, First Edition. E. von Schmilowski, R. H. Swanton.
© 2012 John Wiley & Sons, Ltd. Published 2012 by John Wiley & Sons, Ltd.

EPIC
EPILOG
EPISTENT
EXCEL
FAME
FINESSE
FIRE
FLEXI-CUT
HORIZONS AMI
INNOVATE-PCI
ISAR-DIABETES
ISAR-LM
ISAR-REACT-3
ISAR-TEST-4
LE MANS
LEADERS
LESSON-1
MAIN-COMPARE
MORTAL
NORDIC I, NORDIC III
NORDIC complex bifurcation study
OASIS 5
OAT
OCTOPUS
PEPCAD V
PETAL
PLATINUM
PLATO
PRE-COMBAT
PRISON II
PROSPECT
PROXIMAL
RAPTOR
RAVEL
REACT
REMEDIA
REMEDIAL
RESORB
RITA-2
RITA-3
RRISC
SAFER
SCAAR
SEA-SIDE
SHOCK

SORT OUT II
SOS
SPIRIT IV
SYNERGY
SYNTAX
TAPAS
TIMACS
TOSCA 2
TRANSFER-AMI
TRITON-TIMI 38
TYCOON
TYPHOON

ESC Guidelines for Percutaneous Coronary Interventions
ACC/AHA Guidelines for Percutaneous Coronary Interventions
Consensus Bifurcation Club 2009
Consensus CTO Club 2008

List of scores and classifications:
GRACE score
MBS score
SYNTAX score
EUROscore
MEDINA classification
MADS classification
NHLBI classification
In-stent restenosis angiographic patterns classification
Contrast Induced Nephropathy risk score

References

Expanded references and list of scores and classifications are available on the website www. wiley.com/go/essentialangioplasty.com.

Trials

ABSORB
Serruys PW, Ormiston JA, Onuma Y, et al. A bioabsorbable everolimus-eluting coronary stent system (ABSORB): 2-year outcomes and results from multiple imaging methods. Lancet 2009;9667:897–910.

ACCELL-AMI
Jeong YH, Hwang JY, Kim IS, et al. Adding cilostazol to dual antiplatelet therapy achieves greater platelet inhibition than high maintenance dose clopidogrel in patients with acute myocardial infarction. Results of the adjunctive cilostazol versus high maintenance dose clopidogrel in patients with AMI (ACCEL-AMI) study. Circ Cardiovasc Interv 2010; 3:17–26.

ACCELL-RESISTANCE
Jeong YH, Lee SW, Choi BR et al. Randomized comparison of adjunctive cilostazol versus high maintenance dose clopidogrel in patients with high post-treatment platelet reactivity: Results of the ACCEL-RESISTANCE (Adjunctive Cilostazol Versus High Maintenance Dose Clopidogrel in Patients With Clopidogrel Resistance) randomized study. J Am Coll Cardiol 2009;53:1101–1109.

ACME
Parisi AF, Hartigan PM, Folland ED. Evaluation of exercise thallium scintigraphy versus exercise electrocardiography in predicting survival outcomes and morbid cardiac events in patients with single- and double-vessel disease. Findings from the Angioplasty Compared to Medicine (ACME) Study. J Am Coll Cardiol 1997;30:1256–1263.

ACUITY
Stone GW, Bertrand ME, Moses JW, et al. Routine upstream initiation vs deferred selective use of glycoprotein IIb/IIIa inhibitors in acute coronary syndromes: the ACUITY Timing trial. JAMA 2007;297:591–602.

ARRIVE SVG
Brilakis ES, Lasala JM, Cox DA, et al. Outcomes after implantation of the TAXUS paclitaxel-eluting stent in saphenous vein graft lesions. Results from the ARRIVE (TAXUS

Essential Angioplasty, First Edition. E. von Schmilowski, R. H. Swanton.
© 2012 John Wiley & Sons, Ltd. Published 2012 by John Wiley & Sons, Ltd.

Peri-Approval Registry: A Multicenter Safety Surveillance) program. J Am Coll Cardiol Intv 2010;3:742–750.

ASSENT IV
ASSENT-4 PCI Investigators Primary versus tenecteplase-facilitated percutaneous coronary intervention in patients with ST-segment elevation acute myocardial infarction (ASSENT-4 PCI): randomised trial. Lancet 2006;367:569–578.

AVIO
Colombo A. AVIO: a prospective, randomized trial of intravascular ultrasound guided compared with angiography guided stent implantation in complex coronary lesions. Paper presented at the Annual Meeting of Transcatheter Cardiovascular Therapeutics, September 25, 2010, Washington, DC.

BARI
The BARI Investigators. The final 10-year follow-up results from the BARI randomized trial.J Am Coll Cardiol 2007;49:1600–1606.

BBC ONE
Hildick-Smith D, de Belder AJ, Cooter N, et al. Randomized trial of simple versus complex drug-eluting stenting for bifurcation lesions: The British Bifurcation Coronary Study: old, new, and evolving strategies. Circulation 2010;121:1235–1243.

BENESTENT
Serruys PW, de Jaegere P, Kiemeneij F, et al. A comparison of balloon-expandable-stent implantation with balloon angioplasty in patients with coronary artery disease. Benestent Study Group. N Engl J Med 1994;331:489–495.

BRANCH
Sakata K, Koo BK, Nakatani D, et al. First-in-man IVUS findings using the Medtronic bifurcation stent in patients with coronary bifurcation lesions. J Am Coll Cardiol 2010;55:A199.

BRAVE
Kastrati A, Mehili J, Schlotterbeck K, et al. Multicenter randomized trial to assess reteplase+abciximab versus abciximab before primary PCI for acute MI. JAMA 2004;291:947–954.

CABRI
The CABRI Trial Participants. First year results of CABRI (Coronary Angioplasty versus Bypass Revascularization Investigation). Lancet 1995;346:1179–1184.

CACTUS
Colombo A, Bramacci E, Sacca S, et al. Prospective, randomized multicenter study, to assess crush technique versus provisional side branch stenting. Circulation 2009;119:71–78.

CARDia
Kapur A, Hall RJ, Malik IS, et al. Randomized comparison of percutaneous coronary intervention with coronary artery bypass grafting in diabetic patients: 1-year results of the CARDia (Coronary Artery Revascularization in Diabetes) trial. J Am Coll Cardiol 2010;55:432–440.

CARE

Solomon RJ, Natarajan MK, Doucet S, et al. Cardiac angiography in renally impaired patients (CARE) study: a randomized double-blind trial of contrast-induced nephropathy in patients with chronic kidney disease. Circulation 2007;115:3189–3196.

CARESS-IN-AMI

Di Mario C, Dudek D, Piscione F, et al. Immediate angioplasty versus standard therapy with rescue angioplasty after thrombolysis in the Combined Abciximab REteplase Stent Study in Acute Myocardial Infarction (CARESS-in-AMI): an open, prospective, randomised, multi-centre trial. Lancet 2008;371:559–568.

CAVEAT II

Lefkovits J, Holmes DR, Califf RM, et al for the CAVEAT-II Investigators. Predictors and sequelae of distal embolization during saphenous vein graft intervention from the CAVEAT-II trial. Circulation 1995;92:734–740.

CHAMPION – PCI

Harrington RA, Sone GW, McNutty S, et al. Prospective, randomized, double blind multi-center trial to compare Cangrelor versus Clopidogrel in patients undergoing PCI for ACS. N Engl J Med 2009; 361:2318–2329.

CLASSICS

Bertrand ME, Rupprecht HJ, Urban P, et al. Investigators for the CLASSICS Trial: double-blind study of the safety of clopidogrel with and without a loading dose in combination with aspirin compared with ticlopidine in combination with aspirin after coronary stenting: the clopidogrel aspirin stent international cooperative study (CLASSICS). Circulation 2000;102:624–629.

COGENT

Bhatt DL. The COGENT trial. Paper presented at Transcatheter Cardiovascular Therapeutics 2009, September 24, 2009, San Francisco, CA.

COURAGE

Boden W, O'Rourke RA, Teo KK, et al. Randomized trial: comparison of Medical Therapy with or without PCI for stable coronary disease. N Engl J Med 2007;356:1503–1516.

CREDO

Steinbuhl SR, Berger PB, Mann JT III, et al. Multcenter, randomized double blind, placebo controlled trial to evaluate early and sustained therapy with clopidogrel and aspirin following PCI. JAMA 2002;288:2411–2420.

CURE

Mehta SR, Yusuf S, Peters RJ, et al. Effects of pre-treatment with clopidogrel and aspirin followed by long-term therapy in patients undergoing percutaneous coronary intervention: the PCI-CURE study: Clopidogrel in Unstable angina to prevent Recurrent Events trial (CURE). Lancet 2001;358:527–533.

DIABETES

Jimenez-Quevedo P, Sabate M, Angiolillo DJ, et al. Long-term clinical benefit of sirolimus-eluting stent implantation in diabetic patients with de novo coronary stenoses: long-term results of the DIABETES trial. Eur Heart J 2007;28:1946–1952.

DIVERGE

Verheye S, Agostoni P, Dubois CL, et al. 9-Month clinical, angiographic, and intravascular ultrasound results of a prospective evaluation of the Axxess Self-Expanding Biolimus A9-eluting stent in coronary bifurcation lesions. The DIVERGE (drug-eluting stent intervention for treating side branches effectively) study. J Am Coll Cardiol 2009; 53:1031–1039.

EMERALD

Nikolsky E, Stone GW, Lee E, et al. Correlation between epicardial flow, microvascular reperfusion, infarct size and clinical outcomes in patients with anterior versus non-anterior myocardial infarction treated with primary or rescue angioplasty: analysis from the EMERALD trial. Eurointervention 2009;5:417–424.

ENDEAVOR

Kandzari DE, Leon MB, Popma JJ, et al. ENDEAVOR III Investigators Comparison of zotar-olimus-eluting and sirolimus-eluting stents in patients with native coronary artery disease: a randomized controlled trial. J Am Coll Cardiol 2006;48:2440–2447.

EPIC

Mak KH, Challapalli R, Eisenberg MJ, et al for the EPIC Investigators. Effect of platelet glycoprotein IIb/IIIa receptor inhibition on distal embolization during percutaneous revas-cularization of aortocoronary saphenous vein grafts. Am J Cardiol 1997;80:985–988.

EPILOG

Tcheng JE, Lincoff AM, Miller DP, et al. Benefits of abciximab accrue in the full spectrum of coronary interventional patients: insights from the EPILOG trial. J Am Coll Cardiol 1997;29(Suppl):276A.

EPISTENT

EPISTENT Investigators. Enhancement of the safety of coronary stenting with the use of abciximab, a platelet glycoprotein IIb/IIIa inhibitor. Lancet 1998;352:87–92.

EXCEL

Han Y, Jing Q, Xu B, et al. Evaluation of efficacy of biodegradable polymer-coated sirolimus-eluting stents in real world practice. J Am Coll Cardiol 2009;2:303–309.

FAME

Tonino PAL, De Bruyne B, Pijls NHJ et al. Fractional flow reserve versus angiography for guiding percutaneous coronary intervention. N Engl J Med 2009;360;213–224.

FINESSE

Ellis SG, Armstrong P, Betriu A, et al. Facilitated percutaneous coronary intervention versus primary percutaneous coronary intervention: design and rationale of the Facilitated Intervention with Enhanced Reperfusion Speed to Stop Events (FINESSE) trial. Am Heart J 2004;147:E16.

FIRE

Stone GW, Rogers C, Hermiller J, et al. Randomized comparison of distal protection with a filter-based catheter and a balloon occlusion and aspiration system during percutaneous intervention of diseased saphenous vein aorto-coronary bypass grafts. Circulation 2003; 108:548–553.

FLEXI-CUT
Dahm JB, Ruppert J, Hartmann S, et al. Directional atherectomy facilitates the interventional procedure and leads to a low rate of recurrent stenosis in left anterior descending and left circumflex artery ostium stenoses: subgroup analysis of the FLEXI-CUT study. Heart 2006;92:1285–1289.

HORIZONS AMI
Mehran R, Brodie B, Cox DA, et al. The Harmonizing Outcomes with RevasculariZatiON and Stents in Acute Myocardial Infarction (HORIZONS-AMI) Trial: study design and rationale. Am Heart J 2008;156:44–56.

INNOVATE-PCI
Rao S. INNOVATE-PCI. A randomized, double-blind, active controlled trial to evaluate intravenous and oral PRT060128 (eli-nogrel), a selective and reversible $P2Y_{12}$ receptor inhibitor vs. clopidogrel, as a novel antiplatelet therapy in patients undergoing non-urgent percutaneous coronary intervention. Paper presented at the Annual Meeting of European Society of Cardiology 2010 Congress, August 30, 2010, Stockholm, Sweden.

ISAR-DIABETES
Dibra A, Kastrati A, Mehili J, et al. Paclitaxel-eluting or sirolimus-eluting stents to prevent restenosis in diabetic patients. N Engl J Med 2005;353:663–670.

ISAR-LM
Mehilli J, Kastrati A, Byrneet RA, et al. Single center, randomized trial to assess sirolimus- versus paclitaxel-eluting stents for unprotected left main coronary artery disease. J Am Coll Cardiol 2009;53:1760–1768.

ISAR-REACT-3
Kastrati A, Neuman FJ, Mehili J, et al for the ISAR-REACT 3 Trial Investigators. Bivalirudin versus unfractionated heparin during percutaneous coronary intervention. N Engl J Med 2008;359:688–696.

ISAR-TEST-4
Kufner SF, Byrne RA, Schulz S, et al. Comparative antirestenotic efficacy of biodegradable polymer and permanent polymer drug-eluting stents: the angiographic follow-up results of the ISAR-TEST-4 randomized trial. J Am Coll Cardiol 2010;55:A193.

LE MANS
Buszman PE, Buszman PP, Kiesz RS, et al. Early and long-term results of unprotected left main coronary artery stenting: the LE MANS (left main coronary artery stenting) registry J Am Coll Cardiol 2009;54:1500–1511.

LEADERS
Wykrzykowska JJ, Garg S, Girasis C, et al. Value of the SYNTAX score for risk assessment in the all-comers population of the randomized multicenter LEADERS (Limus Eluted from A Durable versus ERodable Stent coating) trial. J Am Coll Cardiol 2010;56:272–277.

LESSON-1
Raber L. LESSON-I. Long-term comparison of everolimus-eluting and sirolimus-eluting stents for coronary revascularization. Paper presented at the Annual Meeting of the European Society of Cardiology 2010 Congress, September 1, 2010, Stockholm, Sweden.

MAIN-COMPARE
Park DW, Seung KB, Kim YH, et al. Long-term safety and efficacy of stenting versus coronary artery bypass grafting for unprotected left main coronary artery disease: 5-year results from the MAIN-COMPARE (revascularization for unprotected left main coronary artery stenosis: comparison of percutaneous coronary angioplasty versus surgical revascularization) registry J Am Coll Cardiol 2010; 56:117–124.

MORTAL
Chase AJ, Fretz EB, Warburton WP, et al. Association of the arterial access site at angioplasty with transfusion and mortality: the M.O.R.T.A.L study (Mortality benefit Of Reduced Transfusion after percutaneous coronary intervention via the Arm or Leg). Heart 2008;94: 1019–1025.

NORDIC
Steigen TK, Maeng M, Wiseth R, et al. Prospective, randomized, nonblinded, multicenter trial to compare simple versus complex stenting in bifurcation lesions. Circulation 2006;114:1955–1963.

NORDIC complex bifurcation study
Steigen TK, Maeng M, Wiseth R, et al for the Nordic PCI Study Group. randomized study on simple versus complex stenting of coronary artery bifurcation lesions: The Nordic Bifurcation Study. Circulation 2006;114:1955–1961.

OASIS 5
Mehta SR, Granger CB, Eikelboom JW, et al. Efficacy and safety of fondaparinux versus enoxaparin in patients with acute coronary syndromes undergoing percutaneous coronary intervention: results from the OASIS-5 trial. J Am Coll Cardiol 2007;50: 1742–1751.

OAT
Kruk M, Kadziela J, Reynolds HR, et al. Predictors of outcome and the lack of effect of percutaneous coronary intervention across the risk strata in patients with persistent total occlusion after myocardial infarction: Results from the OAT (Occluded Artery Trial) study. J Am Coll Cardiol Cardiovasc Interv 2008;1:511–520.

OCTOPLUS
Louvard Y, Benamer H, Garot P, et al on behalf of the OCTO- PLUS Study Group. Comparison of transradial and transfemoral approaches for coronary angiography and angioplasty in octogenarians (the OCTOPLUS Study). Am J Cardiol 2004;94:1177–1180.

PEPCAD
Unverdorben M summarizing the B. Braun PEPCAD coronary paclitaxel-eluting balloon clinical studies. Paper presented at Transcatheter Cardiovascular Therapeutics September 22, 2009, San Francisco, CA.

PETAL
Ormiston JA, De Vroey F, Webster MW, et al. The Petal dedicated bifurcation stent. Eurointervention Supplement 2010;6 (Suppl J):J139–J142.

PLATINUM

Stone GW, Teirstein PS, Meredith IT, et al. A prospective, randomized evaluation of a novel everolimus-eluting coronary stent: the PLATINUM (a Prospective, Randomized, Multicenter Trial to Assess an Everolimus-Eluting Coronary Stent System [PROMUS Element] for the Treatment of Up to Two de Novo Coronary Artery Lesions) trial. J Am Coll Cardiol 2011;57:1700–1708.

PLATO

Cannon CP, Harrington RA, James S, et al. Randomized double blind study to establish the effectiveness of Ticagrelor versus Clopidogrel in PCI in patients with ACS. Lancet 2010; 375:283–293.

PRE-COMBAT

Park SJ, Kim JH, Park DW, et al. Randomized trial of stents versus bypass surgery for left main coronary artery disease. N Engl J Med 2011;364:1718–1727.

PRISON

Suttorp MJ, Laarman GJ, Rahel BM, et al. Primary stenting of totally occluded native coronary arteries II (PRISON II): a randomized comparison of bare metal stent implantation with sirolimus-eluting stent implantation for the treatment of total coronary occlusions. Circulation 2006;114(9):921–928.

PROSPECT

Maehara A, Mintz GS, Cristea E, et al. Even after percutaneous coronary intervention of angiographically significant lesion, IVUS-defined high-grade stenoses are common. A baseline IVUS analysis from the PROSPECT trial. J Am Coll Cardiol 2010;55.

PROXIMAL

Mauri L, Cox D, Hermiller J, et al. The PROXIMAL Trial: proximal protection during saphenous vein graft intervention using the Proxis embolic protection system. A randomized, prospective, multicenter clinical trial. J Am Coll Cardiol 2007;50:1442–1449.

RAPTOR

Schaufele TG, Grunebaum JP, Lippe B, et al. Radial access versus conventional femoral puncture: Outcome and resource effectiveness in daily routine. The RAPTOR trial. Paper presented at the Scientific Sessions of the American Heart Association 2009, Orlando, FL.

RAVEL

Fajadet J, Morice MC, Bode C, et al. Maintenance of long-term clinical benefit with sirolimus-eluting coronary stents: Three-year results of the RAVEL Trial. Circulation 2005;111:1040–1044.

REACT

Harris S, Gershlick AH, Stephens-Lloyd A, et al for the REACT Trial Investigators. Rescue angioplasty after failed thrombolytic therapy for acute myocardial infarction. N Engl J Med 2005;353:2758–2768.

REMEDIA

Burzotta F, Trani C, Romagnoli E, et al. Manual thrombus-aspiration improves myocardial reperfusion. The randomized evaluation of the effect of mechanical reduction of distal embolization by thrombus-aspiration in primary and rescue angioplasty (REMEDIA) trial. J Am Coll Cardiol 2005;46:371–376.

REMEDIAL
Briguori C, Airoldi F, D'Andrea D, et al. Renal insufficiency following contrast media administration trial (REMEDIAL): a randomized comparison of 3 preventive strategies. Circulation 2007;115:1211–1217.

RESORB
Kaluza GL. The REVA tyrosine-derived polycarbonate bioresorbable scaffold: Long-term outcomes using multimodality imaging. Paper presented at Transcatheter Cardiovascular Therapeutics, 2010, San Francisco, CA.

RITA-2
Henderson RA, Pocock SJ, Clayton TC, et al. 7 year randomized trial to compare coronary angioplasty versus medical therapy. J Am Coll Cardiol 2003;42:1161–1170.

RITA-3
Fox KA, Poole-Wilson P, Clayton TC, et al. Multicenter randomized trial studying the long term outcome of an interventional strategy in non ST elevation acute coronary syndrome BHF Rita-3 trial. Lancet 2005;366:914–920.

RRISC
Vermeersch P, Agostoni P, Verheye S, et al. Randomized double-blind comparison of sirolimus-eluting stent versus bare-metal stent implantation in diseased saphenous vein grafts: six-month angiographic, intravascular ultrasound, and clinical follow-up of the RRISC Trial. J Am Coll Cardiol 2006;48:2423–2431.

SAFER
Cohen DJ, Murphy SA, Baim DS, et al. The SAFER Trial Investigators. Cost-effectiveness of distal embolic protection for patients undergoing percutaneous intervention of saphenous vein bypass grafts: Results from the SAFER trial. J Am Coll Cardiol 2004;44:1801–1808.

SCAAR
James SK, Stenestrand U, Lindbäck J, et al. Long term safety and efficacy of drug-eluting versus bare-metal stents in Sweden. N Engl J Med 2009;360:1933–1945.

SEA-SIDE
Burzotta F, Trani C, Todaro D, et al. Prospective randomized comparison of sirolimus- or everolimus-eluting stent to treat bifurcated lesions by provisional approach. J Am Coll Cardiol 2011; 4:327–335.

SHOCK
Sanborn TA, Sleeper LA, Webb JG, et al. Correlates of one-year survival in patients with cardiogenic shock complicating acute myocardial infarction: Angiographic findings from the SHOCK trial. J Am Coll Cardiol 2003;42:1373–1379.

SORT OUT
Lassen JF, Rasmussen K, Galløe A, et al. SORT-OUT III: A prospective, randomized comparison of zotarolimus-eluting and sirolimus-eluting stents in patients with coronary artery disease. Paper presented at Transcatheter Therapeutics, October 16, 2008, Washington, DC.

SOS

Brilakis ES, Lichtenwalter C, Banerjee S et al. Randomized controlled trial of a paclitaxel-eluting stent versus a similar bare-metal stent in saphenous vein graft lesions: The SOS (Stenting Of Saphenous Vein Grafts) trial. J Am Coll Cardiol 2009;53:919.

SPIRIT

Stone GW, Midei M, Newman W, et al. SPIRIT III Investigators Comparison of an everolimus-eluting stent and a paclitaxel-eluting stent in patients with coronary artery disease. A randomized trial. JAMA 2008;299:1903–1913.

SYNERGY

Mahaffey KW, Tonev ST, Spinler SA, et al on behalf of the SYNERGY Trial Investigators. Obesity in patients with non-ST-segment elevation acute coronary syndromes: Results from the SYNERGY trial. Int J Cardiol 2010;139:123–133.

SYNTAX

Serruys P, Morice MC, Kappetein AP, et al. Multicenter randomized trial to compare PCI and CABG for treating previously untreated 3 vessel and or left main coronary artery disease. N Engl J Med 2009;360:961–972.

TAPAS

Svilaas T, Vlaar PJ, van der Horst IC, et al. Thrombus aspiration during primary percutaneous coronary intervention. N Engl J Med 2008;358:557–567.

TIMACS

Mehta SR, Granger CB , Boden WE, et al for the TIMACS Investigators. Early versus delayed invasive intervention in acute coronary syndromes. N Engl J Med 2009;360:2165–2175.

TOSCA 2

Buller CE, Dzavik V, Carere RG, et al. Primary stenting versus balloon angioplasty in occluded coronary arteries : the total occlusion study of Canada (TOSCA). Circulation 1999;100:236–242,

TRANSFER-AMI

Cantor WJ, Fitchett D, Borgundvaag B, et al. Trial of Routine ANgioplasty and Stenting After Fibrinolysis to Enhance Reperfusion in Acute Myocardial Infarction (TRANSFER-AMI) – Six Month Outcomes. Circulation 2008;188(Suppl 2):S1075.

TRITON-TIMI 38

Montalescot G, Wiviott SD, Braunwald E, et al. Prasugrel compared with clopidogrel in patients undergoing percutaneous coronary intervention for ST-elevation myocardial infarction (TRITON-TIMI 38): double-blind, randomised controlled trial. Lancet 2009;373: 723–731.

TYCOON

Tanzilli G, Greco C, Pelliccia F, et al. Effectiveness of two-year clopidogrel + aspirin in abolishing the risk of very late thrombosis after drug-eluting stent implantation (from the TYCOON Study). Am J Cardiol 2009;104:1357–1361.

TYPHOON

Spaulding C. Four year follow-up of the TYPHOON study, a multicenter, randomised, single-blind trial to assess the use of the Cypher sirolimus eluting stent in acute myocardial infarction patients treated with balloon angioplasty. Paper presented at EuroPCR, May 19, 2009, Barcelona, Spain.

Guidelines

ACC/AHA/SCAI 2005 guideline update for percutaneous coronary intervention

King SB III, Smith SC, Hirshfeld JW, et al. 2007 focused update of the ACC/AHA/SCAI 2005 guideline update for percutaneous coronary intervention: a report of the American College of Cardiology/American Heart Association Task Force on Practice Guidelines (2007 Writing Group to Review New Evidence and Update the 2005 ACC/AHA/SCAI Guideline Update for Percutaneous Coronary Intervention). J Am Coll Cardiol 2008;51:172–209.

ACC/AHA Guidelines for the Management of Patients With ST-Elevation Myocardial Infarction

Kushner FG, Hand M, Smith SC et al. 2009 Focused Updates: ACC/AHA Guidelines for the Management of Patients With ST-Elevation Myocardial Infarction (Updating the 2004 Guideline and 2007 Focused Update) and ACC/AHA/SCAI Guidelines on Percutaneous Coronary Intervention (Updating the 2005 Guideline and 2007 Focused Update): A Report of the American College of Cardiology Foundation/American Heart Association Task Force on Practice Guidelines. J Am Coll Cardiol 2009;54:2205–2241.

Consensus from the European Bifurcation Club

Hildick-Smith D, Lassen JF, Albiero R, et al. Consensus from the 5th European Bifurcation Club meeting. Eurointervention 2010; 6:34–38.

Consensus from the EuroCTO Club

Di Mario C, Werner G, Sianos G, et al. European perspective in the recanalisation of Chronic Total Occlusion (CTO): consensus document from the EuroCTO Club. Eurointervention 2007;3:30–43.

European Guideline on Myocardial Revascularization

Wijns W, Kolh P, Danchin N, et al. Guidelines on myocardial revascularization. The Task Force on Myocardial Revascularization of the European Society of Cardiology (ESC) and the European Association for Cardio-Thoracic Surgery (EACTS) Developed with the special contribution of the European Association for Percutaneous Cardiovascular Interventions (EAPCI). Eur Heart J 2010;31:2501–2555.

Other Resources

Antman EM, Cohen M, Bernink PJ, et al. The TIMI risk score for unstable angina/non-ST-elevation MI: a method for prognostication and therapeutic decision making. JAMA 2000;284:835–842.

Barbeau GR, Letourneau L, Carrier G, et al. Right transradial approach for coronary procedures. J Invasive Cardiol 1996;8 (Suppl D).

Cuisset T, Valgimigli M, Mudra H et al. Rationale and use of antiplatelet and antithrombotic drugs during cardiovascular interventions: May 2010 update. Eurointervention 2010; 6:39–45.

Dudek D, Mielecki W, Dziewierz A et al. The role of thrombectomy and embolic protection devices. Eur Heart J Supplements 2005;7 (Supplement I):I15–I20.

Gibson M, Cannon CP, Daley WL et al. for the TIMI 4 Study Group. TIMI frame count. A quantitative method of assessing coronary artery flow. Circulation 1996;93:879–888.

Gonzalo N, Escaned J, Alfonso F et al. Is refined OCT guidance of stent implantation needed? EuroIntervention 2010;6 Suppl G:G145–153.

Goss JE, Chambers CE, Heupler FA et al. Systemic anaphylactoid reactions to iodinated contrast media during cardiac catheterization procedures. Cath Cardiovasc Diag 1995;34:99.

Granger CB, Goldberg RJ, Dabbous O et al. Predictors of hospital mortality in the Global Registry of Acute Coronary Events. Arch Intern Med 2003;163:2345–2353.

Ellis SG, Ajluni S, Arnold AZ et al. Increased coronary perforation in the new device era. Incidence, classification, management, and outcome. Circulation 1994;90:2725–2730.

Ho PM, Maddox TM, Wang L et al. Risk of adverse outcomes associated with concomitant use of clopidogrel and proton pump inhibitors following acute coronary syndrome. JAMA 2009;301:937–944.

Jokhi P, Curzen N. Percutaneous coronary intervention of ostial lesions. EuroIntervention 2009;5:511–514.

Kandzari DE, Colombo A, Park SJ et al. on behalf of the American College of Cardiology Interventional Scientific Council. Revascularization for unprotected left main disease: Evolution of the evidence basis to redefine treatment standards. J Am Coll Cardiol 2009;54;1576–1588.

Luz A, Hughes C, Fajadet J. Radial approach for percutaneous coronary intervention. EuroIntervention 2009;5:633–635.

Maluenda G, Pichard AD, Waksman R. Is there still a role for intravascular ultrasound in the current practice era? EuroIntervention 2010;6 Suppl G:G139.

Mehran R, Aymong ED, Nikolsky E et al. A simple risk score for prediction of contrast-induced nephropathy after percutaneous coronary intervention: Development and initial validation. J Am Coll Cardiol 2004;44:1393–1399.

Mintz GS. Atlas of Intracoronary Ultrasound. Taylor & Francis, Abingdon UK, 2005.

Mintz GS, Weissman NJ. Intravascular ultrasound in the drug-eluting stent era. J Am Coll Cardiol 2006;48:421–429.

Neumar RW, Otto CW, Link MS et al. 2010 American Heart Association Guidelines for Cardiopulmonary Resuscitation and Emergency Cardiovascular Care. 2010 American Heart Association Guidelines for Cardiopulmonary Resuscitation and Emergency Cardiovascular Care Science. Circulation 2010;122:S729–S767.

Nguen T, Hu Dayi, Saito S, et al. Practical Handbook of Advanced Interventional Cardiology. Wiley-Blackwell, Chichester UK, 2nd edn, 2003.

Orford JL, Lerman A, Holmes DR et al. Routine intravascular ultrasound guidance of percutaneous coronary intervention: A critical reappraisal. J Am Coll Cardiol 2004;43:1335–1342.

Papadopoulou SL, Girasis C, Girasis C. Invasive functional testing. EuroIntervention 2010;6 Suppl G:G72–G78.

Papers presented at: Annual Meeting of European Society of Cardiology (2008–2010), American College of Cardiology (2008–2010), Transcatheter Cardiovascular Therapeutics (2007–2010) and EuroPCR (2007–2010).

Sherman TF. On connecting large vessels to small. The meaning of Murray's law. J Gen Physiol 1981;78(4):431–453.

Werner GS, Ferrari M, Heinke S, et al. Angiographic assessment of collateral connections in comparison with invasively determined collateral function in chronic coronary occlusions. Circulation 2003;107:1972–1977.

www.pcronline.com

www.tctmd.com

Index

Note: page numbers in *italics* refer to Figures and Tables.

Essential Angioplasty, First Edition. E. von Schmilowski, R. H. Swanton.
© 2012 John Wiley & Sons, Ltd. Published 2012 by John Wiley & Sons, Ltd.